GLOBAL CASE STUDIES
in Maternal and Child Health

EDITED BY
Ruth C. White, PhD, MPH, MSW
Assistant Professor
Department of Anthropology, Sociology, and Social Work
Seattle University
Seattle, WA

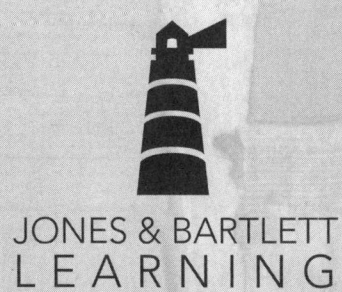

World Headquarters
Jones & Bartlett Learning
5 Wall Street
Burlington, MA 01803
978-443-5000
info@jblearning.com
www.jblearning.com

Jones & Bartlett Learning books and products are available through most bookstores and online booksellers. To contact Jones & Bartlett Learning directly, call 800-832-0034, fax 978-443-8000, or visit our website, www.jblearning.com.

Substantial discounts on bulk quantities of Jones & Bartlett Learning publications are available to corporations, professional associations, and other qualified organizations. For details and specific discount information, contact the special sales department at Jones & Bartlett Learning via the above contact information or send an email to specialsales@jblearning.com.

Copyright © 2014 by Jones & Bartlett Learning, LLC, an Ascend Learning Company

All rights reserved. No part of the material protected by this copyright may be reproduced or utilized in any form, electronic or mechanical, including photocopying, recording, or by any information storage and retrieval system, without written permission from the copyright owner.

Global Case Studies in Maternal and Child Health is an independent publication and has not been authorized, sponsored, or otherwise approved by the owners of the trademarks or service marks referenced in this product.

Some images in this book feature models. These models do not necessarily endorse, represent, or participate in the activities represented in the images.

This publication is designed to provide accurate and authoritative information in regard to the Subject Matter covered. It is sold with the understanding that the publisher is not engaged in rendering legal, accounting, or other professional service. If legal advice or other expert assistance is required, the service of a competent professional person should be sought.

Production Credits
Publisher: Michael Brown
Managing Editor: Maro Gartside
Editorial Assistant: Chloe Falivene
Production Assistant: Alyssa Lawrence
Senior Marketing Manager: Sophie Fleck Teague
Manufacturing and Inventory Control Supervisor: Amy Bacus
Composition: Paw Print Media
Cover Design: Michael O'Donnell
Cover Image: © Pokaz/ShutterStock, Inc.
Printing and Binding: Edwards Brothers Malloy
Cover Printing: Edwards Brothers Malloy

Library of Congress Cataloging-in-Publication Data
White, Ruth C.
  Global case studies in maternal and child health / Ruth C. White.
    p. ; cm.
  Includes bibliographical references and index.
  ISBN 978-0-7637-8153-8 (pbk.)—ISBN 0-7637-8153-3 (pbk.)
  I. Title.
  [DNLM: 1. Maternal Welfare. 2. Child Welfare. WA 310.1]

362.1982—dc23
                        2012025273

6048

Printed in the United States of America
16 15 14 13 12   10 9 8 7 6 5 4 3 2 1

Dedication

This book is dedicated to all the mothers to be, mothers, newborns, and children around the world. It is also dedicated to all the people who donate money, time, energy, commitment, and passion to making the world a healthier place, especially for mothers, newborns, and children everywhere.

Contents

Foreword xiii
Acknowledgments. xvii
Contributors. xix
Introduction. xxiii

PART I	TRADITIONAL BIRTH ATTENDANTS/ TRADITIONAL MIDWIVES	1

Chapter 1	The Local, the Global, the NGO-ization of Birth in Southern Belize 5

Amínata Maraesa

Background 6
The Region 7
Toledo Traditions. 8
Childbirth in the Belizean Medical System 9
Generations of Traditional Birth Attendants 11
The NGO-ization of Birth. 12
Persistent Patterns 18
An Enduring Misunderstanding. 19
Conclusion. 21
Discussion Questions 22
Notes 22
References 23

CONTENTS

Chapter 2	**Weaving Traditional and Professional Midwifery** . . . **25**	
	Jennifer Foster, Jennifer Houston, Ann C. Davenport,	
	Angela Anderson, Virginia M. Lamprecht, and Gal Frenkel	
	Background	26
	Beginnings	28
	Ixmucané as Clinical Practice Model	30
	Training Traditional Midwives	34
	Monitoring and Evaluation of Training	38
	Intertwine with the Ministry of Health	43
	Unraveling and Closure	44
	Lessons Learned	45
	Fabric for the Future	46
	Discussion Questions	48
	Notes	48
	References	49
PART II	**SAFE MOTHERHOOD**	**51**
Chapter 3	**Sing Safe Motherhood: A Story of the Women of Chiwamba, Malawi**	**55**
	Daima Thyangathyanga, Mary Kambewa,	
	Rose M. Kershbaumer, and Joyce E. Thompson	
	Introduction	56
	Background	57
	The Story: Teaching and Learning Safe Motherhood	58
	Adult Functional Literacy Training	65
	Training in Business and Income-Generating Activities	66
	Reflections on the CBSMA Story:	
	Keeping Volunteers Volunteering	66
	Lessons Learned	69
	Summary	71
	Discussion Questions	71
	References	72
Chapter 4	**Maama Omwaana: Community Building for Safe Motherhood in Njeru, Uganda**	**73**
	Ruth C. White and Katherine Camacho Carr	
	Introduction	74

Contents

           Maama Omwaana Safe Motherhood Initiative........ 76
           Community Assessment and Mobilization........... 77
           Implementation Year Two: 2006 79
           Outcomes 82
           Discussion 82
           Conclusion..................................... 85
           Endnote....................................... 86
           Discussion Questions............................ 86
           References 86

Chapter 5   **Behavior Change Initiative in an Integrated Community Health Project** **89**
           Gerda Pohl

           Background.................................... 90
           Nepal and Humla 90
           History.. 92
           The Problem 92
           The Plan 93
           The Solution 95
           Outcomes 97
           Lessons Learned................................ 97
           Discussion Questions............................ 98
           References 98

PART III   **THE IMPACT OF WAR**   **99**

Chapter 6   **Integrating Child Spacing with Maternal Care in Postconflict Timor-Leste**..................... **103**
           Susan Thompson and Mary Anne Mercer

           Background 104
           Health in the Democratic Republic of Timor-Leste... 105
           Integrating Child Spacing into a Maternal and
              Newborn Program........................... 109
           Key Findings 112
           Challenges 114
           Lessons Learned................................ 117
           Conclusion.................................... 118
           Discussion Questions........................... 118
           References 119

CONTENTS

Chapter 7	**LifeLine Community Healthcare Program: Reducing Maternal and Infant Mortality in Liberia** 121	

Lucy November

Background 122
The Players 122
Becoming a Midwife 123
Childbirth in Liberia 124
Training Traditional Birth Attendants 124
War 125
Going Home 126
Building a Clinic 127
Joining LifeLine 129
Discussion Questions 130
References 131

Chapter 8   **Rape as a Weapon of War: Stories from the Democratic Republic of Congo** 133

Elaine Dietsch and Luc Mulimbalimba-Masururu

Background 136
The Story 139
Lessons Learned 144
About the Authors 145
Discussion Questions 146
Acknowledgments 147
References 147

PART IV   SUPPORT GROUPS   149

Chapter 9   **Enhancing Outcomes for At-Risk Moms: The Moms Mentoring Moms Program** 153

Blythe Shepard, Meg Kapil, and Lara Shepard

Introduction 154
Fetal Alcohol Spectrum Disorder 155
The Moms Mentoring Moms Program 156
Overall Effect of Program on Participants 159
Meeting Program Objectives 160

Contents

| | Lessons Learned and Recommendations 165
| | Summary 167
| | Discussion Questions............................. 167
| | References 168

| PART V | **BIRTHING CENTERS** | **171** |

| Chapter 10 | **Maison de Naissance: A Community Birthing Home in Haiti** 175
| | *Whitney A. Smith, Natasha Massoudi, and Stanley G. Shaffer*
| | Case Study................................... 175
| | Background 176
| | Purpose 177
| | Formative Research 177
| | Methods...................................... 179
| | Supporting Technology 181
| | Monitoring and Evaluation 182
| | Results...................................... 183
| | Discussion 184
| | Case Study Review............................. 185
| | Discussion Questions.......................... 186
| | References 186

| Chapter 11 | **Providing a Safe Space for Birth in Warkworth, New Zealand**............................. 187
| | *Liz Smythe, Deborah Payne, Sally Wilson, and Sue Wynyard*
| | Introduction.................................. 187
| | The Case 189
| | Summary..................................... 206
| | Discussion Questions.......................... 206
| | References 207

| PART VI | **THE CULTURE OF MATERNITY** | **209** |

| Chapter 12 | **Maternal–Infant Care in the Brazilian Amazon** 213
| | *Louis C. Forline and Helena dos Santos*
| | Introduction.................................. 213

CONTENTS

The Brazilian Amazon: Regional Ecology, History, and Development 215
Study Results, Community Feedback, and Reflections ..217
Reflections and Recommendations................. 225
Concluding Remarks 227
Discussion Questions........................... 228
References 229

Chapter 13 Mbyá Grandmothers, Mothers, and Granddaughters......................... 231
Carolina Remorini

Introduction.................................... 232
Mbyá Children and Women: Health Conditions and Their Access to Sanitary Services and Programs ..233
Background of Mothers and Wives: Mbyá Women in the Ethnographic Literature.................. 235
Different Stories, the Same Culture: Intracultural Variability and Generational Changes 237
Lessons Learned 249
Acknowledgments 253
Discussion Questions........................... 253
Notes 254
References 254

Chapter 14 Introducing Nursing Students to Childbearing Practices in Rural Guatemala.................. 257
Catherine A. Carr and Amy Levi

Background 258
Cultural Competency Versus Cultural Humility 258
Service Learning to Reduce Health Disparities....... 259
Practical Strategies for Service Learning and Teaching ...260
Learning about Global Maternal Health Care through Service Learning 268
Discussion Questions........................... 269
References 269

PART VII	MEDICAL INTERVENTIONS IN BIRTH 271
Chapter 15	Saving Newborns at the Community Level 275
	Christina Lagos Triantaphyllis
	Background 276
	Public Health System 280
	The MINI Story: Leading the Way in Community-Based Care for Neonates in Nepal ... 282
	Lessons Learned 298
	Notes 300
	Discussion Questions 300
	References 301
Chapter 16	The Nonpneumatic Anti-Shock Garment in Nigeria: The Tension Between Research and Implementation 303
	Oladosu A. Ojengbede, Elizabeth Butrick, Hadiza Galadanci, Imran Oludare Morhason-Bello, Carinne Brody, Titi Duro-Aina, Adetokunbo Fabamwo, and Suellen Miller
	Background 304
	The Project 306
	Results and Reactions 308
	Challenges 310
	Lessons Learned 313
	Discussion Questions 314
	References 314
	Index **317**

Foreword

Birth is remarkable, unique, essential—and intrinsically dangerous. In the modern world it is hidden behind green drapes and IV drips, safe but secret, removed from daily life and sometimes from conscious awareness.

Ruth White's *Global Case Studies in Maternal and Child Health* brings descriptions of birth from around the world in all its wonder, pain, and danger. It is an ingenious and intriguing way to make readers and students think about this most profound and dramatic of all events. Professor White gathers wonderfully vivid writers from Belize, Malawi, Timor-Leste, New Zealand, Haiti, Liberia, and even the jungles of the Amazon to tell the story of birth, of traditional birth attendants and skilled midwives, the security of birthing homes and the chaos of delivery in an environment torn by war.

Global Case Studies in Maternal and Child Health is designed to both engage and help the reader. It can stand alone, or it can supplement and enrich more conventional training material by providing real-life examples. It also contains excellent theoretical and conceptual perspectives not easily found elsewhere.

Birth is powerful, mysterious, and perhaps magical, but in an almost sinister way. We put a newborn baby on YouTube, but usually not the birth canal. Birth is not something we usually make jokes about, although the comedian Gracie Allen succeeded with her quip, "When I was born I was so surprised I didn't speak for a year and a half."

Birth is an obvious metaphor for the creation of the world. Great sages are often reported as having unusual births. It is said that one Sufi poet was born through his mother's hand. Mithra arrived in a burst of light. In some Rabbinic texts, Moses is said to have been born already circumcised and able to walk. In the Old Testament, Sarah, mother of Isaac, was 175 years old when he was born, and in the New Testament Jesus is delivered normally but conceived abnormally.

Sadly, even today, some religions have a strongly patriarchal streak. Birth is sometimes framed as polluting, as in the Old Testament (Leviticus 12:1–8) where *"A woman who becomes pregnant and gives birth to a son will be ceremonially unclean for seven days."* Moreover, as women are so often defined as inferior to men, the Biblical law goes on: *"If she gives birth to a daughter . . . then she must wait sixty-six days to be purified from her bleeding."* Until well into the 20th century, the Churching of Women was a Catholic and an Episcopalian rite, and it still sometimes takes place in the Eastern Orthodox church. It signifies that in some evil way birth must be polluting, demanding a ritual purification before a new mother can fully enter a church.

The true story of the evolution of human birth is much more surprising and revealing than the musings of ancient mystics, edicts of misogynist priests, or maneuverings of U.S. state and federal legislators. Let's circle back to a fundamental question: Why is human childbirth so dangerous?

Between 1785 and 1812, Martha Ballard, a midwife in New England, kept a careful diary.[1] She attended women in labor, as midwives have done for hundreds of thousands of years, but she had no way to deal with obstructed labor, postpartum hemorrhage, or puerperal fever. One in 200 of her mothers died, which was probably the natural maternal mortality rate before modern obstetrics.

The biology of becoming a mammal did have a reproductive downside for females. A cock bird can help the hen incubate the egg and feed the fledglings, and many birds are monogamous. But when mammals began to lactate there was no way that lactation in the male could be synchronized with birth, even if that male had fathered that baby. The evolution of lactation left women literally holding the baby. Most mammals are polygamous or promiscuous, and males often grow big to compete with one another for access to females.

Then life got more difficult for one set of mammals. The primates began to develop bigger and bigger brains, and then there was a problem pushing the baby out of the pelvic canal.

Finally, one species of primate began to walk on two legs, and the pelvic ring had to become even stronger. If the human pelvis were large for easy birth, women would waddle like ducks. If the human pelvis were narrow enough so women could run well, the baby could not be delivered. The current birth canal is an unsatisfactory compromise. When it comes to the burden of reproducing, Darwinian evolution has placed a colossal asymmetry on women: childbirth is difficult and dangerous because while it has been a huge advantage to evolve the big brain that characterizes our species, it is costly for women.

If, as the story of evolution tells us, having a big-brained baby is so important that until the advent of modern obstetrics 1 in 200 parturient women died, then surely we should use that big brain to make the wonder of childbirth as safe as possible for all women—whether in the forests of the Amazon or a friendly birthing house in New Zealand. We should use that brain to listen to the wisdom of traditional birth attendants, which all too often is lost. We should use that brain to respect women and not let men try to overrule a woman's choice as to whether and when to have a child. Both professionals and students alike should read and discuss Ruth White's *Global Case Studies in Maternal and Child Health*.

I feel privileged to contribute to this groundbreaking volume. As a medical student, I wanted to be a neurologist—until I saw my first birth. Today, as a physician and a biologist who has worked all over the world, I feel even more privileged that the first birth I saw turned me into a male obstetrician—a male midwife.

Global Case Studies in Maternal and Child Health puts that experience on paper, and it has the potential to change the perspective of some readers so they use their big brains—whether female or male—to make birth a joyful, wanted, and safe process for the mother and baby.

—Malcolm Potts, MB, BChir, PhD, FRCOG
University California, Berkeley

NOTE

1. Ulrich, L. T. (1990). *A midwife's tale: The life of Martha Ballard, based on her diary 1785–1812.* New York, NY: Alfred A. Knopf.

Acknowledgments

This book started as an idea for my sabbatical project. I placed one call for proposals on a Listserv, and the call went viral. Thanks to all the people who read the call and responded, even if they did not submit a chapter, and even if they did and the chapter was rejected. I would like to express my deepest gratitude to the contributors and the publisher for their support and patience as life, work, death, and illness got in the way of me completing the manuscript in a timely manner. Without the support of my friends, family, and colleagues, I would not have made it through the challenging personal and professional moments of this project and the life challenges I faced during the process. Thank you to all the people of Njeru, Uganda, and the people who work with the Maama Omwaana project who taught me lessons in community collaboration and gracious hospitality that will forever inform my work in community-based public health. They were the inspiration for this book. And finally, a heartfelt thank you to Dr. Nap Hosang and Dr. Malcolm Potts—two of my health professors at UC Berkeley—who made a public health professional out of a social worker.

Contributors

Angela Anderson, CNM, DNP
Director
Intermountain Nurse-Midwives
Adjunct Faculty
University of Utah
Salt Lake City, UT

Carinne Brody, DrPH
Assistant Professor
Touro University
Vallejo, CA

Elizabeth Butrick, NSW, MPH
Bixby Center for Global Reproductive Health
The University of California, San Francisco
San Francisco, CA

Catherine A. Carr, CNM, DrPH
Senior Maternal Health Advisor
Jhpiego, MCHIP program
Washington, DC

Katherine Camacho Carr, PhD, ARNP, CNM, FACNM
Professor and N. Jean Bushman Endowed Chair
Seattle University College of Nursing
Seattle, WA

Ann C. Davenport, RN, MA
Consultant
Metcalfe & Davenport/Matronas
Eagle, CO

Elaine Dietsch
School of Nursing, Midwifery and Indigenous Health
Charles Sturt University
Albury, New South Wales
Australia

Helena dos Santos, PhD
Centro Universitario do Estado do Para (CESUPA)
Nazaré, Belém
Brazil

Titi Duro-Aina, MBBS, MHSc
Pathfinder International
Agidingbi, Ikeja
Lagos, Nigeria

Adetokunbo Fabamwo, MBCLB
Department of Obstetrics and Gynecology
Lagos State University Teaching Hospital
Lagos, Nigeria

xix

CONTRIBUTORS

Louis C. Forline, PhD
Associate Professor
Department of Anthropology
University of Nevada, Reno
Reno, Nevada

Jennifer Foster, CNM, MPH, PhD
Assistant Professor of Nursing
Associate in Anthropology
Center for Maternal-Newborn Survival
Lillian Carter Center for Global Health and Social Responsibility
Nell Hodgson Woodruff School of Nursing
Emory University
Atlanta, GA

Gal Frenkel, MPH
Atlanta, GA

Hadiza Galadanci, MBBS, MSc
Department of Obstetrics and Gynecology
Aminu Kano Teaching Hospital
Kano, Nigeria

Jennifer Houston, CNM, MS
Executive Director
Midwives for Midwives
Catskill, NY

Mary Kambewa, MRN, MRM, CHN
Chief Nursing Officer
Public Health Nurse
Linlongwe, Malawi

Meg Kapil, MA
University of Victoria
Victoria, British Columbia
Canada

Rose M. Kershbaumer, EdD, CNM, MMS
Administrator
Medical Mission Sisters
Assistant Director
Teacher Education Program for Nurses & Midwives
University of Pennsylvania School of Nursing
Philadelphia, PA

Virginia M. Lamprecht, RN, MSPH, MA
Senior Evaluation and Research Specialist
Office of Learning, Evaluation, and Research
Bureau for Policy, Planning and Research
Silver Spring, MD

Amy Levi, CNM, WHNP-BC, PhD
Clinical Professor and Director
Interdepartmental Nurse-Midwifery Education Program
University of California San Francisco
San Francisco, CA

Aminata Maraesa, PhD
City University of New York
Queens, NY

Natasha Massoudi, MPH

Mary Anne Mercer, DrPH
Senior Lecturer
Department of Global Health
University of Washington
Health Alliance International
Seattle, WA

Contributors

Suellen Miller, PhD, CNM
Bixby Center for Global Reproductive Health
University of California, San Francisco
San Francisco, CA

Imran Oludare Morhason-Bello, MBBS
Department of Obstetrics and Gynecology
University College Hospital
Ibadan, Nigeria

Luc Mulimbalimba-Masururu, MD, ND
Medical Director
Mission in Health Care and Development
Kenya

Lucy November, RM, MPH
LifeLine Network International
Dagenham, Essex
England

Oladosu A. Ojengbede, MBBS
Department of Obstetrics and Gynecology
University College Hospital
Ibadan, Nigeria

Deborah Payne, RN, BA, MA, PhD
Centre for Midwifery & Women's Health Research
Faculty of Health & Environmental Sciences
Auckland University of Technology
Auckland, New Zealand

Gerda Pohl, MRCGP, MRCOG, DTMPH

Malcom Potts, MB, BChir, PhD, FRCOG
Professor and Fred H. Bixby Chair
Population and Family Planning
School of Public Health
University of California, Berkeley
Berkeley, CA

Carolina Remorini, PhD
Universidad Nacional de la Plata
Consejo Nacional de Investigaciones Cientificas y Tecnicas
Buenos Aires, Argentina

Stanley G. Shaffer, MD
Pediatrics
St. Luke's Perinatal Center
Bethlehem, Pennsylvania

Blythe Shepard, PhD
Faculty of Education
University of Lethbridge
Lethbridge, Alberta
Canada

Lara Shepard, BA
University of Victoria
Victoria, British Columbia
Canada

Whitney A. Smith, BA
Albert Einstein College of Medicine
Yeshiva University
Bronx, NY

CONTRIBUTORS

Elizabeth Smythe, PhD, RM, RGON
Associate Professor
Auckland University of Technology
Auckland, New Zealand

Joyce E. Thompson, DrPH, CNM, FAAN

Susan Thompson, MPH
Technical Advisor for Monitoring and Evaluation
Health Alliance International
Seattle, WA

Daima Thyangathyanga, MS, MRN, MRM
Commissioner
Health Services Commission
Malawi

Christina Lagos Triantaphyllis, MSc
Cambridge, MA

Ruth White, PhD, MPM, MSW

Sally Wilson, RM, RN, AND
Midwife Director
Warkworth Birthing Centre
Warkworth, New Zealand

Sue Wynyard, RM, RN
Midwife Director
Warkworth Birthing Centre
Warkworth, New Zealand

Introduction

I was talking to my daughter's paternal aunt in Uganda the night before I left after a 5-week visit in 2004. Right before I left she asked if I could help her with a clinic that had been started in her community about 2 years prior. I asked her to send me the annual report and I would go from there. She went into her room and brought me a two-page document that summarized everything the clinic had done and wanted to do. I told her that when I returned to Seattle I would do some research and see how I could help.

Upon my return to Seattle, my research into how to work with this clinic was very challenging. There were lots of research reports about strategies that worked for specific health outcomes, but no easily accessible case study that could help me problem solve about how to work with this community. Where to start? What to do? What *not* to do? What worked? What didn't? Of course, each community is different, and thus each solution is different. However, like everything in life, we need not learn the same lessons repeatedly, and sometimes the analytical focus of research does not allow for broader strategies. It is due to this dearth of examples that I proposed this book because I could not find a book like it. There were case studies in mental health, community organizing, and every other aspect of health, but I could only find one other book of stories from the field of maternal and child health. It took me much longer to write this book than I planned, but here it is.

Global health is a growing field in the area of public health, medicine, nursing, and other health professions. In the public health arena, maternal and child health is one of the most popular specializations and is regaining traction as an important aspect of development that explicitly includes two of the ten Millennium Development Goals (MDG)—maternal

INTRODUCTION

health and child health—but it also implicitly includes other MDGs, such as gender equality and HIV/AIDS.

Although the focus on women and children has been part of the global health strategy for many decades, particularly in the field of microfinance with the success of the Grameen Bank, the new initiatives from the U.S. government spearheaded by Hillary Clinton have explicitly made this area of public health the focus for all USAID funding for years to come.

Professionals in the area of global health find the telling of stories to be useful because stories go beyond the theoretical and into the practical. Practical applications of theory that are grounded in research help us to explore and understand some of the salient issues we should consider when developing and implementing a new program or trying to evaluate the factors that contribute to the success or failure of an existing one.

This book was developed for anyone who has ever considered working in a setting outside of his or her own cultural environment. Though there are no explicit cultural guidelines suggested in any of the examples outlined in this book, the various locales force us to consider important contextual issues that apply outside of specific cultural settings. These case studies present the reader with ethical, practical, and theoretical challenges that develop critical thinking and analytical skills, as well as provide examples that can inform future work.

The success, failure, or cost-effectiveness of the case studies was not a consideration for inclusion in the book. Instead, there was a focus on variability in contexts, program goals, financing, and strategy. The goal is not to provide models for replication but to inspire creativity, develop ethical standards, and reflect on the role of self in the context of global health. With regard to the latter, it is hoped that readers will begin to consider the varied roles they can play in the promotion of the wellbeing of mothers, newborns, and children. Though it may seem adventurous and glamorous to travel internationally to be engaged in global maternal and child health, it can also be highly effective (and cost efficient) to take a hands-off approach that develops human capacity on the ground without direct intervention from abroad. This is becoming much easier than it used to be with the help of technology.

The case studies in this book were gathered through several rounds of Listserv announcements that seem to travel the world in several cycles over a year. It was a challenging exercise to find a standard for each case study because each story is different and each story is told uniquely in a way that not only reflects the author, but also the message of the story. These case studies are meant for medical and allied health professionals, and will bring to life theoretical and conceptual ideas discussed in primary texts through the analysis of lived stories of maternal and child health programs around the world. Ethical, practical, and theoretical questions will develop critical and analytical thinking skills and provide students with practice models they can use in their present or future work.

SOME GENERAL LESSONS FROM THE STORIES

You Don't Need a Degree to Solve Public Health Problems

Solutions are not located only in the capitals of the north or towers of ivory. People who live with public health problems often have public health solutions, but they are rarely asked what they think or for their collaboration. Addressing challenging maternal and child health issues does not require one to build a program in an office in Washington, DC, London, New York, or Geneva and then work with local people on a foreign idea.

There Is No One Solution to a Problem

For every problem in maternal and child health there are many solutions that are shaped by culture, location, resources, and people. We know what works well in many places, but there are few solutions that work everywhere. Immunizations are a solution that works everywhere. Getting someone to get that shot is different in different places. Furthermore, we don't always need new solutions; sometimes we just need to fix what went wrong the first time.

Money Isn't Everything

A lot of the money spent on public health projects that transcend national boundaries is spent on crossing borders—airfare, mailings, translation, transportation, and dual administration. A lot of the money pays northern salaries for southern projects, where southern staff members make a fraction of their northern partners. There is much underutilized human capacity in the south because northern grants come with northern staff.

INTRODUCTION

I remember being at Makerere University's social science department and seeing old computers, while the budgets of their affiliates included laptops for research. Foreign researchers were all over the country, while local academics who were trained at some of the top universities in the world had a hard time finding money to do the same work in their own country.

Indigenous Voices Must Have a Place in Academia

Like most texts with a global scope, the voices in this text are—in all but three cases—those of the highly educated foreigners and outsiders who work with the marginalized and oppressed populations of the world. Granted, they are writing for an audience that reflects who they are, but the stories they tell would be different if told from the perspective of the people who the readers of this text intend to work with. Although I explicitly asked for submissions to be coauthored with people whose stories populated the papers, the dominance of north over south in terms of authorship is striking, and yet it is understandable given that academic Listservs were the primary way of requesting submissions. I will accept responsibility for the way in which this limited my desired audience.

Indigenous voices are rare in academia. Our academic lens filters experiences in very specific and structured ways. It is my hope that as technology expands our ability to present information, we help expand the diversity of voices that are legitimated in the academic sphere, whether through YouTube, Twitter, blogs, or Skype. This will not only change what we learn, but also how we learn, how we engage with our world, and most importantly, the strategies we choose to utilize in solving some of the world's most challenging health issues.

PART I

Traditional Birth Attendants/Traditional Midwives

In poor countries one of the leading causes of maternal and child mortality and morbidity is the insufficient number of trained staff to attend labor and delivery. Data in this area of global health is notoriously unreliable for poor countries because much of this morbidity and mortality occurs outside of official health systems. Improving these outcomes has also been a difficult challenge for many countries, for many complex reasons, some of which will be explored in the case studies.

Because of brain drain, poor countries have a hard time retaining the nursing and midwifery staff they do train, and even those numbers are often inadequate. Furthermore, women tend to want to give birth in the comfort of their homes for many reasons. Sometimes travel is difficult for the women, especially when they are in labor, whether it is because they live in remote areas that are hard to traverse in the best of times or because transportation is costly or slow and uncomfortable during labor, such as on the back of a bicycle. In addition, some hospital labor rooms are overcrowded (e.g., 30 laboring women in one large room with one midwife), understaffed, ill-equipped, and lack privacy or a place to accommodate supportive family members. Under these conditions it is difficult to convince women to leave the comfort of their homes to give birth, despite having untrained (or traditionally trained) attendants such as relatives or traditional birth attendants (TBAs) to assist them.

Despite their lack of training, TBAs serve a vital function in the health of mothers and children around the world. The challenge is that they are independent health workers that do not usually have official oversight, yet they are much more accessible than clinics and hospitals. Because they are local, the women also trust them because they know them. And they usually charge less than government or private hospitals, so it is not difficult to understand why women around the world, particularly rural women, often choose to use TBAs to assist them in their labor and delivery.

Some countries have decided to integrate TBAs into the healthcare system by giving them training and monitoring them, but other countries marginalize them by promoting clinic and hospital-based births, where women in labor and delivery can be monitored by medical professionals. Published research on the role of TBAs spans the globe. Their role as a community-based healthcare provider precedes formal medical training, and despite their limited skills, they are still the provider of choice for millions of women.

PART I Traditional Birth Attendants/Traditional Midwives

The goal of health interventions linked with TBAs has been to promote the use of skilled care—whether through additional training of TBAs or by promoting formally trained medical professionals. Organizations such as the White Ribbon Alliance work with governments, nongovernmental organizations (NGO), and communities to increase access and utilization of skilled birth attendants who have been formally trained because this reduces the risk of morbidity and mortality of both the mother and the child.

CHAPTER 1

The Local, the Global, the NGO-ization of Birth in Southern Belize

Amínata Maraesa, PhD

Location: Toledo District, Belize, Central America

Name of Program/Project: Traditional birth attendant (TBA) training program undertaken by Giving Ideas for Tomorrow (GIFT),[1] a U.S.-based international nongovernmental organization (NGO) with a long history of childbirth and midwifery activism and affiliation with the alternative childbirth community in the United States

Sponsoring Organization (and Funders): UNICEF and GIFT

Target Population: Rural-dwelling women throughout the Toledo District; although ethnicity was specified, the majority of the rural-dwelling population and TBA trainees are Mopan- and Kekchi-speaking Maya

Project Goal: Childbirth attended to by a trained birth attendant, high-risk hospital referrals, and lower mortality rates

Project Objectives: Train rural-dwelling community members to provide trained assistance for perinatal care and high-risk referrals

CHAPTER 1   The Local, the Global, the NGO-ization of Birth in Southern Belize

BACKGROUND

The Belizean Ministry of Health has consistently demonstrated a great interest in participating in international maternal and child health initiatives and was one of the first countries in the world to initiate a TBA training program in 1957 with funding from UNICEF. In the 1990s, TBA funding diminished worldwide; however, GIFT was able to obtain funding from UNICEF for a pilot TBA project in Southern Belize based on a need-assessment/rural health survey conducted by UNICEF in 1998–1999. In two rounds of training from 2000–2001, GIFT trained 19 rural-dwelling women and 3 rural-dwelling men in the Toledo District to provide TBA services to their respective communities.

* * *

The head of Maternal and Child Health Services narrowed her eyes as she surveyed the group of traditional birth attendants gathered in the hospital conference room, and with a flip of her wrist she provocatively exclaimed, "Where are all *my* TBAs? Where are the women *I* trained?" It was true that I had only invited to this meeting the TBAs on whom my research initially focused—those that had been trained by GIFT, an international NGO. And Nurse Lee was aware of this fact. However, I was to interpret this guarded reaction as an explicit testament to her many years of active service to the women in her community. Moreover, it was an implicit warning to outsiders—like myself—to be mindful of local ways of dealing with local affairs.

Despite substantial international involvement in training TBAs as a strategy for lowering maternal mortality worldwide, there may good reason to express doubt and even hostility when Belizean procedures are ignored by well-meaning foreigners who lack a connection to the local protocols governing social relations. Tacitly referencing a deep-seated divide between Belizean cultural practices and foreign development initiatives, Nurse Lee's suspicious inquiry sheds light on a new way to understand how TBA programs are actualized in on-the-ground practice.

Previous anthropological research of TBAs has focused on those trained by the various ministries of health in developing nations (Brink, 1982; Cosminsky, 1986; Hunte, 1981; Jordan, 1978/1993; Pigg, 1995, 1997). This literature suggests that these training programs have not helped to reduce mortality rates primarily due to cultural barriers during the training process. Basing my research thesis on these previous analyses, I hypothesized that the TBAs trained by an outside agency professing a grassroots ideology and unilateral teaching methods would be better trained and have more successful birth outcomes than the TBAs trained by the Belizean Ministry of Health. However, I found that whether these TBAs may or may not have acquired the necessary skills to successfully attend births, most remained inactive or underutilized—hence ineffective. Nurse Lee's emotional response suggests a possible explanation (Bradley & McAuliffe, 2009; Woolfrey, 2002).

This chapter looks closely at how cultural, structural, and interpersonal factors affected GIFT's development initiative and how these factors have shaped the perceptions about and practices of TBAs in the Toledo District. This chapter begins with an overview of the district's demography, cultural beliefs about childbirth, and the maternity services provided by the Ministry of Health. A historical look at the implementation of TBA training and a retelling of GIFT's TBA training program qualitatively frame the quantifiable assertion that the presence of more TBAs has done little to alter reproductive behaviors in the region. This chapter closes with the outcome of the aforementioned meeting with TBAs and hospital personnel that exemplifies the kinds of enduring misunderstandings that impede the success of TBA training programs, yet it offers insight into areas for potential development.

THE REGION

Toledo is the southernmost district in Belize. Its one urban center, the seaside town of Punta Gorda, is surrounded by numerous landlocked rural villages that spread throughout the foothills of the Maya Mountains and along the eastern border of Guatemala. Forming a part of the Central American rainforest ecosystem, Belize is hot, humid, and prone to heavy rains and hurricanes, with Toledo receiving the highest annual rainfall in the country.[2] The many potholed dirt roads that crisscross the district's landscape are often flooded by the overflowing rivers that pour onto roadways and bridges, causing difficulties in both basic and emergency transportation, effectively isolating rural inhabitants from the rest of the country. Concomitantly, Toledo is marked by the worst economic and social indicators countrywide—the greatest poverty, the lowest education levels, the least access to safe water supply, and the greatest difficulty in obtaining emergency medical services (Government of Belize, 2004; Pan American Health Organization, 2001; Statistical Institute of Belize, 2007).[3] It has the highest fertility rate[4] and the highest rate of maternal mortality for the most recent 6 years for which statistics are available (2000–2006), averaging 203.08 deaths per 100,000 live births as compared to 84.58 for the country as a whole.

CHAPTER 1 The Local, the Global, the NGO-ization of Birth in Southern Belize

Table 1-1 Place of birth and attendant (2002)

District	Total births	Total OHDs*	OHD by MTP†	OHD by TBA	OHD by UT‡
Corozal	597	148 (24.8%)	65 (43.9%)	79 (53.4%)	4 (2.7%)
Orange Walk	1,495	463 (31.0%)	280 (60.5%)	182 (39.3%)	1 (0.2%)
Belize	2,089	271 (13.0%)	251 (92.6%)	19 (7.0%)	1 (0.4%)
Cayo	1,766	417 (23.6%)	300 (71.9%)	97 (23.3%)	20 (4.8%)
Stann Creek	852	244 (28.6%)	87 (35.7%)	137 (56.1%)	20 (8.2%)
Toledo	754	278 (36.9%)	2 (0.7%)	90 (32.4%)	186 (67.0%)
Total	7,553	1,821 (24.0%)	985 (54.3%)	604 (33.3%)	232 (12.8%)

* Out-of-hospital delivery
† Medically trained personnel
‡ Untrained birth attendant

Source: Data from Smith, C., and Klima, C. (2004). A Country Report on Women's Health, Belize, Central America. University of Illinois at Chicago College of Nursing and World Health Organization (WHO) Collaborating Centre for International Nursing Development in Primary Health Care. Chicago, IL.

Recent statistics show that the majority of births countrywide take place in a hospital (76.0%), while 87.6% of those that occur outside of a medical facility are assisted by a medically trained attendant (medical officer, nurse–midwife) or a TBA (see **Table 1-1**). However, these national averages flatten the statistical anomalies found in the Toledo District where a substantially larger number of births take place in the home setting (36.9%), of which 67.0% occur without a trained attendant. Presumably this has adversely influenced mortality rates and the influx of development projects such as GIFT's TBA training.

TOLEDO TRADITIONS

The population of Belize is a melting pot of diverse racial and ethnic groups that emphasize their distinct cultural attributes while embracing a Belizean national identity. Although the Toledo District is similarly mixed, the majority of the population draws from ethnic groups known throughout the rest of the country for safeguarding the traditional ways of its inhabitants. The region is dominated by the rural inhabitants from two major ethnic groups (Kekchi- and Mopan-speaking Maya) who maintain their linguistic distinctions and ethnic clothing styles against the creolization of the national culture and the heavy influence of imported cultural practices evident with the omnipresence of satellite television shows, music, and sneakers imported from the United States.[5] A part of these persistent cultural traditions includes reproductive behaviors, such as the practice of childbirth within the confines of the home with limited extrafamilial assistance.

Among both the Kekchi- and Mopan-speaking Maya, attending to one's wife[6] during childbirth is considered one of the duties a husband is expected to perform. A husband is informally trained through observing his mother or mother-in-law at the birth of his wife's first child. From this experience, it is expected that he learn how to physically and emotionally support his wife throughout the labor process and cut the umbilical cord after the delivery of the placenta. Complications are purportedly dealt with through prenatal assessment by the Ministry of Health nurses—who often recommend a hospital delivery to obviate risk—or by ritual specialists known in local parlance as *bush doctors*.[7]

In Toledo, bush doctors are ritual specialists who administer bush (herbal) medicine, massage, and prayer to heal a variety of illnesses and physical ailments. Although their healing repertoire includes limited maternity services, bush doctors do not consider themselves to be midwives or to be practicing midwifery. With few exceptions, bush doctors do not attend births, nor do they care for the pregnant woman or the newborn during the labor and postpartum periods. Instead, they are called upon in times of maternal distress to ameliorate the condition that is causing discomfort or danger. One of the most oft-cited services provided by a bush doctor is to ascertain and ensure a vertex fetal presentation. When the position of a fetus is determined to be "good," the bush doctor leaves the pregnant woman with her kinship support network and returns only after the birth if help is needed to expel a retained placenta through abdominal massage or herbal preparations. Indeed, it was repeatedly emphasized throughout my inquiries into the practices of bush doctors that "only people with problem [*sic*] go to bush doctor." The same cultural logic influences the use of mainstream medical services.

CHILDBIRTH IN THE BELIZEAN MEDICAL SYSTEM

The Belizean government under the direction of the Ministry of Health currently provides all public health services, including maternal and child care. In

CHAPTER 1   The Local, the Global, the NGO-ization of Birth in Southern Belize

the Toledo District, free and comprehensive prenatal services are available at the medical centers located in town and in the larger villages as well as at the mobile clinics that service the rural areas. Because there are no obstetricians or gynecologists permanently stationed in the district, nurse midwives provide all maternity care including labor and delivery. Pregnant women in Toledo have been socialized to attend the prenatal clinics with regularity; however, they do not always comply with risk-reducing protocols, including the increasing push for hospital birth.

In Toledo, there is one hospital located in the town of Punta Gorda.[8] It has a shared maternity ward and a separate delivery room with one delivery table. Here, the practices of nurse midwives conform to the highly medicalized and authoritative procedures characteristic of modern obstetric practice. Medication is often administered to augment labor and hasten contractions; however, epidural anesthesia is not available. Women giving birth for the first time (primiparas) are given an episiotomy, and all deliveries are conducted on a flat delivery table in the lithotomy (supine) position with the feet secured in stirrups. And the Kristeller technique of applying fundal pressure to expel the baby is routinely utilized. These procedures may contribute to the prevalent belief in the Toledo District that childbirth "hurts more" in the hospital than at home—a belief that was often cited when discussing why women preferred to stay home for childbirth. In addition, I heard many complaints from women who have given birth at the hospital about the treatment they received at the hands of the nurse midwives. They were often "scolded" for crying out during labor or outright ignored when requesting care.

Despite the general dislike of these attitudes and practices, women who live in town—regardless of ethnic group or previous cultural practice—give birth at the local hospital because there is a general understanding that partaking of the urban modernity entails birth in the hospital. Indeed, I heard of no instances where women returned to the villages to birth in a home setting. Moreover, the hospital is easily accessible. For women living in the rural villages, however, distance, transportation difficulties, and environmental factors are all cited as justifiable reasons to stay home for the birth, and homebirth remained a "cultural tradition" tolerated by the Ministry of Health nurses who instead placed greater emphasis on risk prevention during prenatal care and seeking the assistance of a trained TBA, whose training is recognized as a factor in official recommendations and subsequent TBA activity.

GENERATIONS OF TRADITIONAL BIRTH ATTENDANTS

As early as 1952, the World Health Organization (WHO) advocated for the training of what would become known in international public health parlance as the *traditional birth attendant* or *TBA*. Identified as "the untrained or partially trained indigenous midwife" (World Health Organization, 1952, as cited in Oakley & Houd, 1990, p. 175), standardized midwifery training programs were initiated worldwide with the belief that so-called traditional behaviors of lay birth attendants were an impediment to the modernization process and that maternal and child health outcomes in poor and developing nations could be ameliorated through a training and certification process that emphasized biomedical risk assessment and institutional referral. Belize, which has consistently demonstrated a great interest in participating in international maternal and child health initiatives, was one of the first countries in the world to initiate a TBA training program in 1957, made possible by funding from UNICEF. Individuals already known to be practicing midwifery were invited through formal letters of invitation to participate in a 6-month training program originally known as Practical Midwifery Course for Nannies to augment their skills through practical training in the main hospital in Belize City. Contained within the files of the Ministry of Health's main office were yellowing copies of these invitation letters, the tone of which corresponds to Nurse Lee's sentiments described at the outset of this chapter: a language of participatory healthcare characteristics of the early public health movement and the assertion of local directives under a burgeoning anticolonial movement and fledgling independence.

Despite these enthusiastic beginnings, the country's limited economic and human resources have meant that the number of TBAs trained by the Ministry of Health has always been small. By 1989, UNICEF's funding for TBA training programs had dwindled, and the WHO began to question the value of these types of programs (World Health Organization, 1997). With the already small number of TBAs aging or dead, the recent disinterest of global funding organizations to cosponsor TBA training programs and the persistent environmentally harsh and isolating conditions of the Toledo District meant that significant numbers of pregnant women were without easy access to a skilled birth attendant. Although a few TBAs were later to be individually trained by Ministry of Health nurses who took it upon themselves to apprentice individuals from the rural areas, the

CHAPTER 1   The Local, the Global, the NGO-ization of Birth in Southern Belize

majority of the villages in the Toledo District, where home birth remains the norm, were without a trained TBA.

In July 1998, the Belize office of UNICEF conducted a survey of the rural areas to determine what the people themselves believed to be their biggest problems related to childbirth. It is unclear from the report who actually answered the questions: "What are the problems associated with deliveries in your community?" and "What do you think can be done to solve the problems?" However, the answers from the 25 villages surveyed overwhelmingly cited that a lack of emergency transportation could be ameliorated by the presence of a nurse or TBA stationed in the community. Although bush doctors are widely used to ameliorate certain perinatal emergencies, their position within the indigenous system of medical care is not officially recognized by the Ministry of Health. The survey does not explicitly state what additional services it was hoped could be provided by a TBA in case of an emergency, but it may have been thought that a trained birth attendant would be capable of handling emergencies on-site or that the presence of a ministry-approved liaison could facilitate a smooth transition from home to hospital care.

As a development NGO, GIFT had already been active in southern Belize since the mid-1980s with a health and nutrition program based on soy protein and environmentally sound, sustainable agricultural practices. Since GIFT's parent organization is associated with a birth center and a direct-entry midwifery training program in the southern United States, when local representatives learned about the results of UNICEF's survey it made sense that GIFT should mobilize its maternal health network to assist the people in the Toledo District. GIFT approached UNICEF with a proposal that addressed the concerns highlighted in the survey, whereupon UNICEF agreed to fund the first phase of GIFT's TBA training project.

THE NGO-IZATION OF BIRTH

Prior to embarking on long-term fieldwork in Belize, I met with Samantha Wood, the program coordinator and first midwife instructor to lead Phase I of GIFT's TBA training project in Belize, to discuss training methods, goals, and her perception of the program's outcome. During our interviews, Wood expressed her awareness of Toledo women's cultural differences, lack of basic education, and literacy impediments, and she described the ways through which she sought to convey information to the TBA trainees that was accessible both culturally and with limited literacy. Consistent with the types of anthropological analyses that informed my thesis, she described the Ministry of Health approach as "telling someone what to do." As an alternative, Wood "wanted to encourage decision making, because situations will arise when the TBA would need to use her own understandings. She cannot rely only on the scenarios she was explicitly told." Wood also believed that her preference for "village" life—which is how she described her small community in the United States—allowed her to gain trust and create mutual understanding among the rural population of TBA trainees. In fact, one of the more literate and outspoken TBAs trained by Wood has continued to write letters to Wood about her experiences—usually to complain about the treatment she receives by hospital personnel who she believes do not recognize her as having been adequately trained to attend birth.

Wood's commitment to the rural population was apparent. In a rickety Jeep, she traveled alone or, at times, with a translator to numerous villages throughout the rural areas of the Toledo District to meet face to face with village leaders and discuss what she referred to as "the village midwife project" at community meetings where she could solicit individuals for training. A total of 14 women, representing 11 of the villages surveyed, were identified to participate in Phase I of the project. Seven were Mopan-speaking and six were Kekchi-speaking Maya; one was Mestizo living in a village of predominantly Mopan-speaking Maya. Six of the women had previous experience attending births, one woman's husband was a bush doctor, and three of the women were single without children.

Well aware of the critiques from local residents about "the gringos' fascination with Mayans" and the attention and money given to this ethnic community at the expense of others, Wood spoke of the poverty and racism that she believed disproportionately affected this community. Although tourist guidebooks, websites, and even some academic ethnographies (McClaurin, 1996; McClusky, 2001)—including my own (Maraesa, 2009)—speak of relatively harmonious ethnic and race relations within the Toledo District, Wood contends that she witnessed firsthand the discrimination to which the Maya populations are subjected by other groups. According to Wood, the way in which Maya women were attended to in the maternity ward by the predominantly "black" nurse midwives was "horrendous." She insisted, "I wanted to train them for birth in the villages to keep them from this treatment."[9] Moreover, it was UNICEF's intention to direct funds to the communities with the highest level of need and living in the villages with the least access to medical services. Thus, Wood found herself turning down requests for TBA training from

CHAPTER 1 The Local, the Global, the NGO-ization of Birth in Southern Belize

women of various ethnic identities who lived in town or areas close to the town center due to a perceived lack of relative need.

Unfortunately, I entered the field a number of years after GIFT's training program had ended. Despite this shortcoming, I offer the following description of the initial training sessions based on my interviews with Wood and the TBAs she trained in 2000. As opposed to the small-scale, individualized, finite 6-month training intensives previously undertaken by the Belizean Ministry of Health, GIFT had proposed a project to train one or two TBAs from each village for a period of 6 months with a provision for continuing education and follow-up skills training. Wood explained that community members in the various districts of Toledo had expressed reservation about foreign NGO involvement in local affairs because they had grown accustomed to surveyors who would leave with information but never act on the requests made. Wood stated that she "did not want to let the population down" and convinced UNICEF to fund an extended program in which the rural-dwelling trainees would assemble for classes at a location in or around Punta Gorda once a week for the 6-month duration of the training. She envisioned the entirety of the project to span three phases, each of which would train 10 to 12 TBAs until every village in the Toledo District was covered.

The sessions followed an internationally acclaimed training manual written for cross-cultural use that included informational drawings helpful for non-English-speaking or illiterate populations (Klein & Miller, 1995). For one of the trainees who could not read or write but was married to a Spanish-speaker from Guatemala, Wood obtained a Spanish version of the book. The training was conducted using a combination of didactic methods and materials including lecture, demonstration and practice with dolls and anatomic models, group discussion, role play, and birth videos. After watching the first film, all of the women admitted that it was the first time they had ever seen a baby emerge from the vagina because most women who give birth at home remain clothed in the long skirts that are characteristic of their traditional dress. Mindful of these types of cultural sensitivities, Wood did not emphasize vaginal examinations to monitor cervical dilation; however, she taught that "from time to time they needed to go and look, even if that meant to take a peek once in a while to see if the cord is wrapped around the neck."

At the end of this theoretical training, each of the TBAs was to spend 3.5 days at the local hospital to observe prenatal examinations as conducted by the nurse midwives and assist during the labors and deliveries of women in the hospital's maternity ward. While undergoing their practical training, the TBAs slept in a room adjacent to the maternity ward. When I conducted my fieldwork, nearly

5 years after the last practical session had ended, the typed sign that said "Please wake us for a birth. TBAs are inside to serve you" remained affixed with adhesive tape to the door of this same room, which was now used to store medical supplies and equipment. One of the nurses on duty at the maternity ward explained to me that "GIFT mi put up the paper when they mi have their TBA trainings, but they no have TBAs sleeping inside again [any more]."[10] Presumably, since it was GIFT that directed the program and put up the sign, it was GIFT's responsibility to remove it when they were finished.

Indeed, the continued presence of this sign is an index of the disjuncture between the maternal health services provided by the Ministry of Health (MOH) and the TBA training program undertaken by GIFT that began when Wood commenced her work among the rural populations in 2000 and lasted into the present, as evidenced by Nurse Lee's reactionary position toward the absence of "her" TBAs at the meeting I orchestrated during my fieldwork in 2006. Although UNICEF's survey indicated a community desire for village-level maternity care, neither GIFT (nor UNICEF) approached the MOH to find a solution. Instead, the MOH was assumed to be at blame for neglecting the needs of the rural populations in the Toledo District. Both Wood and MOH officials mentioned the project proposal drafted by GIFT and submitted to UNICEF for funding, which explicitly cited the MOH as failing to adequately provide services to the rural areas. According to Wood, GIFT's program would succeed where the ministry had purportedly failed. However, local ministry personnel interpreted the proposal as a personal indictment leveled by Wood and felt blamed for the implicit risk to which the women in the rural areas were subjected when they gave birth in their villages without the presence of a trained birth attendant. Although GIFT's project proposal did not call out individual nurses in the Toledo District by name, they were too few in number to go locally unidentified in what was perceived as a blatant disregard for their personal involvement with early public health outreach campaigns and the training of a limited number of TBAs who were often partnered with and directly supervised by a rural health nurse with whom the apprenticeship was ongoing. Prior to GIFT's involvement, UNICEF had funded TBA training through the Belizean Ministry of Health. Now, this crucial international funding was being redirected into a foreign institution—already distrusted by locals because of the perceived lack of understanding for their actual needs and further suspect due to having made enemies before the project even commenced.

CHAPTER 1   The Local, the Global, the NGO-ization of Birth in Southern Belize

Belizeans in the Toledo District are also quick to point out the many development initiatives that were not sustainable and were ultimately deserted once the outside funding sources ran dry. Throughout the region, abandoned buildings with cracking façades, solar panels overrun by rainforest vegetation, and faded, peeling posters stand as testaments to the many development projects implemented with the good intentions of foreigners that ultimately ceased to function in the absence of continued international involvement. Likewise, the region is constantly bombarded with medical aid programs. At the time I conducted my fieldwork, there were six medical teams from North America that had registered with the MOH to provide services in the rural communities in Toledo.[11] According to the director of Health Education at the district hospital, there are also the many medical teams or religious missions that come down without local authorization, "and we no know what they di do until they done do it!"[12] According to MOH personnel, many of these aid organizations are not aware of the existing Belizean medical system and ultimately do more harm than good by providing unnecessary or inappropriate medical services for which locals ultimately pay by draining their non-recompensable resources: their land, their time, and their bodies (O'Neil, 2006).

Although Wood had much experience as a practicing midwife at a freestanding birth center in the United States and with development projects in different parts of the world, her experiences in places like Guatemala were radically different from what she would encounter in the Toledo District of Belize. According to Wood, "The government in Guatemala really didn't care what we did. So the idea of getting permission from the authorities was kind of foreign to me, and I went into it ignorant, thinking to a great degree that it would not even matter that much. It seemed like we had done what we needed to do . . . And UNICEF Belize was funding me." Indeed, most midwives have historically practiced outside of medical authority, and, by definition, NGOs are not governmental bodies. From Wood's point of view, she had obtained funding from an internationally recognized health and welfare agency and did not need to involve the local MOH personnel in her training program. Furthermore, she wanted to differentiate herself from the kinds of MOH training models critiqued in scholarly journals that Wood summarized as "pretty racist . . . The women had not learned anything. They just slept through the class!"

However, it was not long into the training program when Wood realized that her work was ruffling the feathers of the MOH. She was summoned to a meeting at the local hospital:

> Luckily a representative from UNICEF came to the meeting with me to back me up and not let them eat me alive. But one of the things that got said at that meeting was that they see over the years all of these NGOs come down and that nothing changes, so to them the money gets basically wasted. But if that money got put into some decent equipment that the hospital needs, "If that money got put into us, then maybe we can save some lives." Well, I thought, if you miraculously had an attitude change... (Samantha Wood, 2005)

Wood explained that when she had tried to involve some of the local nurses, they would not show up when invited or would "show up late or come unprepared." Rather than seeing their disinterest in the context of the historically all too familiar fly-by-night development ventures, Wood perceived their lack of interest in GIFT's present project as being deliberately unhelpful. The misunderstanding between the local ministry personnel and GIFT extended to include the distrust of the TBAs that GIFT trained.

When Phase I of the project was completed, a graduation ceremony was held "Belizean style." School children sang the national anthem, refreshments were served, and GIFT invited Nurse Lee to be the master of ceremonies. While she personally shook the hands of all the graduates as they received their diplomas, she would later refuse to acknowledge their credentials. Wood explained:

> One of the things we felt was that because the Ministry of Health nurses were not involved in the training, they had no ownership of the project, no personal involvement in the project. So if the midwives showed up at the hospital, they would not treat them well because they didn't know them. If one of the nurses had trained them with their own blood, sweat, and tears, then maybe when one of these women arrived they would say, "Oh, we know you," and they would be more likely to be supportive of them. That was part of the learning process that it was important to have the Ministry of Health involved. So we tried to make up for it in the next phases of the project. (Samantha Wood, 2005)

After the completion of Phase I, UNICEF ceased to fund GIFT's program. Nonetheless, Phase II commenced in 2001 with the NGO's own financial resources and a different midwife coordinator who tried to repair GIFT's relationship with the ministry. According to Wood, "One of the big jobs she had was to make friends with the MOH and be a different person than me." GIFT asked the advice of local ministry personnel in selecting eight new trainees, and Nurse Lee was asked to lead the theoretical instruction with assistance from GIFT's midwife who would "fill in the gaps" and act as a "liaison or facilitator." To further help bridge the disconnect, many of the trainees in the second group were already affiliated with the MOH in some way as community health workers or rural health post caretakers.

CHAPTER 1   The Local, the Global, the NGO-ization of Birth in Southern Belize

After this second phase, a total of 22 TBAs from 19 of the 50 or so rural villages in the Toledo District had been trained. Some areas remained without a trained TBA, and the MOH suggested that GIFT facilitate additional trainings according to its method of the last 50 years: by funding 6-month internships at the hospital. However, this arrangement was never pursued by either party, and Phase III of GIFT's project metamorphosed into a series of continuing education workshops and related services such as basic first aid and CPR training, as well as literacy skills instruction for the TBAs it had already trained. Phase III ended in 2004 when monetary and human resources dried up, and while GIFT continues to work on development projects in the Toledo District, it is no longer involved in TBA training or continuing education for the TBAs. In many ways, this disassociation has contributed to local pessimistic expectations of foreign-led initiatives and suspicion of program quality, thus reproducing an old cycle.

PERSISTENT PATTERNS

By 2002, there were a total of 28 trained TBAs available to attend to births in the rural areas of the Toledo District: 22 birth attendants trained by GIFT, two of the older nannies trained by the MOH, and four TBAs who had apprenticed with rural health nurses in the mid-1990s. However, the vast majority of the births occurring in the home setting continued to take place without a trained attendant (Table 1-1). A closer analysis of more recent data sorted by place of birth and birth attendant for one section of the rural population in the Toledo District confirms this statistical trend (**Table 1-2**).

According to the delivery records for the San Juan village catchment area (covering 13 villages in Toledo with a population of approximately 5,150) that are kept by the rural health nurse at the health post in San Juan and the delivery records kept at the local hospital, I found that in 2003, 75 percent of all births for women residing within the catchment area took place outside the hospital. In 2004 and 2005, this number fluctuated down to 70.8% and up to 72%, respectively. Of the 13 villages included in this statistical analysis, 7 had TBAs trained by GIFT, and the TBA trained by the MOH continued to work alongside the rural health nurse in San Juan until some time in 2005 when she moved to another district. Yet, among the births conducted at home in the villages, the use of a TBA remained steady but was still significantly lower than the percentage of births delivered without formally trained assistance. In other words, throughout the period 2003–2005, close to 70% of the births that took place in the home in

Table 1-2 Rural health center data for the San Juan catchment area (2003–2005)

Place of delivery and attendant for births within the San Juan catchment area	2003	2004	2005
Punta Gorda Hospital	47 (25.0%)	38 (29.2%)	35 (28.0%)
Village (at home)	141 (75.0%)	92 (70.8%)	90 (72.0%)
Village birth with trained TBA	42 (29.8%)	29 (31.5%)	27 (30.0%)
Village birth with family member	97 (68.8%)	62 (67.4%)	60 (66.7%)
Village birth with nurse-midwife	2 (1.4%)	1 (1.1%)	3 (3.3%)
Grand total of births from the catchment area	188 (100.0%)	130 (100.0%)	125 (100.0%)

Source: Data from San Antonio Rural Health Center (2006). Medical delivery records, Jan 2003–Dec 2005.

this large rural area were delivered with family members who had never received any formal midwifery training (mothers, mothers-in-law, husbands), or women delivered their babies alone. Moreover, these numbers changed little from the previous decade when a much earlier health survey conducted by the Belizean government found that from the time period 1994–1999 about 75% of deliveries that occurred at home in the rural villages were conducted without a trained birth attendant (Central Statistical Office, 2001; Woolfrey, 2002).

AN ENDURING MISUNDERSTANDING

After I had conducted individual interviews with the TBAs trained by GIFT and amassed a fair amount of statistical data, I found certain indexical consistencies—namely inactivity and an enduring misunderstanding between the TBAs and MOH personnel that I believed contributed to the TBAs' inability to implement their training. In an attempt to bridge the gap, I organized a meeting where the TBAs could interact as a group with the public and rural health nurses in charge of providing government-sponsored maternity care. I hoped that the meeting would provide a venue for both sides to air their grievances and create a means through which to create the types of collaboration alluded to in the UNICEF survey that had prompted GIFT's program in the first place. Because I had also spent a significant amount of research time at the

CHAPTER 1   The Local, the Global, the NGO-ization of Birth in Southern Belize

hospital-based prenatal clinic—where I often heard the MOH personnel making disparaging remarks about the TBAs—I was able to arrange for the meeting to take place in the hospital conference room. And after Nurse Lee voiced her opinion about the attendees—or lack thereof—the meeting continued with a TBA's retelling of a controversial incident that reached a conciliatory solution, albeit one that never manifested.

Two days before the meeting, one of "Wood's TBAs" had a confrontation with the nurse–midwife on duty when a woman she had brought to the hospital as a transfer patient was ready to deliver. Filomena, the TBA, had been summoned by a man living in her village whose wife had been in labor for a few hours with no apparent progress. Acting in accordance with her training that emphasized detection of high risk and referrals, Filomena brought the woman into the hospital "just in case." Filomena stayed with the woman in the maternity ward until it became apparent that the woman would soon deliver because she began to feel the urge to push. Filomena looked for the on-duty nurse–midwife. When she could not find her in the maternity ward, Filomena decided to bring the woman into the delivery room where she assisted her onto the delivery table. As Filomena was putting on the white delivery smock and latex gloves to prepare for the delivery, the nurse–midwife entered the delivery room and began to "cuss her out" for doing what Filomena believed to be her job as a birth attendant. At this point in the story, Nurse Lee sent for the nurse–midwife, who corroborated the story and added that a TBA is not allowed to perform a hospital delivery without a nurse's supervision. Filomena, however, asserted her belief that she was acting in the best interest of the woman who was ready to push and could not wait until the nurse–midwife, who had apparently strayed from her post, was found. Nurse Lee ended the discussion by asserting that Filomena had endangered the life of the laboring woman through her disregard for hospital policy. Meanwhile, no official mention was made of the nurse's "cussing" or of her disappearance from the maternity ward. The meeting then concluded with a date set for an entire one-day workshop to be held for the TBAs, hospital nurses, and public health officials to discuss protocols. Unfortunately, it was discovered a few weeks later that the Inspector of Nurse Midwives from the country's capital city was not available on this date. A few days later a tragic roadway accident involving a MOH vehicle left two members of a local public health official's family dead, and the importance of holding a TBA meeting fell by the wayside. Shortly thereafter, I concluded my fieldwork in Belize and, according to ongoing communications with local colleagues, this meeting has never happened.

CONCLUSION

Throughout this analysis I have highlighted the various environmental, structural, and cultural challenges posed by the Toledo District vis-à-vis development initiatives that have influenced women's reproductive behaviors and the statistical trend toward home birth. The Belizean MOH is aware of the need for trained attendants and has provided small-scale training consistent with its limited financial means. Because many of the rural areas of the Toledo District remained without a trained attendant, GIFT initiated a larger-scale program to provide culturally sensitive maternity care that adhered to internationally recognized conventions of maternal and child health. Although the training of TBAs appears to be one solution to the problem of unattended home births, their underutilization obviates their NGO-initiated presence.

Undeniably there are many factors that influence the ability of the TBAs trained by GIFT to effectively implement their midwifery skills. However, this chapter has focused on an aspect of the training program that may not be obvious without a situated analysis. Despite the apparent dedication of GIFT's personnel to the rural communities and an awareness of traditional cultural values, a lack of sensitivity to larger cultural hierarchies between local and global levels, as manifested in the interpersonal misunderstandings between GIFT and MOH personnel, proved damaging to the integration of many of the NGO-trained TBAs with the national healthcare system. Without this integration, nurse midwives are unlikely to recognize their qualifications as capable maternity care providers. This chapter concluded with a recent example of the kind of mistrust that has characterized GIFT's training program from the outset, further suggesting that GIFT's TBAs will remain underutilized by the larger community without serious attention to rebuilding their relationship with the MOH. GIFT's good intentions, the WHO-approved agenda, and the network recruitment of local trainees could not compensate for the slight they caused to national and regional protocols of birth.

CHAPTER 1 The Local, the Global, the NGO-ization of Birth in Southern Belize

> **Discussion Questions**
>
> 1. How do you think the traditional role of Maya husbands in childbirth influences the process of birth for the mothers and the interaction with health personnel?
> 2. Discuss the push for hospital births in this context with the demand for home births in the United States and other rich countries.
> 3. Why should funding be given to NGOs instead of the Belizean government? Do you agree with the reasons given in this chapter? Why or why not?
> 4. Discuss possible reasons why there is a shift away from training traditional birth attendants.
> 5. Develop at least one strategy or policy that would coordinate foreign medical aid to the Toledo region (or any other service region in a poor country). Is this coordination necessary? Why or why not?

NOTES

1. Pseudonyms are used throughout to protect the identity of all private organizations and individuals.
2. In 2005, the year before I conducted my fieldwork, the annual rainfall countrywide was 84 inches. In the Toledo District, it was 199.9 inches, almost four times higher than any of the other meteorological readings from the rest of the country (Central Statistical Office, 2006).
3. In the Toledo District, the percentage of the population classified by the Central Statistical Office as poor is 79.0, while the countrywide total is 33.5% (2004).
4. The most recent statistics indicate that the total fertility rate for the Toledo District is 5.59, while the rate is 3.97 countrywide (Central Statistical Office, 2001).
5. The Kekchi- and Mopan-speaking Maya represent 65.4% of the population of the Toledo District (Central Statistical Office, 2006).
6. In the Toledo District, it is common to refer to all cohabitating domestic partners, both legally married and common-law unions, as husband and wife.
7. North American interest in the Maya, indigenous therapies, and herbal medicine has brought about the use of a nobler title—traditional healer—to refer to bush doctors (Arvigo, 1994). However, Belizeans in Toledo often laugh at this "foreign" way of referring to their local practitioners because they see nothing pejorative about the term "bush doctor."

8. A second hospital, located in the largest rural village, was completed in 2009. Future research will be needed to determine if women will deliver in a hospital now that one is located nearer to their homes.
9. Later in our interview, Wood relayed a story told to her by a "black" woman from town who complained to her that the nurses at the local hospital were mean. Wood then clarified that it is not just the Maya who are mistreated, "but that all of the women complain about the treatment that they get at that hospital."
10. A common Belize Creole linguistic structure is the copular variant "mi" (pronounced "mee"), which signifies the past tense of the Standard English verb "to be" (Escure, 1992). For example, "I mi see it" means "I was seeing it" or "I saw it."
11. Information supplied by Health Education and Community Participation Bureau (HECOPAB).
12. "Di" (pronounced "dee") signifies the present tense of the Standard English verb "to be" (see footnote 10).

REFERENCES

Arvigo, R. (1994). *Sastun: My apprenticeship with a Maya healer*. New York, NY: Harper San Francisco.

Bradley, S., & McAuliffe, E. (2009). Mid-level providers in emergency obstetric and newborn health care: Factors affecting their performance and retention within the Malawian health system. *Human Resources for Health, 7*, 14.

Brink, P. (1982). The traditional birth attendants among the Annang of Nigeria. *Social Science and Medicine, 16*, 1883–1892.

Central Statistical Office. (2001). *Belize family health survey: Females*. Belmopan, Belize: Ministry of National Development.

Central Statistical Office. (2004). *Environmental statistics for Belize: 2004*. Belmopan, Belize: Ministry of National Development.

Central Statistical Office. (2006). *Abstract of statistics for Belize: 2006*. Belmopan, Belize: Ministry of National Development, Investment and Culture.

Cosminsky, S. (1986). Traditional birth practices and pregnancy avoidance in the Americas. In A. Mangay Maglacas & J. Simons (Eds.), *The potential of the traditional birth attendant* (Publication No. 95, pp. 75–89). Geneva, Switzerland: World Health Organization.

Escure, G. (1992). Gender and linguistic change in the Belizean Creole community. In K. Hall, M. Bucholtz, & B. Moonwomon (Eds.), *Locating power: Proceedings of the Second Berkeley Women and Languages Conference* (pp. 118–131). Berkeley, CA: University of California.

Government of Belize. (2004). *The convention on the rights of the child: Periodic report* (Addendum December 2004). Retrieved from http://www.unhchr.ch/tbs/doc.nsf/0/6e69cc12b9a f5f3ec1256f6a005ae3ba/$FILE/Belize.doc.

Hunte, P. (1981). The role of the dai (traditional birth attendant) in urban Afghanistan: Some traditional and adaptational aspects. *Medical Anthropology 5*(1), 17–26.

Jordan, B. (1993). *Birth in four cultures: A crosscultural investigation of childbirth in Yucatan, Holland, Sweden, and the United States*. Prospect Heights, IL: Waveland Press. (Original work published 1978.)

CHAPTER 1 The Local, the Global, the NGO-ization of Birth in Southern Belize

Klein, S., & Miller, S. (1995). *A book for midwives: A manual for traditional birth attendants and community midwives*. Palo Alto, CA: Hesperian Foundation.

Maraesa, A. (2009). *"I no 'fraid for that": Pregnancy, risk, and development in Southern Belize* (Doctoral dissertation, Department of Anthropology, New York University).

McClaurin, I. (1996). *Women of Belize: Gender and change in Central America*. New Brunswick, NJ: Rutgers University Press.

McClusky, L. J. (2001). *"Here, our culture is hard": Stories of domestic violence from a Mayan community in Belize*. Austin, TX: University of Texas Press.

Oakley, A., & Houd, S. (1990). *Helpers in Childbirth: Midwifery Today*. New York: Hemisphere Publishing Corporation. Published on behalf of the World Health Organization, Regional Office for Europe.

O'Neil, E. (2006). *Awakening Hippocrates: A primer on health, poverty, and global service*. Chicago, IL: American Medical Association.

Pan American Health Organization. (2001). Country health profile. Retrieved from http://www.paho.org/english/sha/prflbel.htm.

Pigg, S. L. (1995). Acronyms and effacement: Traditional medical practitioners (TMP) in international health development. *Social Science and Medicine, 41*(1), 47–68.

Pigg, S. L. (1997). Authority in translation: Finding, knowing, naming, and training "traditional birth attendants" in Nepal. In R. E. Davis-Floyd & C. F. Sargent (Eds.), *Childbirth and authoritative knowledge: Cross-cultural perspectives* (pp. 233–262). Berkeley: University of California Press.

Smith, C., & Klima, C. (2004). *A country report on women's health, Belize, Central America*. Chicago, IL: University of Illinois at Chicago College of Nursing and World Health Organization Collaborating Centre for International Nursing Development in Primary Health Care.

Statistical Institute of Belize. (2007). Labour force survey. Retrieved from http://www.statisticsbelize.org.bz/default.asp.

Wood, S. (2005). Personal interview.

World Health Organization (WHO). (1997). Strengthening Midwifery within Safe Motherhood. Report of a Collaborative ICM/WHO/UNICEF Pre-Congress Workshop, Oslo, Norway, May 23–26, 1996. Geneva, Switzerland: WHO, Division of Reproductive Health.

Woolfrey, J. (2002). *Safe motherhood: A matter of life and death for women in Belize (an exploratory study on pregnancy related death, illness and disability in Belize: Its causes, and how to address them)*. Washington, DC: Pan American Health Organization.

CHAPTER 2

Weaving Traditional and Professional Midwifery

The Story of Midwife, Birth Center, and the Empowerment of Midwives in Guatemala

Jennifer Foster, CNM, PhD
Jennifer Houston, CNM, MSN
Ann Davenport, RN
Angela Anderson, CNM, DNP
Virginia Lamprecht, RN, MPH
Gal Frenkel, MPH

Location: Antigua, Guatemala, Central America

Name of Project: Ixmucané Women's Health and Birth Center; Midwives for Midwives (MFM) Training Program

Sponsoring Organization: Midwives for Midwives

Target Population: Traditional midwives (training); women

Project Goals: To improve the skills and knowledge of traditional midwives; to provide prenatal care, well-woman gynecology care, contraception, childbirth classes, and birth services (Ixmucané)

CHAPTER 2   Weaving Traditional and Professional Midwifery

To be trained by a professional midwife who understands what midwifery is made the difference in the training. They respected our role in the community and understood what we need to be better midwives and serve our communities.

—JELIN YADIRA CARRANZA GIRON,* GUATEMALAN TRADITIONAL MIDWIFE

BACKGROUND

Each of us were compelled to contribute to this case study because of our commitment to improving the lives of women, their newborns, and families. Some of us are midwives (Jenna, Jenny, Ann, and Angela), and others are international public health professionals (Virginia and Gal). Our calling to serve in Guatemala began by observing women's reproductive lives there, simply because we took the time to hear women and feel the fabric of their daily reality. We learned that traditional midwifery in Guatemala is central to a community's sense of itself and is integral to a cultural context that may or may not interlace with biomedical culture, and that the midwifery model is vital for women's empowerment.

Traditional midwives, *comadronas* in Guatemalan Spanish,[1] attend approximately 71% of births to indigenous women (United States Global Health Initiative, 2010). They construct the fiber of social and personal health of Guatemalan society. They are eager to receive more clinical skills training. However, many political and economic forces outside of those midwives' control determine who pays for and defines that education.

In this case study, we explain the story of the Ixmucané [pronounced ISH-MOO-KA-Né] birth center and the Midwives for Midwives (MFM) training program from 1997 to 2004. We weave together Guatemalan traditional values, professional midwifery modeling in knowledge acquisition and skills competency, biomedical intervention when appropriate, and respect for women's rights. We entwine all this with the challenges we confronted to sustain nonprofit health services for the poor—challenges we eventually could not overcome.

The Guatemalan Context

The traditional midwives (comadronas) of Guatemala live and work in a country where maternal and infant mortality rates rank among the highest in the Western hemisphere; only Bolivia, El Salvador, and Haiti have higher mortality

---

*Pseudonym

rates, although none of these countries have confirmable measurement systems in place for counting their dead mothers and newborns (World Health Organization [WHO], 2007). The maternal mortality rate in Guatemala in 2007 was 139/100,000 live births (Pan American Health Organization [PAHO], 2011). In contrast, the maternal mortality rate in the United States was 24/100,000 (PAHO, 2011).

Guatemala's population of about 14 million (United States Central Intelligence Agency [CIA], 2012) is expected to double by 2050. The total fertility rate (the average number of children born to a woman during her lifetime) is 3.18, and the contraceptive prevalence rate is 43%, with an unmet need for family planning of 28%, and higher in rural areas (United Nations, 2011). Although abortion is illegal in Guatemala, except to save a woman's life, unsafe abortions result in a high annual rate of hospitalization for complications (8/1,000 women) (Singh, Prada, & Kestler, 2006). Abortion is the third leading cause of maternal death (Guatemala, 2003). These statistics demonstrate a great need for women's reproductive health improvements among the general Guatemalan population, but the situation among the indigenous Mayan population is far worse. Two principal cultural groups define the fabric of the Guatemala population: Ladinos, who are of both Spanish and Mayan descent (about 59% of the population), and the indigenous Mayans (about 41% of the total population) (CIA, 2012). The Ladinos dominate the economic and political systems and are collectively wealthier and better educated than the indigenous population.

Most of the indigenous population lives in rural areas far from government health care or hospitals. They lack transportation to travel long distances to access emergency care, and 54.5% of them suffer from chronic malnutrition (PAHO, 2011). Only 17% of indigenous women give birth with a skilled birth attendant, as defined by the World Health Organization (WHO), compared to 41% of the nonliterate Ladino population (Instituto Nacional de Estadísticas, 1995). Traditional midwives do not meet the WHO or UNICEF definitions of "skilled attendants," and in rural Guatemala these are the women who attend the vast majority of births. In some areas, the traditional midwives attend 95% of all births. Even though 41% of all births in Guatemala are reportedly attended by "skilled attendants" (UNICEF, 2003), there is wide variation in staff distribution and competency of those "skilled attendants." In our experience, there are rural indigenous areas where the traditional midwives attend 95% of all births.

In addition to gender inequality, discrimination and illiteracy are additional burdens of the poor and indigenous. The maternal mortality rate for nonliterate women is three times the rate of their literate counterparts (Guatemala, 2003). Nonliterate women tend to marry early (as young as 13 or 14 years old) and have little knowledge of their own reproductive systems, and they do not have access to information about reproduction services or choices (which are usually written). Thus, they become pregnant sooner, and most of their reproductive lives are spent either lactating or pregnant, increasing their health risks with every pregnancy.

Men make most of the reproductive healthcare decisions for women and children. Women have very little voice or choice regarding their own reproductive rights. Women in all cultural and economic groups suffer from gender discrimination, and many are victims of increasing violence; rape and incest, particularly prevalent in marginalized groups (MSPAS, 1993). The women who came to the Ixmucané Women's Health and Birth Center complained of infidelity, fear of being exposed to sexually transmitted infections including HIV, forced sexual relations, domestic violence, and husbands who they said would "*never* use a condom." Many women told us that their husbands "won't give me permission to use contraception."

Discrimination is not limited to the privacy of the family. Many poor women, particularly indigenous women, report crude treatment and discrimination from hospital staff. Mistrust of Guatemala's public healthcare system may in part be a legacy of the 35-year history of civil war and five centuries of colonial domination of indigenous peoples. Two or three generations of Mayan indigenous and rural poor have a social history of being "disappeared" by government forces; thus to go into the government healthcare system for a normal process such as pregnancy or birth is counterintuitive.

In ancient Mayan society, men and women had equally important roles in society, and neither was considered to be a whole person without the other. The domination of the Spanish- and later U.S.-sponsored business interests marginalized Mayan traditions and practices (Nelson, 1999). Traditional sustainable agricultural rituals, diet, and healing arts that encompassed plant medicine and Mayan rituals for pregnancy, childbirth, and newborn care do continue, but they are eroded because of the hegemony of Western influences (Cosminsky, 1975, 1982).

BEGINNINGS

The Ixmucané Birth and Women's Health Center opened in 1997 in Antigua, a historic and beautiful town near Guatemala City and one of UNESCO's cultural world heritage sites. Jenna Houston (a certified nurse–midwife from the United

States with many years of home birth, hospital, and birth center experience) and Hannah Friewald, a German resident of Antigua and a graduate from Maternidad La Luz midwifery school in El Paso, Texas, worked together to open the birth center in Antigua.

The center was named in honor of Ixmucané, described in the primary Mayan text *Popol Vuh* as the grandmother of all Mayans and the entire human race. She is the feminine goddess, the protector of women, and the vessel maker (Goetz, Morley, & Recinos, 1950). Ixmucané is the midwife for all midwives. The Ixmucané Birth and Women's Health Center (Centro de Partos y Salud de la Mujer Ixmucané) opened in a large old hacienda in the center of Antigua.

A year after Ixmucané opened, Jenna's and Hannah's interests diverged. Hannah moved on to start a birth center in Guatemala City and worked with a more affluent population. Jenna stayed at Ixmucané in Antigua, drawn to her connections with the local traditional midwives and eager to learn more about indigenous birthing practices. Jenna soon discovered that the local midwives were required to attend monthly meetings facilitated by a government-trained nurse. What happened at one of those meetings forever changed the direction of Jenna's work.

About 40 traditional midwives came to the meeting from the small towns and remote areas in the Department of Sacatepéquez, dressed in traditional woven *traje* (skirts and woven blouses with sashes). Most wore shoes, some were barefoot, some brought children. While seated in a circle, the midwives spoke in turns, shared their stories and problems, asked questions, and voiced their concerns. Although many spoke from the heart, the nurse seemed dismissive of their comments. One comadrona stood to speak. She began quietly and carefully, as if finding it difficult to share what she had to say. Looking downward, she told this story:

> I attended a birth two months ago and the mother died. I see the family every day and am so sad. The husband cried at the birth, and the children are now all motherless. I too cry and go to church every day. On my knees, I ask God for forgiveness. I know it is God's will, but maybe I did something wrong. I can't work anymore, because they took my *carnet* (license) away, and I feel guilty and very, very sad. I want to know what happened and what I could have done. (Antonia Son Xanic,* 1998)

All the midwives sat in silence for a moment. The nurse facilitating the meeting then said, "Alright. Next?"

---

*Pseudonym

CHAPTER 2   Weaving Traditional and Professional Midwifery

The loss and pain in the traditional midwife's story left Jenna shocked. The tender and personal plea for assistance was ignored, and the enormous anguish and courage of this midwife to share her story with the group was dismissed. At the meeting's end, so moved by what she had heard and by the nurse's response, Jenna offered to start a midwifery support group and invited the midwives to come to a meeting at the Ixmucané birth center. Thus a relationship between the local traditional midwives and MFM began, as well as an attempt to intertwine them within the Ministry of Health system.

The next day, 19 midwives arrived at the doorstep of Ixmucané. Jenna was astounded by their eagerness to learn and connect. During that very first meeting, they suggested the idea of a support group of midwives, by midwives and for midwives. Soon thereafter, the nonprofit organization Midwives for Midwives formed and gave birth to Ixmucané Women's Health and Birth Center, which became a place where women could receive care, a clinical practice site for midwifery students from other countries, and a place where traditional midwives could bring clients from their communities for consultation and care. Ixmucané Women's Health and Birth Center became the living representation for the midwifery model of care.

The birth center sought clients who spanned a wide economic range, including clients who could subsidize those who could not pay. However, many more poor women than wealthy women accessed Ixmucané's services. MFM needed to constantly conduct fundraising activities to support the midwives and the birth center because very few clients had the means to pay for the operational costs of the clinic.

IXMUCANÉ AS CLINICAL PRACTICE MODEL

The Ixmucané Women's Health and Birth Center provided prenatal care, well-woman gynecology, contraception, childbirth classes, and birth services. A trusting, respectful relationship between midwife and woman, through confidence building, information sharing, and childbirth preparation, became fundamental to service provision. Unhurried prenatal visits included husband and family participation, nutritional counseling, lifestyle changes to encourage rest and appropriate activity, and early problem identification. Women felt cared for in the homey, relaxing environment of Ixmucané, where they regularly met with other women, borrowed books from the extensive library, and attended classes.

Jenna recounted the following:

During labor we encouraged relaxation and movement, nourishment, and hydration. We provided an environment with music, massage, privacy and support, all of which encouraged spontaneous labor and birth in most cases. We monitored the mother and baby in a calm, attentive way. All emergency equipment was well within reach, but out of view. We offered water birth and encouraged delivery in any position the mother desired. We promoted the participation of any support person the mother wanted and provided protection from overbearing in-laws at the mother's request. We treated the mother and the birth process with great respect and sacredness. Women felt safe and cared for. Babies stayed with their mothers continually. Mother, baby, and partner had uninterrupted time for taking in the deep satisfaction and joy of a conscious birth. (Jenna Houston, 2000)

Ixmucané staff expected the local midwives to remain with their clients and encouraged them to participate in their clients' care. The staff used every opportunity to work with local midwives and encouraged information sharing and teamwork. Support and camaraderie defined the atmosphere among the midwives and volunteers at Ixmucané. Every birth became a unique teaching opportunity for the traditional midwives and international midwifery students, a time to observe good birthing management and apply the skills they already knew or wanted to learn. Ixmucané provided an environment not only for a respectful interface and exchange of ideas, but also for hands-on skills practice for the traditional midwives. Ixmucané's large, comfortable waiting room transformed into a learning center after clinic hours, equipped with a library, pelvic models, and videos on midwifery practice.

During our provision of comprehensive women's health care, we faced firsthand the vast social inequities in Guatemala. For example, international travelers who had read about Ixmucané (Gorry, 2001) sought and paid for emergency contraception with us, and Ladina Guatemalans drove to Antigua from Guatemala City in search of personalized and humane maternity care at Ixmucané. Wealthy, informed women chose and paid for their gynecologic care. Most of the care, however, was given to poor local women brought in by the traditional midwives.

Having heard of the professional and caring attention at Ixmucané by word of mouth, the traditional midwives brought young pregnant girls, undernourished women, overworked grand multiparas (women who have borne five or more children), and others to Ixmucané for treatment of complications due to infection, hemorrhage, obstructed labor, or anemia. Sometimes the poor and illiterate just came to access a safe place, a place where neither the traditional midwife nor her pregnant woman would face ridicule or shame.

Jordan articulated a concept of "fruitful accommodation" (1993, p. 136) in which professional practitioners attending births would combine the best of knowledge from the Western scientific model of obstetrics with the intuitive and cultural knowledge learned through the experience of generations of birthing women. Ixmucané became a place where accommodation could be put into action; it was an environment where both effective science and nonharmful traditional practices could coexist (Sesia, 1997) and the authority of both thrived (Lukere, 2002).

MFM and the Ixmucané clinic provided a unique opportunity for professional midwives to learn about Guatemalan rituals and observe their knowledge and skills. Because the center provided rich fieldwork experience to midwifery apprentices and international students in women's studies, public health, and anthropology, Ixmucané received hundreds of requests from volunteers and students who were interested in the center as a clinical practice site. For many students, Ixmucané offered experiences that they would never have encountered anywhere else. As one apprentice said, "I was interested in learning midwifery unrestricted by institutional protocols that are often established for litigation issues and not necessarily in the woman's best interest."

Another said, "There are so few places in the U.S. where one can study 'true' midwifery, to take time and give one-on-one care throughout the entire childbearing process."

The midwifery model at Ixmucané encouraged the presence of students and apprentices, people who brought enthusiasm, new ideas, and fresh ways of seeing things. The model valued intergenerational exchanges and offered students knowledge and skills often lacking in formal midwifery educational systems based on hospital care. The MFM model for midwifery training became a powerful educational tool.

Student midwives input at Ixmucané and their dedication to documenting outcomes truly benefited the center. In 2004, for her graduate thesis, a nurse–midwife student reviewed all births at the center that were attended by professional midwifery students who had complete perinatal data (99 births) between October 1997 and July 2002. She compared these outcomes with those of a home birth service of professional midwives serving a primarily immigrant Latina population in Chicago (Romano, 2004). She selected the home birth service in Chicago because the style of practice and population served were similar to those of Ixmucané and because of its reputation as an exemplary midwifery service.

Her study used the Optimality Index-U.S., a research instrument that evaluates both the outcome itself and the means by which it was achieved. The instrument incorporates a measurement of the frequency of obstetric interventions, with less reliance on interventions themselves, yielding a more optimal score (Murphy & Fullerton, 2001). This is a unique research tool that allows capturing the midwifery model of care within the quantitative analysis of outcomes.

This method excluded women in active labor who transferred to Ixmucané with a traditional midwife if the woman had no recorded prenatal record or medical history. The method also excluded women who required transfer to hospital-based care, because outcome data were not reliably recorded for these women and their newborns. However, the study did provide an important look at the outcomes at Ixmucané and allowed comparison with an exemplary midwifery practice in the developed world.

The study controlled for the effects of social and medical background and for differences in the practice guidelines between the two birth settings. There were no significant differences in the processes and outcomes of professional midwifery care in the two populations, with high optimality scores in both settings. This student nurse–midwife's study supported the claim that the provision of professional midwifery care to a population in Guatemala can yield outcomes similar to those of an exemplary midwifery practice among a similar population in the United States (Romano, 2004).

Due to Ixmucané's unique position as a transfer center for the comadrona clients, the caseload at Ixmucané included a high percentage of primigravidas (women having their first baby), women attempting a vaginal birth after Cesarean (VBAC), and women presenting after prolonged labor and/or rupture of amniotic fluid. Overall, the midwives at Ixmucané attended 262 women between 1997 and 2004. The first birth was a water birth of a healthy female baby, born fully in the amniotic bag, which spontaneously ruptured upon movement of the baby. This is such a rare event that we considered it an auspicious sign. Women brought to Ixmucané by a traditional midwife comprised 56 of the total 262 births. Of those 262 births, 32 were transferred to the referral hospital; of 32 transfers, 25 were resolved with surgery (a Cesarean rate of approximately 10%). There were no maternal deaths between 1997 and 2004, although we did have two neonatal deaths. Both of these neonates had normal fetal heart rates that were closely monitored during labor, but they had very poor Apgar scores following birth. Neither infant responded to vigorous resuscitation efforts, raising the possibility of cardiac anomaly. In both cases, autopsy was offered and encouraged, but the families declined to have it performed.

Although the births studied were those attended by student professional midwives, models of maternity care organizations emphasize a dual role for professional midwives who are working with traditional midwives—that of weaving direct care provision of women with their community-based providers and intertwining it all with the formal healthcare system (International Confederation of Midwives, 2003).

TRAINING TRADITIONAL MIDWIVES

The more the professional midwives learned about comadronas, the Guatemalan healthcare system, and community realities of isolation, poverty, and violence, the more they changed the focus at Ixmucané from that of service provider to that of curriculum development for training the comadronas. These two roles required fundamentally different skills and orientations.

MFM initially worked for 3 years in Sacatepéquez, the department (state) that includes Antigua, providing care to our own clients and attending births with local traditional midwives when they came to Ixmucané for consultation and emergency services. The traditional midwives had a standing invitation to bring in their clients so they could attend their births at Ixmucané, and we had the backup services of a local Guatemalan general physician with hospital privileges. When necessary, the professional midwives transferred emergencies to either a local private hospital or the local national hospital, depending on the economic resources of the woman in labor.

Due to regular monthly support meetings for a core group of traditional midwives and many other traditional midwives coming in and out of the group (depending on their ability to attend classes), MFM had the opportunity to conduct hours of in-depth interviews to understand the traditional midwives' knowledge levels, how they became midwives, and how they acquired their skills.

Traditional midwives throughout Guatemala have very diverse knowledge levels, and as the MFM midwives began to train in other departments in Guatemala, they learned that skills also varied greatly between geographic areas. MFM eventually worked in six different departments and interviewed more than 200 traditional midwives during our 9 years in Guatemala.

Some traditional midwives were literate; however, most were nonliterate or semiliterate. Some had received some form of continuous education about pregnancy and childbirth (from information), but none had received skills training. Some had attended basic nursing courses, some had many years of empirical experience, and some were beginners. A few had attended many births, but the majority of the comadronas we trained had attended 50 or fewer births in their entire career. The majority had attended only two or three births a month.

The following list shows some, but not all, of the average traditional midwives' level of knowledge and skills concerning maternal and newborn health care. The traditional midwives adapted some practices from what the nurses in the public health system taught them, from what they were expected to perform by members of their village, or from practices that were passed on to them by other traditional midwives. There were many areas where traditional midwives did not have the knowledge and skills important for promotion and care of normal pregnancy and birth. Only two practicing traditional midwives (out of approximately 250) knew how to take blood pressures and had the equipment to do it. The following list indicates knowledge gaps for the traditional midwives that were observed. Most traditional midwives could not identify gestational age and did not measure uterine height to compare fetal growth with gestational age. Thus, they did not know about intrauterine growth retardation or if a fetus was too large for dates.

- Other unknown concepts included a woman's current or prepregnancy weight, nutritional counseling, rest, fluid intake, or urine.
- Most traditional midwives did not have the equipment or skills to measure blood pressures or listen to or count fetal heart rates.
- Many traditional midwives identified preeclampsia as swelling, but they did not know the relationship between high blood pressure and preeclampsia. They knew about convulsions, but not the cause, treatment, or medical diagnosis (eclampsia).
- The majority of traditional midwives lacked skills to intervene in cases of hemorrhage or to resuscitate a newborn in distress.
- Most traditional midwives lacked basic skills in birth support and could not identify signs of complications or management of emergencies during labor or childbirth, postpartum, or in the newborn.

- The laboring mother was covered with a heavy blanket during labor and postpartum to accommodate the concept of "warmth" that leads to "down and out" bodily energy movement. The traditional midwives did not encourage walking or position change during labor.
- Almost all traditional midwives use the *umbliguero*—a small cloth to cover the umbilical stump of the newborn, which, if not sterile or changed frequently, may cause infection.
- Many traditional midwives, and women in general, believed that colostrum was "bad milk" that should be expressed and expelled, not given to the newborn. Many thought that babies should be given bottled formula. They began to value formula feeding while watching their upper-class employers feeding their babies that way (many Mayan women work as house cleaners or nannies).

Various nongovernmental organizations (NGOs), church groups, and Ministry of Health nurses have conducted training courses for traditional midwives over the years, courses that last from a few days to a few weeks. None of those courses teach skills, except for the UNICEF courses that teach the Four Cleans: clean hands, clean area, clean cord cutting, and clean baby. Not a single curriculum addresses the difficult issues of sexual rights or humane treatment of women—issues that traditional and professional midwives deal with on a regular basis—such as rape, incest, unwanted pregnancies, and forced sex for procreation. Many participants said they see these problems all the time, but no one ever talks about them, and they do not know how to confront these issues when they occur.

Because the MFM professional midwives listened to the traditional midwives and observed how they attend women, they developed a training curriculum together, weaving scientific evidence, practical skills, and nonharmful traditional methods with nonharmful technological methods. They intertwined what the comadronas wanted to learn with essential lifesaving skills they should have—what nonharmful traditional practices were expected by their clients with basic care skills the midwives should provide for the well-being, safety, and comfort of the women and babies in their charge.

The MFM midwives designed much of the curriculum based on our own experiences as midwives (collectively we had more than 100 years of experience) and drew from the Hesperian Foundation's *A Book for Midwives* (Klein, Miller, & Thomson, 2004). The book is not only well written and organized, but it also speaks to the social issues that midwives confront every day. The MFM midwives began using this book in their initial training, even with nonliterate midwives. As training evolved, literacy became a requirement for participation, and each traditional midwife participant received a copy of *A Book for Midwives* (in Spanish), for personal use as a text and reference.

In addition to the Hesperian book, the course design drew from other important and globally recognized resources for curriculum and reference, including the following:

- The Integrated Management of Pregnancy and Childbirth (IMPAC) manual (WHO, 2000) for integrated management of pregnancy and childbirth
- Checklists for knowledge and skills acquisition and demonstration developed by midwives at the Johns Hopkins Program for International Education in Gynecology and Obstetrics (JHPIEGO), modified for traditional midwives
- ASECSA (Asociación de Servicios Comunitarios de Salud) curricula, selected for relevant and thorough content coverage in Guatemala and because it addresses the underlying social causes and medical consequences of poverty
- Training manuals and guidebooks published by PAHO; Ministries of Health from Guatemala, El Salvador, Nicaragua, and Peru; and other NGO publications based on their work with midwives, including MotherCare and CARE/Peru.

The training course evolved over time. By spring 2005, the course for traditional midwives consisted of 27 one day a week, 6-hour sessions. Most traditional midwives could not attend training full time, and one day a week was the most practical solution. The program used adult learning methodologies and techniques emphasizing participatory interaction, reinforcement of key messages, critical thinking skills, and practical application. Learning formats included minilectures, discussions, role plays, live model demonstrations (with pregnant clients, if available, or within the Sololá hospital prenatal clinic), hands-on skills labs for developing physical assessment techniques, and small group work involving case studies and problem solving. The MFM training curricula focused on three main areas:

- Assessment and care of the pregnant woman and newborn, covering basic reproductive anatomy and physiology; healthy behaviors and nutrition;

prenatal examination; history taking; estimating gestational age and expected date of birth; initiation of breastfeeding; and postpartum evaluation of the mother and baby
- Technical skills, including vital signs; measuring uterine fundal height; palpating for fetal position and presentation; auscultation of fetal heart tones; sterilizing birth kit equipment; active third-stage management and management of postpartum hemorrhage; and neonatal resuscitation
- Critical thinking skills, including categorizing both traditional and modern methods into helpful, harmful, or benign; management of normal labor and birth; assessment and timely identification of danger signs and potential complications; prudent and judicious use of technology; and strategies for ensuring emergency transportation and transfer

The MFM midwives encouraged the traditional midwives to ask themselves, when confronted with new and improved methods or existing cultural practices, whether or not their practices would serve the health of women and the community. In addition, the MFM midwives included discussions on larger cultural constructs, such as machismo and gender-based violence. They challenged the traditional midwives to consider the ways in which cultural traditions contribute to inequities between men and women, they stressed women's reproductive rights as human rights, and emphasized the importance of women working together for change.

The MFM midwives also incorporated effective traditional practices, such as personalized care, presence and support, education, and respect for women as a primary participant in her own process. They created a training model that spoke to the role and everyday work of the community-based traditional midwife.

MONITORING AND EVALUATION OF TRAINING

By June 2005, MFM had trained 239 traditional midwives distributed in five cohorts located in six different departments in the Guatemalan highlands (Sacatepéquez, Chimaltenango, Quetzaltenango, Huehuetenango, Sololá, and Totonicapán). Of the traditional midwives trained, 215 (90%) graduated successfully. However, the question should be asked how success was assessed and documented. Since its inauguration, MFM correctly recognized the need to monitor, evaluate, document, and report its training progress. Processes and outcome evaluations received increasing attention and enhancement as the program matured under the guidance of Virginia Lamprecht, a member of the advisory board and an international reproductive healthcare specialist.

In late 2004, with the help of funding received from American Jewish Worldwide Services (AJWS), MFM hired Gal Frenkel, a public health professional, to further design, develop, and implement MFM's monitoring and evaluation activities and provide the MFM staff, board members, and other stakeholders with a comprehensive report of MFM's training program. The first step in this process was to review all of the evaluation tools and data collected to date; the second step was to analyze those data, provide recommendations for improvement of the training, and enhance (and revise) the monitoring and evaluation design. The following box presents a list of the tools used.

> **BOX 2-1** **Monitoring and Evaluation Tools**
> - Precourse screening interview
> - Pre- and postcourse knowledge assessment
> - Weekly quiz
> - Weekly class written evaluations (by participants and instructors)
> - Weekly class oral discussions
> - Final exam
> - Focus groups and postcourse descriptive evaluations

These tools were under constant development and underwent ongoing revisions and improvements; however, their objective remained the same:

- To characterize the incoming cohort of traditional midwives in terms of their midwifery experience, literacy level, and Spanish comprehension ability
- To assess the traditional midwives' change in knowledge before and after attending the MFM training
- To help the instructors better tailor the content of the training to the needs of each specific cohort and assess the participants' progress
- To evaluate the satisfaction of the traditional midwives who attended the course

The focus groups and postcourse evaluations were consistently and overwhelmingly positive. The traditional midwives expressed a very high level of

CHAPTER 2 Weaving Traditional and Professional Midwifery

satisfaction with the training and the instructors, and they were honored to have had the opportunity to participate in the course. These tools also provided the MFM team with the opportunity to address challenges, in addition to other topics they would have found useful in the training.

The screening tool was extremely useful for selecting traditional midwives at a level appropriate for the training. In the first couple of cohorts, participants varied greatly in their backgrounds and abilities. The youngest participant was 22 years old, and the oldest was 86 years old; some were not active traditional midwives and had no prior experience in midwifery, and the most experienced traditional midwife had 50 years of experience. Among the active traditional midwives, the number of births per month ranged from zero to six. Moreover, approximately one-third of the traditional midwives did not speak Spanish and/or were illiterate. This fact demonstrates that MFM was indeed reaching the targeted population of indigenous midwives or those that were most in need, but at the same time this also proved to be a challenge in administering the training and teaching more complex materials. For example, incorporating blood measurement into the training was challenging for traditional midwives who could not read numbers and found it difficult to comprehend numeric values and the meaning of systolic and diastolic blood pressure. Given the increasing level of comprehension required as the training expanded throughout the years, there was a need to select traditional midwives who were able to understand the concepts taught in Spanish, read the materials provided in the training, recognize numbers, and complete the course successfully.

The final exam and the pre- and postcourse knowledge assessment were the two key quantitative tools designed to demonstrate the level of success of the course participants. Questions were designed in an attempt to address the three core topics of the MFM training: assessment and care of the pregnant woman and newborn, technical skills, and critical thinking skills. The final exam eventually consisted of 195 possible points that covered the range of topics taught in the course, including a clinical section to assess selected clinical skills such as measurement of vital signs and infant resuscitation. The final exam was organized by topic, and participants had to obtain a score of 70% or higher to pass. Clinical skills were assessed using a checklist, and they were scored as pass or fail. The traditional midwives were required to demonstrate every clinical step correctly in order to pass the exam. It should be noted that the content of both the training and the final exam, including the administration of the final exam (i.e., in oral and verbal format) and the score required to pass successfully, changed greatly

Monitoring and Evaluation of Training

> **BOX 2-2**
>
> ## Traditional Midwives and the Final Exam
>
> **Topics Traditional Midwives Struggled with on the Final Exam**
> - Knowledge of what to do during the first prenatal visit
> - Gestational age and its relationship to the size of the uterus
> - Correct blood pressure measurement
> - When not to perform a vaginal exam
> - Knowledge of normal signs during the third stage of labor
> - Sexually transmitted diseases (STDs)
> - Having an emergency plan
> - The importance of keeping the baby warm
>
> **Topics Traditional Midwives Excelled at on the Final Exam**
> - Risk signs and factors
> - Management of postpartum hemorrhage
> - Knowledge of the three signs of a healthy baby immediately following birth
> - Infant resuscitation
> - Advantages of exclusive breastfeeding
> - Knowledge of different contraception methods
> - Focus groups and postcourse descriptive evaluations

throughout the years (e.g., "success" had previously been defined as a score of 50% or higher).

The pre- and postcourse knowledge assessment tool was used for the first time in the third MFM training cohort, which was held in the second part of 2003. Like the final exam, it underwent constant changes and as such was challenging to analyze, especially when different precourse and postcourse versions were administered in the same cohort. One of the major modifications of this tool resulted from the need to clearly establish knowledge indicators. In terms of results, some demonstrated an increase in knowledge, and others demonstrated a decrease in knowledge, an unexpected outcome after having attended and graduated from the course. The latter results, therefore, are a critique on the validity and reliability of this evaluation tool as it is currently designed and administered.

In addition to the outcome evaluation assessed by both the final exam and the pre- and postcourse knowledge assessments, the importance of process evaluation

CHAPTER 2   Weaving Traditional and Professional Midwifery

> **BOX 2-3**
>
> ## Traditional Midwives' Knowledge during the Training
>
> **Topics in Which Traditional Midwives Demonstrated Increased Knowledge from the Beginning to the End of the Training**
> - White vaginal discharge with no other symptoms is normal
> - Equipment must be sterilized
> - How to detect meconium
> - When the placenta is delivered normally
> - Exclusive breastfeeding
>
> **Topics in Which Traditional Midwives Demonstrated Decreased Knowledge from the Beginning to the End of the Training**
> - Correct counseling when there are signs of preeclampsia
> - What to do if the water breaks but labor does not begin after 36 hours
> - What to do with postpartum complications
> - Focus groups and postcourse descriptive evaluations

(in this case, dropout rate) should also be mentioned as another indicator of the challenges that faced the MFM training team and that impacted overall success. The first example is from the fourth training cohort, where 75 traditional midwives attended the training, 65 completed the training, and 62 graduated successfully (i.e., passed the final exam). Another example is from the third training cohort, where 50 traditional midwives attended the third MFM training cohort and 49 graduated successfully. However, when MFM offered a refresher course in the summer of 2004, only 12 traditional midwives showed up. The reasons why only one-quarter of the MFM trained traditional midwives attended this refresher course may vary. However, this example clearly demonstrates the difficulties associated with continued education and reinforcement of new knowledge, attitudes, and practices that may not be sustainable independently in the original communities of the traditional midwives.

To summarize, MFM faced a great challenge when administering this training to traditional midwives. On one hand, the professional midwives identified the unmet need to train the indigenous and most traditional midwives, where infant and maternal mortality were the highest. On the other hand, there were many barriers to successfully implementing the training and sustaining the knowledge acquired in this training. Lessons learned from this experience include the need to clearly define the characteristics of participants in terms of language, literacy, and experience and to tailor the training to meet their level. It could also be beneficial to assess the beliefs and attitudes of the participants toward the new information and address these issues during the training. Finally, it is important to keep in mind that even when course participants demonstrate positive attitudes and increased knowledge upon graduation, the road to incorporation of the new and correct practices and their implementation is very long. Professional and technical support groups and continuing education for these trained traditional midwives are essential.

INTERTWINE WITH THE MINISTRY OF HEALTH

By 2004, MFM's training program had become established enough to be known in Guatemala, particularly by other NGOs, local health facilities, and the Ministry of Health. As the program's success and visibility grew, and after many previous attempts by MFM to work with the Ministry of Health (MOH), some doctors from the MOH approached MFM with the idea of developing a pilot curriculum for traditional midwives that would include a clinical practical component. This request by the MOH signified a major first step on the part of the Guatemalan government to acknowledge the contribution of midwifery and the need to effectively work with and incorporate comadronas into the official health system.

The MOH invited MFM to conduct training in the Department of Sololá, where MFM had been in previous contact with various doctors working with comadronas and began developing a relationship with the medical director of the Sololá hospital—the main public referral hospital in the department. The group we trained in Sololá graduated in June 2005, along with another group from Totonicapán. This latter group included 37 traditional midwives that live in the region around Lake Atitlan. The Totonicapán group did not have the training component that included clinical skills because of transportation and distance problems to the Sololá hospital.

In addition to attending 27 classroom sessions, the Sololá group participated in 10 clinical sessions inside the Sololá hospital, where they worked in collaboration with hospital staff supervised by MFM's training team headed by Melida

CHAPTER 2 Weaving Traditional and Professional Midwifery

Jimenez, an advisor on the MFM board. Ms. Jimenez was uniquely suited to be the clinical supervisor within the public system, given that she is a Guatemalan physician who later moved to Canada, where she graduated from midwifery training. Ms. Jimenez was joined by Cornelia Muhl, a German midwife. The practical component of the training provided clinical experience for traditional midwives, with modeling and supervision by a professional midwife—the first time this had ever happened in Guatemala.

The experience in the hospital was very challenging. Although MFM midwives tried valiantly to orient hospital staff and present the project in a manner that respected their authority, and even with institutional support from the MOH, our presence met with steady and daily opposition. The hospital administrator gave the MFM trainers a large room where they set up a space that allowed for birthing privacy, freedom of movement, and practice of the midwifery model. Although they made many attempts to invite nurses and doctors in the birth room, the MFM midwives were met with ongoing resistance from both. Despite the challenges, the traditional midwives did experience clinical practice under supervision within the hospital, and MFM was able to observe client care provided within a public health system over many weeks, instead of only during an organized tour.

UNRAVELING AND CLOSURE

In November 2004, Ixmucané in Antigua closed. Ixmucané Birth Center and MFM could not maintain sufficient personnel to run a birth center 24 hours a day, seven days a week, and also have enough staff for the training program. We made an organizational decision to focus exclusively on training, rather than trying to incorporate training concurrently with a full-time birth center that included direct care provision. Although many professional midwives expressed interest in, and support for, the work of MFM, experienced midwives were not willing to relocate to Guatemala for extended periods to work with us full time at the birth center. Since no cadre of professional midwifery existed in the country, recruiting professional Guatemalan midwives to run the Ixmucané center was not an option.

Finding continuous funding became another insurmountable challenge to the birth center and the organization. MFM's work came at a point in the history of international development when funding priorities had moved away from training traditional midwives toward training "skilled birth attendants" (in the language of international donors, that means nurses and doctors) and toward improving referral care facilities and health systems. The U.S. Institute of Medicine published a recommendation in 2003 that every delivery be assisted by a skilled birth attendant with access to essential obstetric and newborn care. This recommendation requires a network of good-quality health facilities that provide basic essential obstetric care (BEOC includes the availability supplies, i.e., antibiotics, oxytocics, and anticonvulsants, along with skill sets of practitioners that involve manual removal of the placenta, removal of retained products of conception, and mechanically assisted vaginal deliveries) (Bale, Stoll, & Lucas, 2003).

The traditional midwives of Guatemala had never been integrated into the official health system of the MOH. Even though a meta-analysis on the effectiveness of training traditional midwives urged more evaluation, refinement, and dissemination of promising community-based approaches to care during birth (Sibley & Sipe, 2004, 2006), MFM's experience was that by 2004, the global donor community had already unraveled the prioritizing of such approaches.

From the beginning, the commitment to work with the poor created economic challenges and limited MFM's ability to pay for growing staff needs. Ixmucané and MFM survived as long as it did because of the interest and dedication of volunteers, students, experienced midwives, and others committed to the work. Funds came from clients who could afford to pay for services, small grants from local Guatemalan charities, and individuals who supported the effort. Without funding or sufficient staff, MFM had to close the Ixmucané birth center, and we eventually had to discontinue the training sessions as well.

LESSONS LEARNED

Despite its closure, MFM and Ixmucané made many important contributions to the global midwifery discourse. As MFM looks back at the underlying causes of women's unmet reproductive health needs, it was not difficult to also identify some causes of unmet knowledge and skills needs of traditional midwives, who continue to be blamed by the "skilled birth attendants" for maternal and newborn morbidity and mortality rates in almost every country. The consequences of global economic policies, misuse of power and authority, extreme devaluation of women, and machismo are only some of the reasons why women suffer and maternal and infant mortality remain so high among indigenous populations around the world.

Guatemala has seen developmental organizations and projects come and go over many decades. Despite 9 years of MFM and Ixmucané Women's Health and Birth Center presence in Guatemala, and regardless of very favorable relationships with local midwives, it would have taken many more years and much more financial support to build a strong enough organizational structure to have the necessary influence over public policy that might have enabled the kind of social change needed to improve reproductive health care for women.

Another important lesson from the MFM experience is that communication between professional providers and traditional midwives, along with interfacility (clinic to hospital, birth center to hospital) communication, needs to be clear, respectful, and continuous. When midwives are excluded from the hospital system, continuity of care suffers, trust from the community is lost, and women and children die.

Regarding specific work with traditional midwives, the MFM training experience shows that to improve their knowledge and skills, traditional midwives must be able to read and write and that governmental or charitable literacy programs need to include traditional midwives.

MFM's experience also shows that professional midwives who can model midwifery care to traditional midwives (and other skilled birth attendants) are essential for improving healthcare provision and outcomes. Working side by side and building relationships with the midwives was not only based on theoretical concepts (Jonsdottir, Litchfield, & Pharris, 2004; Kennedy, 2000), but also an essential and practical training strategy.

FABRIC FOR THE FUTURE

Midwifery care and midwifery training should be local, accessible, and personal. A traditional midwife needs to be respected, enabled, and included in reproductive health policy and training design. Studies have shown that what midwives need in their training, and what they do not receive from governmental programs, include a solid knowledge base, clinical experience for skills practice, and ongoing support with follow-up over months or years (MacLean, 2003). Midwifery training needs to focus on building critical thinking skills, enhancing self-esteem, understanding the root causes of maternal morbidity, and teaching and practicing lifesaving skills to effectively meet the needs of women and newborns.

Midwives from developed countries have the opportunity to help traditional midwives organize themselves and create a group identity. These organized midwives can and do advocate for health policies that respect the important role of women in their communities. Traditional midwives could participate in national training programs based on MFM's midwifery model, a model that empowers women, incorporates both knowledge acquisition and skills competence, and promotes social change.

In some places in Guatemala, midwives have organized. The exclusion that traditional midwives experienced from hospital personnel, witnessed over and over again by MFM, has changed in places where midwives can enter with the mother and continue their relationship as a trusted provider (Maupin, 2008; Schooley, Mindt, Wagner, Fullerton, & O'Donnell, 2009). Yet the role of the midwife has shifted; Maupin has noted that the recruitment, education, practice, and authority of the midwife is changing, based on the influence of the national priority of the Sistema Integral en Atención en Salud (SIAS), which links traditional midwives with the goals to significantly reduce maternal and infant mortality. The reshaping of the midwife role, however, is as community advocate and source of referral, *not as birth attendant*. Institutional delivery is the national emphasis (Maupin, 2008).

Nine years of MFM in Guatemala have enabled many students of midwifery, anthropology, and public health to profoundly understand the differences between indigenous health and governmental public health systems; establish close relationships with traditional midwives; understand the level of knowledge, skills, discrimination, and obstacles traditional midwives face; and determine what a traditional midwife needs to become a knowledgeable, capable community-based healthcare provider. MFM learned what is possible given effective training based on a midwifery model; we tested that model in practical settings (in the Ixmucané center and the Sololá government referral hospital) and in training (throughout six departments within Guatemala), and we came away not only with some highly positive results, but with a solid conviction that the midwifery model contributes much to improving the health of mothers and newborns.

CHAPTER 2   Weaving Traditional and Professional Midwifery

> **Discussion Questions**
>
> 1. How would you describe the relationship between the traditional midwives and the staff of Ixmucané?
> 2. How do you think the participation of student midwives influenced the client–provider relationship and the quality of care at Ixmucané?
> 3. Describe the socioeconomic and health systems implications of a skills-based, literacy-dependent curriculum. Consider the community, the traditional midwives, and the clients of the traditional midwives.
> 4. What do you think were the causes of the conflict between the MFM and traditional midwives in the Sololá hospital? How do you think it could have been prevented?
> 5. What were the challenges presented by international funding priorities on training skilled attendants in a country such as Guatemala?

NOTES

1. A point of clarification is warranted here about the nuances in the language of midwifery. Today's Guatemalan midwives are categorized in official World Health Organization language as traditional birth attendants, or TBAs (WHO, 1992). Midwives for Midwives (MFM) declined to adopt the TBA label. This term diminishes the role and significance of traditional midwives. The word "midwife" means "with woman," referring to the way women have accompanied women during childbirth throughout history. MFM referred to the indigenous Guatemalan practitioners who attend births as they refer to themselves, *comadronas*, or simply *midwives*. We use the term *traditional midwife* interchangeably with term *comadrona*. A generic definition offered by medical anthropologist Shelia Cosminsky (1977) became the alternative that felt realistic for MFM to use for midwives: "The term 'midwife' refers to a position which has been socially differentiated as a specialized status by the society. Such a person is regarded as a specialist and a professional in her own eyes and by her own community."

REFERENCES

Bale, J., Stoll, B., & Lucas, A. (2003). *Improving birth outcomes.* Washington, DC: National Academies Press.

Cosminsky, S. (1975). Changing food and medical beliefs and practices in a Guatemalan community. *Ecology of Food and Nutrition, 4,* 183–194.

Cosminsky, S. (1977). Childbirth and midwifery on a Guatemalan finca. *Medical Anthropology, 1*(3), 69–104.

Cosminsky, S. (1982). Knowledge and body concepts of Guatemalan midwives. In M. Kay (Ed.), *Anthropology of human birth* (pp. 233–252). Philadelphia, PA: F. A. Davis.

Goetz, D., & Morley, S. G. (1950). *The Popul Vuh, the sacred book of the Mayas* (A. Recinos, Trans.). Tulsa, OK: University of Oklahoma Press.

Gorry, C. (2001). *Guatemala.* Melbourne, Australia: Lonely Planet.

Guatemala. Ministerio de Salud Pública y Asistencia Social (MSPAS). (2003). *Línea basal de mortalidad materna para el año 2000.* Guatemala City, Guatemala: MSPAS.

Instituto Nacional de Estadística, et al. (1995). *Encuesta nacional de salud materno infantil 1995.* Guatemala City, Guatemala: INE.

International Confederation of Midwives. (2003). *The essential competencies of midwifery practice.* Geneva, Switzerland: Author.

Jonsdottir, H., Litchfield, M., & Pharris, M. D. (2004). The relational core of nursing practice as partnership. *Journal of Advanced Nursing, 47,* 241–250.

Jordan, B. (1993). *Birth in four cultures: A cross-cultural investigation of childbirth in Yucatan, Holland, Sweden, and the United States* (4th ed.). Prospect Heights, IL: Waveland Press. (Original work published 1978.)

Kennedy, H. P. (2000). A model of exemplary midwifery practice: Results of a Delphi study. *Journal of Midwifery and Women's Health, 45,* 4–19.

Klein, S., Miller, S., & Thomson, F. (2004). *A book for midwives.* Berkeley, CA: Hesperian Foundation.

Lukere, V. (2002). Native obstetric nursing in Fiji. In V. Lukere & M. Jolly (Eds.), *Birthing in the Pacific* (pp. 100–124). Honolulu, HI: University of Hawaii Press.

MacLean, G. (2003). The challenge of preparing and enabling "skilled attendants" to promote safer childbirth. *Midwifery, 19,* 163–169.

Maupin, J. N. (2008). Remaking the Guatemalan midwife: Health care reform and midwifery training programs in Highland Guatemala. *Medical Anthropology, 27*(4), 353–382.

Ministerio de Salud Pública y Asistencia Social. (1993). *Programa mujer, salud y desarrollo.* Guatemala City, Guatemala: Author.

Murphy, P., & Fullerton, J. (2001). Measuring outcomes of midwifery care: Development of an instrument to assess optimality. *Journal of Midwifery and Women's Health, 46*(5), 274–284.

Nelson, D. (1999). *A finger in the wound.* Berkeley, CA: University of California Press.

Pan American Health Organization. (2011). *Health situation in the Americas: basic health indicators 2011.* Retrieved from http://new.paho.org/hq/index.php?option=com_content&task=view&id=2470&Itemid=2003.

CHAPTER 2   Weaving Traditional and Professional Midwifery

Romano, A. (2004). *Obstetric and perinatal outcomes of a professional midwifery service in Guatemala: A retrospective cohort study measuring optimality* (Unpublished master's thesis). Yale University School of Nursing, New Haven, CT.
Schooley, J., Mindt, C., Wagner, P., Fullerton, J., & O'Donnell, M. (2009). Factors influencing health care-seeking behaviours among Mayan women in Guatemala. *Midwifery, 25*(4), 411–421.
Sesia, P. (1997). Women come here on their own when they need to. In R. Davis-Floyd & C. Sargent (Eds.), *Childbirth and authoritative knowledge* (pp. 397–420). Berkeley, CA: University of California Press.
Sibley, L. M., & Sipe, T. A. (2004). What can a meta-analysis tell us about traditional birth attendant training and pregnancy outcomes? *Midwifery, 20*(1), 51–60.
Sibley, L. M., & Sipe, T. A. (2006). Transition to skilled birth attendance: Is there a future role for trained traditional birth attendants? *Journal of Health, Population, and Nutrition, 24*(4), 472–478.
Singh, S., Prada, E., & Kestler, E. (2006). Induced abortion and unintended pregnancy in Guatemala. *International family planning perspectives, 32*(3). Retrieved from http://www.guttmacher.org/pubs/journals/3213606.html.
UNICEF. (2003). At a glance: Guatemala. Retrieved from http://www.unicef.org/infoby country/guatemala_statistics.html#18.
United Nations. (2011). World Contraceptive Use 2011. Retrieved from http://www.un.org/esa/population/publications/contraceptive2011/contraceptive2011.htm.
United States Central Intelligence Agency. (2012). World Factbook. Retrieved from https://www.cia.gov/library/publications/the-world-factbook/index.html.
United States Global Health Initiative, Guatemala Strategy. (2010). Retrieved from http://pdf.usaid.gov/pdf_docs/PDACR172.pdf.
World Health Organization. (1992). *Traditional birth attendants: A Joint WHO/UNICEF/UNFPA statement.* Geneva, Switzerland: Author.
World Health Organization. (2000). *Managing complications in pregnancy and childbirth handbook.* Geneva, Switzerland: Author.
World Health Organization, UNICEF, UNFPA, and The World Bank. (2007). Maternal mortality in 2005. Estimates developed by WHO, UNICEF, UNFPA, and The World Bank. Retrieved from http://www.who.int/maternal_child_adolescent/documents/9789241596213/en/.

PART II

Safe Motherhood

Safe motherhood is a worldwide campaign to improve the outcomes of pregnancy, labor, and delivery. The initiative was started in 1987 by the World Health Organization (WHO) and other international organizations. In the past 24 years, many countries have been able to improve their birth outcomes, but at the same time the inequalities between and within countries are also growing; those who have access to quality health care reap the benefits and those who are poor or living in remote areas are unable to take advantage of these improvements.

According to WHO (Oct 2007 Bulletin), there are at least 3.2 million stillborn babies, 4 million neonatal deaths, and more than half a million maternal deaths per year globally. These data suffer from issues of validity because few poor countries have accurate data about maternal and newborn morbidity and mortality. According to WHO, the scant attention paid to data and monitoring means that programs are often implemented without evidence-based information or program evaluation.

Progress that has been made through improvements in healthcare service delivery is being challenged by the impact of malaria and HIV. Most maternal deaths occur in the post-natal period and obstetric complications explain a little more than half of neonatal deaths. Although many women in poor countries make at least one prenatal visit, systematic and regular post-partum care is rare, even if a woman delivers in a healthcare facility.

The requirements for safe motherhood are very basic as can be seen in the case studies that follow, although delivery by a skilled attendant is the most important factor. Knowledge and technology dramatically reduce the rates of mortality and morbidity and are readily available. The primary challenge is to scale up healthcare services and delivery and to educate communities. The easiest part of that challenge is providing institutions, but these institutions and communities need trained staff.

Training healthcare professionals requires teachers, and in some countries class size, for groups of nurses and midwives are so large they are taught in open tents. Upon graduation, these nurses and midwives often go to urban areas and foreign countries where their skills have much higher economic value, leaving poor countries and rural areas dependent on trained community volunteers and, if lucky enough, trained traditional birth attendants.

Other challenges to the implementation of safe motherhood programs include decaying infrastructure; supply chain management of drugs, supplies and equipment; adequate transportation; good management; and political will.

The case studies presented show local innovations that face these challenges. Whether they are idiosyncratic solutions for local situations or can be scaled up for replication is a question to be considered.

CHAPTER 3

Sing Safe Motherhood: A Story of the Women of Chiwamba, Malawi

Daima Thyangathyanga, MS, MRN, MRM
Mary Kambewa, MRN, MRM, CHN
Rose M. Kershbaumer, EdD, CNM
Joyce E. Thompson, DrPH, CNM

Location: Chiwamba, Malawi, Africa

Name of Project: Community-Based Safe Motherhood Advisor program, Penn-Malawi Women for Women's Health project

Sponsoring Organizations: University of Pennsylvania School of Nursing, Malawi Ministry of Health and Population; primary funding from the Rockefeller Foundation

Target Population: Women and men living in Traditional Authority Chimutu (village women and men), Lilongwe District, Malawi, Africa

Project Goal: Promote and improve the health and well-being of women at the village level through activities and partnerships aimed at reducing maternal morbidity and mortality

Project Objective: Design and implement a series of Safe Motherhood training of trainer (TOT) workshops that will prepare village women to carry the messages of Safe Motherhood throughout their communities

CHAPTER 3   Sing Safe Motherhood: A Story of the Women of Chiwamba, Malawi

INTRODUCTION

Women in many developing countries are still dying needlessly from pregnancy-related complications. In the small African country of Malawi, the 2009 estimated maternal mortality ratio was 847 per 100,000 live births (Ministry of Health, 2006). Among major contributors to maternal death are a lack of Safe Motherhood knowledge and cultural misconceptions related to pregnancy, labor, and the postpartum period (Thompson, 2005). For these reasons, strategies to reduce maternal mortality need to include wide dissemination of Safe Motherhood information to community members at the grassroots level. This endeavor is often hampered by a grave shortage of trained health personnel. One trained health worker based at a busy health center with a 10-kilometer radius catchment area cannot leave the health facility to teach in a village. Health workers need to find ways of utilizing community members to teach health in their own communities.

Community-Based Health Education: Key Challenges

There are many details involved in creating and implementing a community-based health education program. First is the selection of a public health model based on determinants of health (Thompson, 2007). Next is to identify and confront the challenges and build on the opportunities for improving the health of childbearing women at the village level, using members of the community as teachers. This story represents successful interventions based on surveying the community to be served and understanding their knowledge of health promotion related to childbearing prior to implementing the program (Gennaro, Thyangathyanga, Kershbaumer, & Thompson, 2001).

One of the major challenges represented in this story relates to the fact that village women were to be trained as health educators in Safe Motherhood, which involves threats to strong cultural traditions that view women as less than men and whose primary value in the community is to bear and raise children and make sure the men are fed (Thompson, 2004). Training women also challenged traditional male authority as the women became trusted, wise counselors beyond their own families. Thus the Community-Based Safe Motherhood Advisor (CBSMA) program took advantage of the opportunity to enhance the status of women by bringing health messages to the men, women, and children of their villages.

A second major challenge in designing and implementing a community-based health intervention in a resource-poor country such as Malawi is the lack of literacy that is often found among village women and young girls who are denied the opportunity to complete primary school. Ideally, training of trainer (TOT) workshops are conducted with individuals who can read and write during their learning and teaching sessions. This case study tells the story of how music and dance were used to meet the literacy challenge in Chiwamba, an area of Traditional Authority (Chief) Chimutu, Lilongwe District, Malawi, Africa, during the implementation of the CBSMA program from 1996 to 2002.

BACKGROUND

The CBSMA program was a direct outcome of the evaluation of the first 5 years of project activities under the umbrella of the Penn-Malawi Women for Women's Health project (1990–2002). The overall goal of the Women for Women's Health project was "To promote and improve the health and well-being of women at village level through activities and partnerships aimed at reducing maternal morbidity and mortality" (Thyangathyanga, 1994). The first 5 years of the project focused on TOT Safe Motherhood workshops for Malawian registered nurse midwives (RNMs) who then taught enrolled nurse midwives how to promote Safe Motherhood. Each RNM was also expected to share the messages of Safe Motherhood in their church meetings and community gatherings when they went to their own villages to check on family, crops, and homes.

An external evaluation of the Penn-Malawi project in 1994 included interviews of village men and women. Consistent feedback during these interviews highlighted how much they had learned from the RNM Safe Motherhood trainers (Thyangathyanga, 1994). A frequent comment from individual women during the interviews was the value of teaching and learning at the village level. "When we go to the clinic it is because I am sick or my child is sick and I am not able to listen to the general talks given in the waiting area. When the nurse gathers us in the village I can listen and ask questions." Mrs. Mary Kambewa also noted that giving life-saving information to women and men in their villages reaches many women who would never go to a clinic. Several women, and some men, said that if the RNMs had come sooner, maybe their sister or wife might not have died in childbirth.

The CBSMA program started in March 1996 in Chiwamba Area Traditional Authority (TA) Chimutu, an undeveloped rural area with no easy access to the district hospital. This area was designated by the Ministry of Health and Population because it was underserved with only one health facility that had one enrolled nurse–midwife serving a population of 35,000. The facility registered

CHAPTER 3 Sing Safe Motherhood: A Story of the Women of Chiwamba, Malawi

40–50 deliveries per month and referred many women with obstetrical complications to Lilongwe District hospital. This TA area accounted for most of the maternal deaths in Lilongwe District, with the major causes being ruptured uteri or postpartum hemorrhage, as confirmed by the chief nursing officer (CNO). The CNO thought that if the CBSMA program was implemented in TA Chimutu, the TOT leaders might be able to identify why this was happening and avoid bad practices in the future. Likewise, Chief Chimutu was very supportive of the CBSMA project. He sadly noted that he was often called to open "grave sites" for young women who had died in childbirth.

Prior to implementation of the TOT workshops for village women, Penn researcher Dr. Susan Gennaro designed a preintervention survey to collect data on the communities' knowledge, attitudes, and practices (KAPs) related to Safe Motherhood. This was followed by a postintervention survey in 1999 that supported the many successes of the Community-Based Safe Motherhood Advisors (CBSMAs) and their health education (Gennaro et al., 2001).

Mrs. Daima Thyangathyanga was hired as the Malawian in-country coordinator of the CBSMA program because of her extensive teaching background, Peace Corps leadership, and commitment to village health. She asked one of the RNM Safe Motherhood trainers, Mrs. Mary Kambewa, also the district community health nurse, to join her in codesigning and implementing the CBSMA program with the support of the Penn codirectors. This is their story of a successful maternal health intervention with village women as the messengers of health.

THE STORY: TEACHING AND LEARNING SAFE MOTHERHOOD

The plan for teaching village women about health and well-being during pregnancy, birth, and postbirth included three TOT 5-day workshops approximately 3 to 4 months apart. The coleaders of the TOT program would visit the women between the workshops to monitor and support the women's teaching efforts. Criteria for graduation from the program included attendance at all workshops and continued teaching in the village.

The TOT Workshops

The primary aim of the program was to provide information, education, and communication skills for behavior change on issues of Safe Motherhood in order to reduce maternal morbidity and mortality in the area. The first TOT workshop in TA Chimutu was conducted in April 1996. As agreed, Chief Chimutu had requested each of his five group village headmen to choose three women who met the selection criteria of well-respected, literate, and willing to volunteer as messengers of Safe Motherhood information. Thirteen women showed up for the first TOT. They were genuine local, indigenous, rural, grassroots women—the kind of women one only sees sitting on the ground or on the bench of the rural clinic listening to the health talk. They looked like everybody else in the community, yet this project was endeavoring to turn these women into the givers of the health talks in their own villages and to empower them to be the agents of positive behavior change for safer motherhood in their communities. The Malawian trainers were excited by the challenge.

The first TOT workshop lasted for one week and was held in a hostel in the capital city, Lilongwe. The group would then go back to the community to teach Safe Motherhood for 3 to 4 months, about one teaching session per week, and then come back for another TOT workshop. Eventually, about 90 women were trained—six groups of 13 to 15 participants per group. Each group attended three Safe Motherhood TOT workshops, along with extra sessions when literacy and income-generating activities were added. Each workshop followed the same content outline, with guest speakers, micro teaching, and lots of singing and dancing.

Overview of Content

The topics covered during the TOT workshops included an introduction to Safe Motherhood, participants' experience with maternal deaths, causes of maternal death and disability in Malawi and Chiwamba Area, and personal health issues related to infection, hygiene, infestations, and prevention of anemia. Much time was also spent on the status of women in Malawi and in the eyes of God, the effects of women's status on maternal and fetal health, and local cultural beliefs surrounding childbearing practices, both positive and negative. Theory and practice related to teaching others, characteristics of a good teacher, and how people learn were also included.

A brief description of how the workshops were conducted follows to illustrate some of the factors for success that were demonstrated on the postintervention survey (Gennaro et al., 2001).

Welcome and Introductions

A prayer was said to open each workshop. Introductions were proposed, and the women spontaneously broke into song, "We are glad we have met." The trainers

CHAPTER 3   Sing Safe Motherhood: A Story of the Women of Chiwamba, Malawi

(we) assumed that these women could at least read and write Chichewa, the Malawian national language. We wanted to be sure that the women understood the voluntary nature of their assignment, so we discussed this with them. We appealed to them to accept the challenge of volunteering to partner with God and health workers in saving lives through community teaching. We also gave them the liberty to withdraw from the training and be taken home if they were not willing to be volunteers. No one left. No one ever left a training session in the 6 years that followed, though of the total, 10 women did not complete their teaching obligations.

Registration was the next exercise. A sheet of paper was passed around so that each woman could write her own name and a few other particulars. Surprise, surprise! Most of the women could not write! Only 2 of the 13 could read and write well enough to fill in all the particulars on the registration form. Some could write their name only, others only their first name. Some could not write anything at all. Self-registration was used in later groups as a means of assessing each woman's literacy level.

Another surprise was the discovery that the women had a hard time understanding Daima's Chichewa accent, and she had trouble understanding the Chiwamba dialect of Chichewa. Luckily, Mary was able to clarify for both sides because her own dialect was closer to that of the women. In addition, Mary had experience talking to women of the same level in this district in her roles as the district community health nurse, the district Safe Motherhood trainer, and the district traditional birth attendant (TBA) trainer. The choice of trainers created a good teaching team!

Creative Teaching Methods

The women's lack of literacy rendered the prepared teaching aids irrelevant and invalid. The flipcharts were hung up, but less than a quarter of the group looked at them. The rest just intently looked at and listened to the speaker. Flyers and handouts were put away into their files without being read. "Our grandchildren will read these to us at home," they said. Even posters were often looked at upside down, sideways, or even diagonally, often with distorted interpretations. We realized the need to use more teaching methods that did not require much reading and writing.

Talking in class is not traditional in Malawi, so it took a lot of effort to get the women to participate in classroom discussions. When they did talk, we learned a lot from their revelations, so we encouraged them to talk. Just as some were too

The Story: Teaching and Learning Safe Motherhood

shy to talk, others were too shy to role play or to comment on the role plays. However, we noted that whenever break time came the women sang and even danced without being asked. Nobody was too shy to sing. And everyone remembered the words of the song, literate or not. Everyone seemed to enjoy the singing, dancing, and ululating! We decided that music would be the major method of teaching and learning in the program. Music would no longer be relegated just to teatime.

During the first TOT workshop microteaching, the CBSMAs used mainly the lecture and discussion method to practice teaching the basic Safe Motherhood messages that they had learned. In the community, they used the same talk method except for the learning song. During the second TOT workshop the CBSMAs were taught other methods of teaching, such as role modeling, role playing, dramas, storytelling, singing, poetry, etc. These methods were chosen because they did not require much literacy on the part of the CBSMA teacher or the learners (village women and men). We capitalized on the women's cultural spontaneity in singing and spent a lot of time developing this method with the women. Singing is entertaining, easy to learn, easy to remember and retain, and to teach. This was illustrated by how those who had been to school could *sing* the alphabet song, but they could not *say* the alphabet. So the women were now ready to use singing to teach Safe Motherhood.

Singing in Class: What Songs and Why
The first song that was sung in class for learning purposes was called "Kuphunzira Nkusintha," which means "to learn is to change." The CBSMAs had been taught how to teach using the lecture and discussion method. They did quite well on lesson planning and lecture delivery, and they even managed some learner involvement during the teaching session. However, most of them had a hard time with assessments of learning. We asked the CBSMAs to evaluate the learning of their fellow CBSMAs during their microteaching and then to explain how they would know the community had learned. The CBSMAs would say, "I have explained clearly, so I am sure my friends have understood," or "If I tell them everything I planned on the lesson, I will know that they know what they should know about this problem."

We thought the women should sing the definition of learning so they would remember to look for positive behavior changes among the learners. Daima used the tune of a popular traditional wedding song that the women knew very well. We asked the women to put in the new words: "What is learning? To learn is to change. We should stop the bad things. We should do the good things. Then

CHAPTER 3   Sing Safe Motherhood: A Story of the Women of Chiwamba, Malawi

we shall save lives." So when one was having a hard time with evaluation we would all sing the learning song so the person would remember to ask questions during the microteaching class. They would say things like, "In the community, I would observe if they are changing, for example, if they are starting antenatal clinic at 3 months instead of at the usual 7 or 9 months." "I would find that they are now delivering in hospital rather than at home." "I shall notice that they are leaving the baby's umbilical cord clean instead of applying cow dung or rat droppings on the cord." The CBSMAs used this same song during their community teaching to let the community realize and remember that change for the better was expected of them after having been taught by the CBSMAs.

The women were asked to compose songs that focused on the specific childbearing problems of Chiwamba. They knew the problems from their own experience and from the presentation we had made to them on the findings of the preintervention survey during the second TOT workshop. The women, however, challenged Daima to compose a song first as an example they could emulate. This was a big challenge for her because she had no prior experience in song composing. In any case, Daima accepted the challenge and composed a song targeting the Chiwamba problem of retained placenta resulting in postpartum hemorrhage, which we had learned of from the preintervention survey and from the women during an early session in the first TOT workshop when each woman had to tell a story about her experience with maternal death in Chiwamba. More than 75% of them told of a retained placenta, hemorrhage, and death. Apparently, a laboring woman is encouraged to push the baby for hours, even before the second stage. Then, after the baby is born, she is asked to just wait for the placenta to fall out and is not asked to push. For some, this results in hemorrhage behind the placenta. The song called "The Placenta Is Retained" went like this: "Help me fellow women, I am in trouble. The baby is born but the placenta is retained. What should I do?" The fellow women tell her to "Put the baby to the breast and push. The placenta will come out and you will save your life." Daima wrote the words and asked the CBSMAs to put a Chiwamba tune to the words so that it could be easily learned in Chiwamba. They put a beautiful "Gule Wamkulu" tune to it, and it worked well. It was gratifying to hear community members singing this song during the postintervention survey as an example of what they had learned from the CBSMAs.

With that example given, the challenge of composing and singing Safe Motherhood songs was repeated to the women. The women's first response to the challenge was a song called "Kantayo," meaning "a small abortion." There is another significant story behind this song. During the preintervention survey there was a question, "Suppose a pregnant woman starts bleeding, is that a problem?" The response almost invariably was, "How many months pregnant?" We would say, "Any gestation. One, two, three, six, seven, any number of months." Both men and women would say, "It depends. One, two, or three months is not a problem." Why is it not a problem? "Because that is just a small abortion. It just comes out without any trouble. We worry if the pregnancy is more than six months on." That was the dangerous misconception targeted by the song, "Kantayo." The song says, "Even a small pregnancy can kill the mother. Do not ignore the small pregnancy. Go to the hospital to get help." A lovely churchlike tune came with this song. We were happy with and proud of the women. Learning had taken place. There was a significant change of behavior! This was group two. So the song-making endeavor continued with the collaboration of each group until, by the end the project, more than 10 songs were composed, adopted, and adapted. Several of these songs were also broadcast over radio in Malawi, reaching women and men in other areas of the country.

Activities Targeted to Raise Women's Status and Self-Concept

The fact that only women were selected to be trained as CBSMAs was a deliberate move to raise the women's status by helping them to believe in themselves and to show the men that the women could teach others. People asked why we were not training men to be CBSMAs. We told them that maybe we would later, otherwise the men would overtake the women and the women would withdraw, then our objective would not be achieved. In fact, the syllabus and curriculum assumed womanhood and the woman's childbearing experience as part of the entering behaviour. This also accorded high status to womanhood and childbirth.

Starting in the first TOT session, a lot of work was done with the women to make them status aware. On the first day of the workshop, a question and answer session was held in the classroom to help the women recognize the low level of their self-concept and explore how socialization had brought that about. The women said they were lower than men; even a young male was more important than an adult female. "Man is the head and woman is the tail." Woman is nothing. "Woman was created just to serve the man and make him happy." We tried to encourage the women to think, "OK, the man is the head but the woman is the neck or the heart." The tail was too low. The women seemed really surprised that we were even suggesting that they had a status higher than that which they accorded themselves. They believed that God intended their low status. "Even the Bible tells us so," they insisted. Besides, God created the man

CHAPTER 3   Sing Safe Motherhood: A Story of the Women of Chiwamba, Malawi

before the woman. That showed that man is the real person and woman was just an afterthought. They couldn't embrace our proposal that maybe God created woman for man because He realized that the man could not manage without the woman, therefore she was very important. Being oppressed and constantly undermined was viewed by the women as their God-created lot.

Having anticipated these perceptions of low self-esteem from the women, we planned for a male church elder to address the women, using the Bible to illustrate to the women that God intended the woman to be a partner or helpmate of the man, not his slave. The elder did this in a session titled "The role and status of women in society in the eyes of God." He particularly used the book of Genesis. This session made quite an impression on the women. They realized they were more significant than they had thought all their lives. This gave them new confidence in themselves. They talked to each other a lot during break times during those first few days. They were surprised that God created them with a positive view but men utilized them negatively. They expressed some anger. For the first time the women realized that they were somehow abused.

During the second TOT session the women reported how obvious the man–woman imbalance was after what they had learned during the first TOT workshop. It was like their eyes had opened wider. This realization strengthened some marriages where the men were pleasantly surprised by their wives' new confidence, but, at least for a while, it shook other marriages where the men felt threatened by the women's change. Learning more, doing more in the community rather than just in the family, dressing better, having soap and body oil to use, and generally looking and feeling better increased the women's confidence further.

Community Recognition of CBSMAs

After attending a minimum of three TOT workshops, a CBSMA was considered to have the minimum abilities required to disseminate Safe Motherhood information in the community. Graduation ceremonies were fun and a day of great celebration. All graduations, except the first one, happened in the village during the dry, cool month of June. The chief and his five group village headmen were present along with the Penn project directors and officials from the Ministry of Health and Population. The village was considered the most suitable venue for graduation because more people could witness the graduation and recognize the women as CBSMAs. The CBSMAs' spouses and families could also be present. The CBSMAs used this day to teach the large gathering about Safe Motherhood through songs and dance. Each group of CBSMAs taught on a selected topic and sang and danced to a Safe Motherhood song. In this way, more community members, especially men, became aware of the project so they could identify and utilize the CBSMA in their area. Speeches were made by the Ministry of Health and Population representative, the Penn-Malawi project directors, and finally Chief Chimutu, who gave both national and international recognition to the CBSMAs and their efforts to promote Safe Motherhood. Finally, certificates were handed out amid cheering and ululating.

ADULT FUNCTIONAL LITERACY TRAINING

By 1999, 5 groups of 15 women each had been trained fully in basic Safe Motherhood and teaching methods. A project extension was announced, and Penn asked us to propose further program content and activities that would renew and expand the volunteers' interest.

Enhancement of the women's literacy and numeracy skills was considered important for the actual performance of their role. Though we wanted them to be literate in the beginning, they were not. Literacy was an important next step. Even though the women had learned methods they could use to teach without reading and writing, there were other tasks in their role that required literacy, such as writing a teaching plan; writing a letter to the village headman to announce a planned Safe Motherhood teaching session in their community; studying to prepare for teaching; reading posters, flyers, and other materials during their teaching sessions instead of asking a participant to read them; counting the number of participants in each teaching session (required for TOT follow-up); writing their evaluation of the lesson; and writing brief reports. The women also wanted to read the Bible in church, write their own letters privately, and read the letters they found in their husbands' pockets.

Everyone who was still volunteering to teach Safe Motherhood was eligible to participate in the literacy program. Participation was at two levels: those who were literate were taught to be literacy trainers, and those who were illiterate gained literacy skills. The Ministry of Gender, Youth, and Community Services agreed to support this literacy effort. The literacy program was conducted in accordance with the ministry's standards and with the ministry's staff. The few literate CBSMAs were trained for 2 weeks to be instructors. They had a 1-week teaching practicum using the illiterate CBSMAs as pupils. Upon completion, the instructors received certificates from the Ministry of Gender, Youth, and Community Services as certified Malawian Adult Literacy Trainers.

CHAPTER 3   Sing Safe Motherhood: A Story of the Women of Chiwamba, Malawi

Continuing literacy classes were held in the community. For those who taught, it was gratifying to see the previously illiterate CBSMAs be able to read and write their names and read the presentation of their community teaching reports. When the program was ending, there was a lot of progress, but there was still a lot of literacy teaching and learning to be done. From our own experience, we recommended to the Ministry of Gender, Youth, and Community Services that a 1- or 2-week workshop was a more manageable setup for literacy classes than the usual 1-day-a-week system in which teachers and students miss lessons because of various home commitments, funerals, weddings, and gardening needs. The literacy program was another incentive to uplift the status of the CBSMAs.

TRAINING IN BUSINESS AND INCOME-GENERATING ACTIVITIES

In 1999, income-generating activities (IGA) were added for the CBSMAs to help them make some money for themselves, since they were volunteers in the project. The women felt they needed to be economically empowered to be good leaders and to be self-reliant to improve health. We collaborated with Community Development Assistants to train the women in the same way that they train other groups.

All the CBSMAs who were still volunteering (about 65) attended the IGA workshops in two groups of about 32 participants. Each of the women received K1,000.00 (equivalent to US$200) from a revolving loan fund sponsored by a Dutch organization working with the Lilongwe District Health Office. The women set up a variety of businesses in the village. Some bought and sold farm produce, fish, sugar, and groceries. Others bought and raised pigs or goats for sale. Some women opened a tea room that was quite successful, at least for a while. The loan repayment rate was quite good. This IGA program was also meant to be an incentive for the women to stay with the project and volunteer to teach Safe Motherhood.

REFLECTIONS ON THE CBSMA STORY: KEEPING VOLUNTEERS VOLUNTEERING

The success of this program was tied to the volunteer efforts of the CBSMAs. Reflecting on possible reasons for continued volunteer service leads to some of the lessons learned from this program. Why did these women, who were still living in their grass-thatched mud huts and were economically hard up, continue teaching Safe Motherhood without any remuneration? After working closely with and listening to the women, the following motivational factors were identified that could be replicated in other community-based projects.

A Trip to the City for Training

The prestige and excitement of taking a trip to town and leading an urban lifestyle for a week was attractive to the women, even without understanding exactly what it was about. The women would shine in the village with tales of their capital city experiences. While in the city, the women had the novel experience of being accommodated in a hostel or motel-like setting. For the first time in most of their lives, they slept in a bed with a mattress and bedding, bathed in showers, used flush toilets, ate a whole quarter chicken at one meal, had animal protein like fish or meat besides vegetables with nsima or rice at two meals a day every day (instead of just vegetables or beans), had tea with bread three times a day, and sometimes had a soda for afternoon tea break. What you and I might regard as the bare minimum lodging and food, was to them a luxury. I noticed women keeping some of the food, especially the meat, chicken, and soft drinks, to take home to their husbands and children. When we followed up with the women between workshops, most CBSMAs asked, "When are we going to the city again for training?" Even husbands would ask, "When are you taking my wife to town again? She comes back looking plump, smooth-skinned, and beautiful."

Gaining New Knowledge

As mentioned earlier, the expected volunteerism was explained to the women during the first TOT workshop, and they were offered transportation home immediately if they did not want to teach as volunteers. But if they stayed and learned, they would be expected to volunteer to teach others what they had learned. Nobody left because they wanted to learn about Safe Motherhood. "The knowledge will help me personally, and I can save the lives of my own children and other relatives besides the other community members. I would rather learn and teach without pay than not learn."

The Friendship, the Mutual Respect, and the Partnership

The experienced trainers let the women know they recognized the following in them: (1) they would do the work that health workers should do (i.e., teach health in the village) but could not because there were too few; (2) after they had learned,

CHAPTER 3   Sing Safe Motherhood: A Story of the Women of Chiwamba, Malawi

the CBSMAs would do the village teaching work better than the health workers because they had the same culture, language, and beliefs as the community members, and therefore they would be more accepted as criticizers of dangerous childbearing practices and more credible introducers of new Safe Motherhood ideas; (3) we saluted them as cohealth workers who would reach the people we could not reach but who really need to be reached; and (4) we related to them as partners of the same level rather than juniors. We were not their bosses. They did not have to do this voluntary work, and we were ever grateful that they were doing it.

The Contact and Follow-Up

The trainers followed up with the CBSMAs in their homes between trainings. The trainers wanted to support their efforts and see how they were doing with the implementation of their 4-month community teaching programs, which they had planned during their previous TOT session. Sometimes we made our visits coincide with their planned teaching session. The women continued to volunteer teach so that when we followed up with them, they would have conducted a number of teaching activities that they proudly reported to us.

The High Status of Being Visited by a Health Worker Traveling by Vehicle

The highlight of the 4-month break between TOT workshops was the visits from Daima or Mary. To have an automobile parked in front of a village woman's house and a town visitor sitting on her veranda was the pride of every CBSMA and the envy of the other villagers. People would come to the woman's home to find out why the car was there. Was it bad news? Was it the police? If it was a Ministry of Health ambulance, was the ambulance bringing a dead body home from the hospital? The CBSMA would happily and proudly say, "There is no problem. This is my teacher (or "These are my teachers" if they both came) of Safe Motherhood. I told you I am now a Safe Motherhood advisor, remember? My teacher is here to supervise me." We would endorse her statements. "Do you believe now that I am a CBSMA?" she would ask with a satisfied laugh. The home visit, even more than a certificate, was visible proof to the villagers that this woman was a CBSMA. After all, not many people could read or understand the certificate, but everyone understood that anyone who had a car visitor was important. Not even the village headman had ever received a car visitor!

I have vivid memories of stopping my little Toyota Corolla in front of the first house in the Jenti compound only to see Letia, the CBSMA, running toward the car, motioning me to drive on past one more hut and park right in front of her hut. I said I could just walk to that house, but she insisted. I drove on and parked my car in front of her house. After having me seated on her veranda she explained that she was one of three wives of Jenti and she wanted everyone to know that she was the particular wife of Jenti being visited by car. "You stopped in front of my cowife's hut. I couldn't accept that!" Thus the CBSMAs continued volunteering so that a car would one day park outside their personal huts and enhance their status in the community.

Attendance of More TOTs in the City

We noticed after first TOT session that the CBSMAs' rate of activity varied from twice a week to once a month or less. We informed them that anyone who did not teach an average of once a month would not be considered experienced enough to learn well in the subsequent TOT workshop and would not be invited to attend. Well, everyone wanted participate in another TOT to learn more Safe Motherhood and to have the town experience again. Besides, if they could not attend the following TOT session, they could not receive a formal certificate.

Work-Related Gifts and Incentives

No gifts had been planned or budgeted at the beginning of the project. However, as the project went on some gifts were worked in that were directly related to the CBSMAs' actual teaching and traveling needs. The women realized that there was a need for them to be presentable as they passed on the Safe Motherhood messages to the communities. Therefore, they asked for incentives that would assist them in their work. They received a cloth bag for carrying teaching materials, a large umbrella with the program logo ("Safe Motherhood, Everyone's Responsibility" in both English and Chichewa) to protect them from sunlight and rain, and 6 meters of cloth for a full chitenje outfit—skirt or wrapper, blouse, head scarf, and neck scarf or shoulder cloth—so they could have at least one decent outfit to wear when teaching. This was received after the third TOT, which was like a revision block, almost 1.5 years into the project for each CBSMA.

LESSONS LEARNED

Several lessons were learned from the program:
- Teaching based on mutual respect: The most important lesson we learned related to how we conducted the teaching sessions based on mutual respect

CHAPTER 3 Sing Safe Motherhood: A Story of the Women of Chiwamba, Malawi

and trust. Mary and Daima let the women know that even though the project was set up to teach them, the truth was that we, the trainers, had to learn from them before we could start to teach them about safe pregnancy, birth, and the postpartum–newborn period. We appealed to them that, at the beginning of each session before we could teach, they had to tell us what was known, believed, and practiced in Chiwamba about that topic. They called us "Teachers" and we called them "Advisors." We were colearners and coteachers. In such a safe environment of mutual respect and mutual learning, they opened up to let us know about their, and the community of Chiwamba's, knowledge and practices surrounding pregnancy and childbirth. This information helped us identify where to jump in and how to correct misconceptions and reinforce positive aspects. The women couldn't wait to come back to another session to teach us some more about their lives in Chiwamba. We could not wait to meet again.

- Flexibility in teaching: Another lesson learned was the value of flexibility in running TOT workshops. Overcoming the literacy challenge was the first step in gaining the trust and respect of the village women. Adding literacy training and IGA activities enhanced both the women's status and their ability to provide for their families.
- Baseline knowledge of community: A third lesson learned was the importance of understanding the preintervention knowledge about pregnancy and childbearing so the content of the TOT sessions would be tailored to the needs of TA Chimutu. Conducting the postintervention study also supported the success of this community effort to improve maternal and child health at the village level.
- Collaboration with existing health systems: The fourth lesson learned was the importance of collaborating with existing ministries and staff to increase the likelihood of sustainability and to maximize resources. The Ministry of Health and Population continued the program for an additional 2 years, primarily because of the efforts of Mary Kambewa, district community health nurse and coteacher of the CBSMAs. Resources were maximized by the collaborative efforts of the Ministry of Health and Population and the Ministry of Gender, Youth, and Community Services.
- Using community members to teach others: The fifth lesson learned was the importance of taking health information directly to the village with knowledgeable individuals from the village as teachers. We used the traditional

tribal system for recruiting the women so they would have the support of the chief and village headmen in their work.
- Enhancing the status of women: The final lesson learned relates to the importance of enhancing the status of women wherever one lives and works. It is now widely accepted that if one invests in women, the women will invest in their families and make communities stronger and healthier. We were honored to be a part of this Safe Motherhood project and humbled by the village women who became CBSMAs and made a real difference in the health of their communities, one village at a time.

SUMMARY

From 1996 to 2002, more than 90 CBSMAs were trained, with a great majority still teaching in the following years. The achievements included reduction of maternal death in the community, increased facility-based deliveries, timely referrals from TBAs, improved nutrition for women and children, and increased status and literacy for women. Follow-up comments from the CNO reported that no women with ruptured uteri came into the hospital after the first year of the program, and Chief Chimutu noted that he had not opened a single grave for a pregnant or newly delivered woman for an entire year.

Discussion Questions

1. Identify at least three strategies for working with women who have low levels of literacy. How do you develop trainers from this sector of the community?
2. How could the Penn partners have been better prepared for the linguistic challenges of this project?
3. Do you think a Safe Motherhood program needs to be for women only? Why or why not?
4. What steps should one take to ensure sustainability of a Safe Motherhood training program for village workers?

CHAPTER 3   Sing Safe Motherhood: A Story of the Women of Chiwamba, Malawi

REFERENCES

Gennaro, S., Thyangathyanga, D., Kershbaumer, R., & Thompson, J. (2001). Health promotion and risk reduction in Malawi, Africa, village women. *Journal of Obstetric, Gynecologic, and Neonatal Nursing, 30*(2), 224–229.

Ministry of Health, Department of Health Statistics. (2006). Maternal mortality ratio estimate 2009. Malawi: Ministry of Health DHS.

Thompson, J. B. (2004). A human rights framework for midwifery care. *Journal of Midwifery and Women's Health, 49*, 3.

Thompson, J. B. (2005). International policies for achieving Safe Motherhood: Women's lives in the balance. *Health Care for Women International, 26*(6), 472–483.

Thompson, J. B. (2007). Poverty, development, and women: Why should we care? *Journal of Obstetric, Gynecologic, and Neonatal Nursing, 36*(6), 523–530.

Thyangathyanga, D. (1994). *Penn-Malawi Women for Women's health project: Evaluation report 1990–1994.* Unpublished report submitted to the Rockefeller Foundation, the Malawi Ministry of Health and Population, and the University of Pennsylvania School of Nursing.

CHAPTER 4

Maama Omwaana: Community Building for Safe Motherhood in Njeru, Uganda

Ruth C. White, PhD, MPH, MSW
Katherine Camacho Carr, PhD, RN, CNM

Location: Njeru, Uganda, Africa

Project: The Maama Omwaana Safe Motherhood Initiative

Sponsoring Organizations (and Funders): Seattle University; Parents of Seattle Country Day School, Seattle, Washington

Target Population: Women of childbearing age; community-based organizations that serve women

Project Goal: Improve the health of mothers, infants, and children by increasing utilization of critical health services

---

This chapter is based on White, R. C., Carr, K. C. (2007). "Strategies for Increasing Utilization of Maternity Services in Njeru, Uganda." *African Journal of Midwifery and Women's Health* 1(1):14-19, republished with kind permission from MA Healthcare Limited.

73

CHAPTER 4 Maama Omwaana

INTRODUCTION

According to the Safe Motherhood initiative (www.safemotherhood.org) a woman dies from pregnancy and childbirth complications every minute of every day, with 99% of these deaths occurring in the developing world. This makes pregnancy-related complications one of the leading causes of death and disability for women aged 15–49 years. Newborn health is also closely linked to the health of the mother during the prenatal period, labor and birth, and postpartum. The death of a woman impacts families and communities because of her caregiving and economic responsibilities, especially in low-resource settings. In the past 10 years, research has shown that small-scale, cost-efficient interventions can significantly reduce the health risks of pregnancy, childbirth, and the postpartum period, with the key ingredients being access to health care during pregnancy, childbirth, and the postnatal period; a skilled birth attendant; and emergency obstetrical services (World Health Organization, 2005). This paper describes the methods, outcomes, and implications of a needs assessment and small-scale intervention to improve the maternal and infant health of the semirural community of Njeru, Uganda.

Uganda is located in Eastern Africa with a population of 24.7 million people and an annual growth rate of 3.4% (Uganda Ministry of Finance, Planning, and Economic Development [UMFPED], 2006). Unlike many of its African counterparts, Uganda has had rapid and sustained economic growth during the past decade, which has resulted in significant declines in poverty in both urban and rural areas (Ssewanyana & Younger, 2005). However, according to the Uganda Ministry of Finance, Planning, and Economic Development (2006), from 1995–2000 there was an increase in infant mortality from 81 to 88 deaths per 1,000 births, which maintained Uganda's status as having among the highest infant mortality rates (IMR) in Africa and the world. According to U.S. Agency for International Development (USAID) statistics from 2004, maternal mortality is also high at 505–880 per 100,000 live births (2005).

These mortality and life expectancy rates compare to African countries with near-collapsed economies or countries that are in the midst of severe conflict, with little or no social service infrastructure (UMFPED, 2006). During the same period, maternal mortality had a minor reduction from 527 to 505 deaths per 100,000 live births. These indicators are important measures of success of the country's Poverty Eradication Action Plan (PEAP) and therefore present a challenge to the economic indicators that are not reflected in the most basic measures of the population's well-being. The government attributes this high rate of maternal and infant mortality and increased morbidities to lack of access to care and chronically underfunded health centers that result in poor-quality care with limited access to drugs and supplies (UMFPED, 2006).

Reducing maternal and infant mortality and morbidity are two Millennium Development Goals (MDGs) that are often linked with poverty reduction, which is another of the eight MDGs (United Nations, 2006). Although Ssewanyana and Younger (2005) argue that improvement in immunizations and general healthcare delivery services can lead to an improvement in infant mortality rates, they argue that the MDG for infant mortality cannot be achieved by Uganda, even under the most optimistic scenarios, due to inadequate human, fiscal, and material resources (Ssewanyana & Younger, 2005).

The Uganda Ministry of Finance, Planning, and Economic Development has established a five-pronged approach to improving maternal and infant mortality rates: malaria control, sanitation, community development, family planning, and improving the quality of healthcare services (2002). Major causes for infant mortality include prematurity and low birth weight (LBW), malnutrition, starvation, diarrhea and dehydration, neonatal tetanus, and HIV/AIDS. Major causes of maternal mortality include hemorrhage (25%), infection (15%), hypertensive disorders (12%), unsafe abortion (13%), and obstructed labor (8%). Major causes of maternal morbidity include anemia, sexually transmitted diseases and HIV, malaria, diabetes, and obstetric fistula (USAID, 2005).

Gender issues also factor into women's health in Uganda. In this patriarchal society, women bear the burden of agricultural and household labor and have very little decision-making power within the home. There is also heavy pressure placed on girls to marry young and, after marriage, to produce many children, with 70% of births occurring to girls younger than age 20 years. Lastly, teenage girls are often the head of orphaned households and are forced to become sex workers to provide financial and other resources for themselves and younger siblings left in their care (UMFPED, 2006).

Trained birth attendants (TBAs) are lacking in Uganda, with only 38% of births attended by a trained healthcare worker. More than 60% of births are attended by a TBA, who may or may not be a skilled birth attendant (USAID, 2005).

CHAPTER 4 Maama Omwaana

MAAMA OMWAANA SAFE MOTHERHOOD INITIATIVE

The Maama Omwaana Safe Motherhood Initiative (MOSMI) is a maternal and child health improvement project based in Njeru, Uganda, a town of 53,000 people living in 36 villages near the convergence of Lake Victoria and the Nile River. Maama Omwaana means "mother and baby" in Luganda—the most widely spoken indigenous language in Uganda. This community is located in a district where more than 500 women and 8,000 children die for every 100,000 deliveries (Mukono District Health Management Information System, 2006).

MOSMI was founded in the summer of 2004 by a retired Ugandan nurse midwife and an extended family member, based in the United States, with public health training. It is managed by the clinical officer in charge at Namwezi Health Center, where the project is based. A retired health inspector serves as community mobilizer at the organizational level. The growing number of partners include Seattle University, Njeru Town Council, Jinja School of Comprehensive Nursing—a public training facility at Jinja Hospital—a regional referral hospital, and St. Francis Health Services (which serves more than 7,000 HIV-positive clients).

As stated by the Uganda Ministry of Finance, Planning, and Economic Development, "sustained reductions in infant and maternal mortality rates requires a series of coordinated, multi-sectoral interventions" (2006, p. 2). This coalition of community partners can move forward in a coordinated, sustained effort to identify needs, obtain resources, and implement community-based interventions to reduce the maternal and infant mortality and morbidity in Njeru.

The goal of the project is to improve quality, access, and utilization of maternal and child health services in Njeru, with a focus on antenatal care, use of a skilled attendant at birth, and appropriate utilization of emergency obstetrical procedures. This combination has been shown to improve maternal and infant outcomes (Save the Children, 2006). Skilled health personnel or skilled attendants include doctors (specialist or nonspecialist) or persons with midwifery skills who can diagnose and manage obstetrical complications and normal deliveries. Skilled health personnel may also have additional skills related to family planning and gynecology.

The primary objectives of MOSMI are as follows: (1) promote the health of mothers during pregnancy in the Njeru Town Council area; (2) increase the number of women seeking skilled care at delivery; and (3) reduce the rate of maternal and infant mortality and morbidity. The promotion of mother's health during pregnancy involves more than traditional prenatal care and blood pressure checks. In equatorial Africa, it involves malaria prophylaxis and use of medicated bed nets. Tetanus vaccination of pregnant women is another important aspect of prenatal health care to prevent neonatal tetanus. In order to increase the number of women seeking skilled care at delivery, a number of elements must be put into place, including TBA training, community-based preparedness for birth, and linkages to the referral centers where emergency obstetrical care may be available. The strategies focus on resource mobilization, community organization and mobilization, and community education.

Measurement of the program objectives include two *quantitative performance indicators* articulated by the Uganda Ministry of Finance, Planning, and Economic Development to monitor performance of the health sector: deliveries in a health unit and outpatient utilization per capita (UMFPED, 2002). In particular, MOSMI focuses on utilization of antenatal services, use of skilled birth attendants, and access to emergency obstetrical care. Nationally, outpatient utilization remained stagnant during the 1980s but increased slightly during the 1990s.

COMMUNITY ASSESSMENT AND MOBILIZATION

In the summer of 2005 a team from Seattle University met with 36 trained volunteer community health workers (CHWs) in Njeru to explore health issues of concern related to maternal and infant health in the community. These volunteers had received 6 months of training from Franciscan nurses, and in return they were required to volunteer at least 1 hour per week in their communities. A community-empowerment model was employed, which required the team to respond directly and immediately to the expressed training and information needs of the group. Simultaneous translation by a retired nurse midwife was provided. At times the large group was divided by geographic region into small discussion groups of five to seven participants.

When the small groups reported back to the larger group about general concerns related to health, the list included HIV/AIDS, ignorance, malaria, poor sanitation, and lack of awareness. Maternal and child health issues included nutrition, sanitation, lack of child spacing, home delivery with a family attendant, and unclean environments. The three priority areas selected by the group were women giving birth at home (and what to do about the umbilical cord and placenta), hygiene (environmental and specific to birth), and lack of breastfeeding.

Table 4-1 Summary of Community Health Workers Discussion of Maternal and Child Health Priorities

Problems	Issues	Solutions
Delivery at home	Anemia and hemorrhage Poor care of umbilical cord Premature baby kept at home Herbal medicines that accelerate labor and lead to ruptured uterus Failure to recognize presentation HIV+ mother Adolescent mothers Lack of referral by TBAs Lack of transport to health facility Culture that prefers home delivery even if antenatal care received at facility Women do not want to be 'cut' or operated on	Educate community about health issues Promote antenatal care
Unclean Environment	No running water No boiling of water Minimal washing of hands	Promote handwashing Encourage landlords to build more latrines Educate community on use of latrines Use dry banana leaves and burn Use pine for bad smell
Failure to breastfeed	HIV+ mother Working mothers Poor nutrition and little drinking water Cosmetic concerns Men want to have sex soon after delivery	Encourage men to support women in breastfeeding Educate community on importance of breastfeeding

In response, the training facilitators had the group members return to their small groups to discuss possible strategies for intervention. These were listed on sheets of newsprint on the wall; the results are outlined in **Table 4-1**.

With regard to delivery at home, CHWs reported that problems associated with this practice included anemia and hemorrhaging, inadequate care of the umbilical cord, obstructed labor, use of herbal medicines that often lead to ruptured uterus, HIV-positive mothers, adolescent mothers, lack of referral by TBAs, lack of transport to health facility when emergency services are needed, and inability to pay for a TBA or midwife. Training focused on empirically based information on hygiene, breastfeeding, and promotion of nutrition. Contraceptive information and the benefits of antenatal care were also briefly discussed to support the CHWs' efforts to mobilize and educate the community. Cord care was raised as an issue with regard to hygiene, and this topic received specific attention with a demonstration on proper cutting and care of the umbilical cord.

CHWs were encouraged to share this information with pregnant women and their families. The CHWs also expressed concern that they were lacking credibility within the community as agents of change because they had no authority from the city administrators to enforce regulations with regard to environmental hygiene. They requested some kind of official badge that would identify them as representing the public health system.

In addition to the CHW session, the team met with 12 TBAs. Again the community-empowerment model was employed, which required the team to respond directly and immediately to expressed training and information needs of the group of TBAs. The training was concurrently translated by a well-respected and highly active CHW with 2 years of nursing training. The TBAs presented the mother and baby problems they handled most frequently and dictated the topics about which they wanted more information. The TBAs listed problems they experienced with mothers or infants during the prenatal period, labor and birth, and the postpartum period. The list included hemorrhage, early delivery, cord care, seizures and other symptoms of preeclampsia, and others. Each issue was addressed with specific strategies for intervention or recommendations for referral. With regard to hemorrhage, which is the leading cause of maternal death in Uganda, a demonstration of external uterine massage was conducted using one of the trainers as a mother. TBAs acknowledged that they did not have any training in the active management of the third stage or utilize any antihemorrhagic medications.

In addition to hemorrhage, the TBAs asked about slow labor, care of the umbilical cord, hygiene, and ways to recognize hypertension prior to an eclamptic seizure. These topics were explored, and the TBAs were given specific intervention strategies to use in the future.

IMPLEMENTATION YEAR TWO: 2006

In 2005, CHWs were given a mandate to mobilize the community around the issues they raised in the training and to use the training to educate the community. In early 2006, each CHW received a laminated name badge with the logos of Njeru Public Health Department and Seattle University at the top, and the

CHAPTER 4 Maama Omwaana

title of Community Health Worker on the bottom. According to Namwezi clinic staff, this greatly increased morale among the group and increased their activity and presence within the community.

In 2006, the main strategy of the initiative continued to be community mobilization and education using CHWs, but this was expanded to include community-based organizations (CBOs); health institutions; village women's groups; and a music, dance, and drama youth development and performance group called Bright Actors, which used performance to educate the community about various health issues.

In 2006, a manual adapted from *Awareness, Mobilization, and Action for Safe Motherhood: A Field Guide*, published by the White Ribbon Alliance for Safe Motherhood (www.whiteribbonalliance.org), was used to train 40 CHWs and 15 representatives of CBOs in Maama Omwaana's Safe Motherhood messages. Prevention and danger sign messages were printed on small (3 by 5 inches) laminated cards in English with copies in Luganda also available. (The latter were on double-sided 8.5 by 11 inch cards due to the longer translation into Luganda). These cards were titled "The Maama Omwaana Safe Motherhood Card," with the subtitle "Preparing for birth because every pregnancy should result in a healthy mother and baby," because they promoted planning for a healthy labor and birth. The prevention messages presented on one side of the card were good nutrition with a focus on anemia prevention, malaria prevention, tetanus toxoid immunization, good hygiene, HIV and sexually transmitted disease prevention through use of condoms, delivery with a skilled attendant, and a plan for transportation with questions such as "Who will take me?" and "How much will it cost?"

On the other side of the card, danger signs focused on both the prenatal and the labor and delivery period. The danger signs for the prenatal period included severe headaches, bleeding, vision problems, vomiting and dehydration, and high fever. The danger signs for the mother during the labor and delivery period included early labor, long labor, excessive bleeding, and dehydration and severe vomiting. The danger signs for the infant included preterm delivery, breathing difficulties, jaundice (yellow coloring), bleeding from the cord, fever or not eating, and lots of mucous and fast breathing. At the bottom of that side of the card was the question "What to do if you see these signs?" and the answer "Transport immediately to the next level of care. Or get medical attention if transport not possible."

These messages were developed using the results of the discussions of TBAs and CHWs in 2005. To respond to resource shortages that often resulted in pregnant women being turned away from some health facilities, Seattle University donated 200 birth kits (in large Ziploc bags) containing cord tape, a one-sided razor, a pair of gloves, a plastic sheet, and an information card to be distributed to women who were least likely to use antenatal care from a skilled attendant at birth. The goal was to provide each woman in her third trimester with a kit, no matter where she went for care, given that patients are often required to bring their own supplies to hospitals or to provide supplies when a TBA cares for them during labor. If any of the items are not needed, the women can return them to Namwezi to be used in clinic-based deliveries.

The objective for the participation of CBOs was to integrate consistent Safe Motherhood messages in their daily activities when presented with women who are pregnant. Health and social services are accessed through various venues in Njeru. The list of CBOs that participated in the training included an adult education center, drug shop operators, HIV/AIDS care providers, and women's groups, among others. Through their participation, women and their partners were exposed to these messages, even if they did not access a health facility specifically for maternal care.

In 2006, Maama Omwaana celebrated its membership in the White Ribbon Alliance for Safe Motherhood with several events that brought the community together to learn about the Safe Motherhood message. In Kasanja village, which had less than 2,000 people, the Bright Actors wore white ribbons while entertaining more than 300 people with a skit promoting antenatal care, good nutrition, and delivery by a trained attendant. A 1-hour radio talk show featured a discussion of Maama Omwaana, Safe Motherhood, Namwezi Health Center services, and the upcoming health fair that was to be the official launch of the Maama Omwaana Safe Motherhood Initiative.

The First Annual Njeru Town Council/Maama Omwaana Health Fair, which received political support at all levels, brought together 12 exhibits from CBOs in health and social welfare, including clinic-based services, drug shop operators, women's groups, and CHWs, as well as more than 100 members of the community who accessed health services such as HIV, blood pressure, and diabetes testing and counseling. The chief guest, Minister of Health Dr. Stephen Mallinga, had to be absent but was represented by Dr. Fred Katumba, head of the reproductive health section. All participants wore white ribbons.

OUTCOMES

In the 2 years of its existence, utilization of antenatal care and the use of a skilled attendant at birth more than doubled at Namwezi Health Center, from 197 antenatal visits in 2003–2004 to 483 visits in 2005–2006 (**Figure 4-1**).

This is striking in the context of a 7.5% increase in total outpatient visits in the same time period (**Figure 4-2**).

Deliveries at the clinic, attended by a trained midwife, for the July 2005 to June 2006 fiscal year (n = 56) outnumber those of the TBAs (n = 43) in the area (Mukono District Health Management Information System, 2006), where most births are attended by a relative or a traditional birth attendant (**Figure 4-3**).

DISCUSSION

Through use of community empowerment methods, the MOSMI has been able to show significant increases in utilization of maternal services when community health workers were mobilized. From anecdotal reports, there has been no similar increase in utilization across the district. We plan to collect data across health facilities in the future to substantiate this finding. There has also been no corresponding reduction in use of hospital-based antenatal care services, as reported by Mukono District, in which Njeru is located.

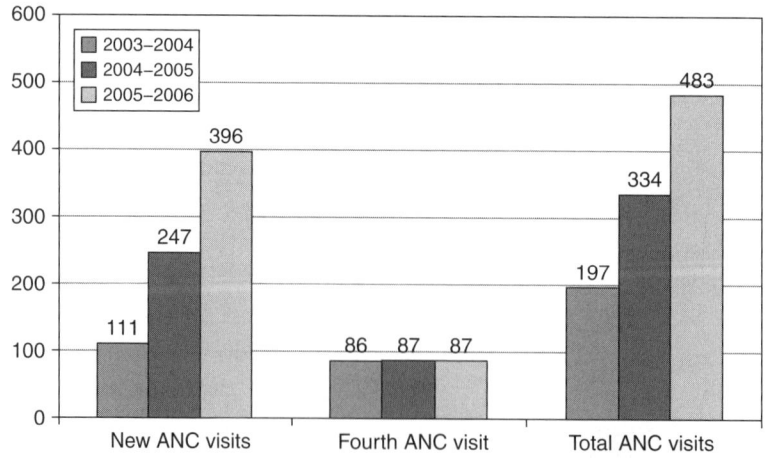

Figure 4-1 Utilization of antenatal care (ANC) services at Namwezi Health Center, 2003–2006.

Discussion

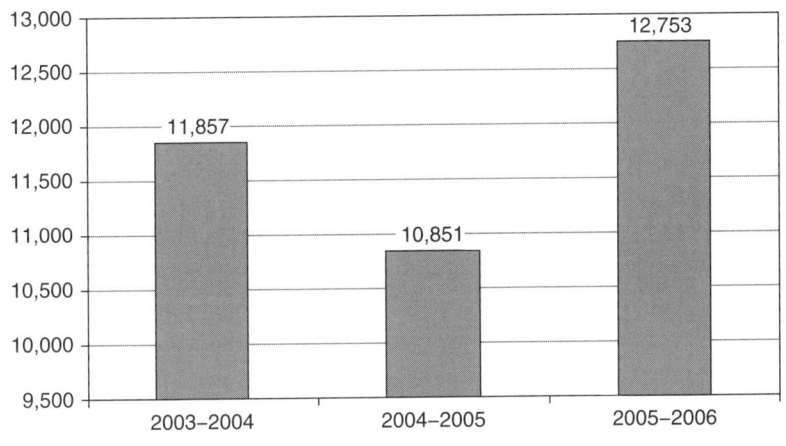

Figure 4-2 Outpatient Attendance at Namwezi Health Center, 2003–2006.

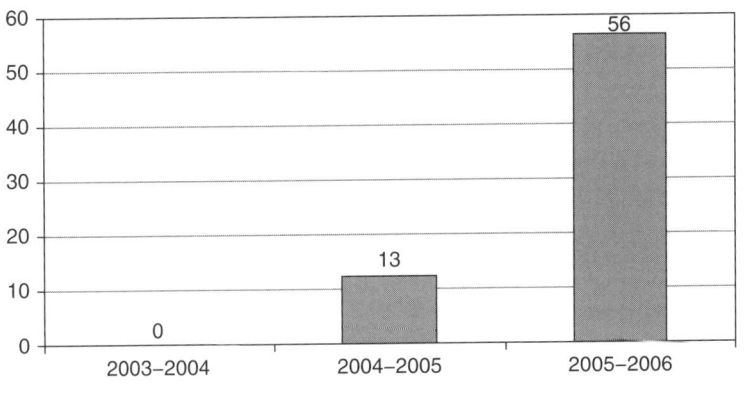

Figure 4-3 Deliveries at Namwezi Health Center 2003–2006.

We acknowledge that having the blessing and support (through donations of supplies, equipment and even curtains and sheets, which were not previously available) of a U.S.-based university may have contributed to the desirability of services at Namwezi Clinic, but the comparison to outpatient services in general reflects that there is an increased awareness about the importance of maternity services to a healthy mother and baby following birth, which is not reflected in broader health service utilization trends.

83

CHAPTER 4   Maama Omwaana

We have not been able to follow-up with TBAs to see how training impacted their practice, and there is no tracking system for referrals to see if they used the knowledge they gained to refer clients to higher levels of care as necessary. This is a limitation of the health service system because TBAs are entrepreneurs with limited official connection to the existing healthcare system. We plan to access the health management information system of the Ministry of Health to examine whether the increase in utilization of maternity services in Njeru is reflected throughout the healthcare system (i.e., in private settings or the referral hospital). Good data collection is an area for future research and implementation as Maama Omwaana grows. Efforts to organize community-based organizations, in collaboration with nongovernmental organizations and public health facilities, will not only improve the assessment of health-related activities in the area, but they will also strengthen the capacity to solve health issues as well as systemic and policy barriers to effective and efficient service delivery.

As requests for MOSMI come in from other areas in the district, there is a need to develop a standardized implementation strategy that allows for maximum flexibility across locales. The key to MOSMI's success is community ownership and leadership of the project. Visits from Seattle University occur only for 2–3 weeks once a year. In the meantime, the faces of the project are male and female members of the community who volunteer in the community and have gained the community's respect. The ideas, issues, and strategies were determined by the clinic staff at the very beginning of their relationship with Seattle University and by community health workers and traditional birth attendants as the project progressed. The budget is small (less than $10,000 in 2006), with a large proportion of it being related to travel costs for one U.S.-based staff member to travel to Uganda.

Sustainability is therefore not limited by regular infusions of cash from outside the country. The local leaders of the project are seeking local support for activities from service clubs, such as Rotary, Lions, Kiwanis, and by one of the nation's largest employers located right in the community, Nile Breweries, which has also come on board with MOSMI through their company-based clinic that provides a wide range of health services to their employees but does not include labor and delivery. Seattle University collaborators will fundraise and seek donations of medical supplies and equipment that focus on maternal health with the hope that Uganda's plan for health system upgrades will eventually make such donations unnecessary. It should be noted that the 56 deliveries conducted between July 1,

2005, and June 30, 2006, were not dependent on Seattle University contributions. It should also be noted that all births were in the healthy range of weight, and there was no morbidity despite a 12% HIV-positive rate among the women who delivered during that period (Mukono District Health Management Information System, 2006).

CONCLUSION

National initiatives to improve health outcomes in heavily rural developing countries are, by their nature, top-down initiatives designed by bureaucrats for implementation by local healthcare providers whose efforts are often hampered by socioeconomic and cultural factors that were not considered when these programs were being designed.

Expecting poor village women in labor to travel on bad or nonexistent roads to a clinic on the back of a bicycle or motorcycle is asking a lot, with regard to her desire and ability to access prenatal care and a skilled attendant at birth. Having community-based (i.e., home-based) maternity services may be a strategy that needs to be explored with regard to maternal services the way it has become institutionalized for HIV/AIDS care. Maama Omwaana is exploring how we can utilize the bicycles donated to the clinic to go beyond outreach in basic care and immunizations to include maternity care. We are also exploring the feasibility of a community-based training program (Home Based Life Saving Skills) for TBAs, family members, and women themselves for basic maternal and infant lifesaving skills.

Nursing schools, such as the Jinja School of Enrolled Comprehensive Nursing, have changed their training strategy to focus on community-based nursing, rather than clinic-based nursing, so that interns are affiliated with a clinic but spend most of their time in the community. Furthermore, their new model of comprehensive nursing training means that all graduates are both nurses and midwives, ensuring that there will be more skilled attendants who can provide maternity services at the community level. With poor infrastructure and a lack of money to facilitate transportation to the clinic, this is a timely strategy that will be reflected in higher utilization rates of maternity services and better outcomes for both mother and baby. As these students graduate with both nursing and midwifery skills, it is hoped that with an education, a bicycle, and a bag, a home delivery will not mean an unsafe delivery.

CHAPTER 4 Maama Omwaana

ENDNOTE

Since the original publication of this paper, the Maama Omwaana project applied for grants from the White Ribbon Alliance that funded 11 quilt panels for the Mothers Memorial quilt project launched at the Women Deliver conference in October 2007 in London. Several of the leaders developed through the project became part of the movement that launched a national secretariat for Safe Motherhood that is one of only 15 (of 150 country members) in the White Ribbon Alliance. In 2008, with utilization of key services still on the rise, the project was successfully transferred to the Uganda Ministry of Health, Mukono District.

> **Discussion Questions**
>
> 1. Discuss the challenges and opportunities presented by community mobilization as a strategy in public health generally, and maternal and child health specifically.
> 2. What are some of the institutional systems of cross-border practice and research that influence research agendas and program development and delivery?
> 3. Explore some of the unintended outcomes related to short-term (e.g., 1–5 years) engagement of highly educated foreigners with local services?
> 4. How was sustainability promoted, and hindered, in the development and implementation of this project?
> 5. Maama Omwaana began because of a personal link between the community in Uganda and Seattle University. How do you think this influenced the engagement process and sustainability?

REFERENCES

Mukono District Health Management Information System. (2006).
Save the Children. (2006). *State of the world's mothers 2006. Saving the lives of mothers and newborns.*
Ssewanyana, S., & Younger, S. D. (2005). *Infant mortality in Uganda: Determinants, trends, and the Millennium Development Goals.* Paper presented at the African Development and

References

Poverty Reduction Conference, Cape Town, South Africa. Retrieved from http://www.saga.cornell.edu/images/wp186.pdf.

Uganda Ministry of Finance, Planning, and Economic Development. (2002). *Infant mortality in Uganda, 1995–2000: Why the non-improvement?* Kampala, Uganda: Author.

Uganda Ministry of Finance, Planning, and Economic Development. (2006). *Infant and maternal mortality in Uganda*. Kampala, Uganda: Author. Retrieved from http://www.finance.go.ug/documents.html.

United Nations. (2006). UN Millennium Development Goals. Retrieved from http://www.un.org/millenniumgoals/.

United States Agency for International Development. (2005). USAID country health statistical report: Uganda. Retrieved from http://pdf.usaid.gov/pdf_docs/PNADF861.pdf.

World Health Organization. (2005). The world health report: Make every mother and child count. Retrieved from http://www.who.int/whr/2005/en/.

CHAPTER 5

Behavior Change Initiative in an Integrated Community Health Project

Gerda Pohl, MRCGP, MRCOG, DTMPH

Location: Humla, Nepal, Asia

Name of Program/Project: Behavior Change Initiative within the Context of an Integrated Community Health Project

Sponsoring Organizations (and Funders): Nepalese Children's Foundation, PHASE Nepal (implementing organization), PHASE Worldwide UK (logistic support)

Target Population: New mothers and newborn babies in Southern Humla; for the wider program, the communities of Maila and Melchham, Southern Humla (total population 5,920), and many more beneficiaries from neighboring communities

Project Goal: Reduce the incidence of puerperal and neonatal infections in the project area by encouraging the provision of a safe and clean environment for new mothers and their babies

Project Objectives: Enable families to house new mothers and newborn babies in a clean and safe environment, thereby reducing the risk of puerperal and neonatal infections

CHAPTER 5 Behavior Change Initiative

> **General:** Improve the health status of the target community, particularly women and children, and reduce the negative impact of poor health on families and communities
>
> **General Program:**
> 1. Provide integrated, accessible and appropriate primary care services to the target population
> 2. Increase demand for and access to family planning and other reproductive health services, including skilled attendance at delivery
> 3. Reduce the impact of diarrheal illness and respiratory infections on child health and improve childhood nutrition in the target area
> 4. Work closely with governmental services and utilize available local and district resources wherever possible
> 5. Increase awareness of health issues and preventive measures and of available health services in the target population

BACKGROUND

PHASE (Practical Help Achieving Self-Empowerment) is a not-for-profit, nonpolitical, and nondenominational, nongovernmental organization (NGO) that is registered in Nepal and works in three different districts of Nepal. The organization mainly tries to implement integrated development programs, targeting health, education, and poverty reduction together. In some areas, only the health component has been implemented so far. In Humla, PHASE was partnering with the Nepalese Children's Foundation, an Irish charitable organization, that works particularly in Humla District.

NEPAL AND HUMLA

Nepal is among the poorest countries in the world; according to the United Nations Development Programme (UNDP), it ranks 157 out of 187, and besides East Timor it is the lowest-ranking country in Asia. Nepal has been shaken by political instability and violent civil conflict for more than 10 years. In the remote areas where PHASE works, access to health services or school education is very limited and often nonexistent.

Nationally, literacy rates are well below 50% for adults (United Nations Development Programme, 2011). Half of children aged 5 years and younger are malnourished, and the mortality for that age group is 54/1,000 (Ministry of Health and Population, 2011). The official figure for maternal mortality is 281/10,000 (but the adjusted UN estimate is 850/10,000) (World Health Organization [WHO], 2007). These national figures have improved recently, but the situation in the remote communities of Humla is much worse.

Humla District is the second-least developed district of Nepal. Since March 2008, PHASE (with initial support from the Nepalese Children's Foundation Ireland) has been working in two of the most remote communities, Maila and Melchham, which have a total population of 5,920. These communities are more than a 2-day walk away from the nearest airports and are more than a week's walk away from the nearest road access.

Because of the extreme remoteness of the area, health service provision is extremely patchy. Government health workers are absent from their posts for several weeks at a time when they have to attend meetings or training at the district headquarters, and the transport of vaccinations and drugs to the village is unreliable and slow. Humla has been suffering real food shortages for years, and in spite of rice distribution by the UN World Food Programme (WFP), malnutrition rates are very high—up to 90% among children aged 5 years and younger were identified as malnourished by a survey PHASE conducted in 2009. In the summer before PHASE started work in Humla, more than 20 adults died from simple diarrhea and dehydration in Maila alone.

PHASE supports the two governmental health posts (which are usually unstaffed) with two well-trained health workers each; the workers provide general services but concentrate on maternal and child health. They have full access to governmental drug supplies, but PHASE supplements this with drugs bought through Mrigendra Samjhana Medical Trust (MSMT) (a not-for-profit distributor) in Kathmandu. PHASE also employs a staff nurse for supervision and support of the auxiliary nurse midwives (ANMs) and to coordinate with the head office and district headquarters.

The projects in Humla are the busiest of all PHASE health projects, with between 40 and 60 patients attending every day. From July 2008 to June 2009, PHASE health workers delivered 38 babies and inserted 58 ring pessaries for uterine prolapse (a common disabling condition among Nepali women).

CHAPTER 5   Behavior Change Initiative

HISTORY

In March 2008, PHASE health workers started work in Maila, and in July 2008 they started work in Melchham. The health workers involved were four ANMs: Rita Karki and Pushpa Basnet in Maila, and Mamita Gurung and Sandhya Bhatta in Melchham, as well as Urmila Adhikari, a staff nurse who supervised both centers.

One of the main tasks of the PHASE health workers was to encourage pregnant women to call for help when they go into labor. The Nepalese national average for skilled attendance in childbirth was only 19% in 2006 (Ministry of Health and Population, 2006), and this is widely accepted to be one of the main factors influencing the high rate of maternal deaths in Nepal.

In Maila and Melchham, there had not been a local skilled birth attendant before PHASE started work, so with very few exceptions (those who left the village for the nearest town before they went into labor), women had no professional help in childbirth. As in all PHASE health projects, the ANMs spent a lot of time in the first few months walking from house to house, trying to get to know the community and conducting a survey of the numbers of pregnant women, children, and older people, as well as rates of malnutrition, vaccination status, toilet use, and other factors.

They talked to all women about family planning and the importance of antenatal care and having skilled help during child birth. They also conducted community meetings and called together the Female Volunteer Health Workers (FVHWs) of the community. These are local women who have received very basic training from the governmental health workers and mainly help in vaccination campaigns and the twice-yearly distribution of vitamin A and albendazole (medication to reduce worm infestation). The FVHWs are very helpful in convincing other women to change their behavior because they are trusted members of the community.

THE PROBLEM

Our health workers quickly saw an increase in the number of women attending for antenatal checkups, and within a few weeks they were called to almost every delivery within a radius of 2–3 hours walking distance (and sometimes farther away!). They found that they were called to attend a childbirth at least once or twice a week. This is very important because two of the main causes of maternal death are hemorrhage and infection, both of which can be prevented or treated if the health workers attend the delivery.

The ANMs were very concerned, however, to find that in this area many families still followed an old Nepalese tradition linked to the Hindu culture. As soon as she goes into labor, a prospective new mother is moved into the cowshed, where she and her newborn baby will stay for a month after the birth. Because childbirth is considered unclean and new mothers (and menstruating women) are believed to contaminate others if they get into close contact with them, these women are treated as untouchable in the period after delivery, that is, they must not touch the food or drink of anybody else, or even the implements used to cook. However, cows are holy and considered clean—their dung is used to "treat" infections and repel or draw out malignant spirits. Therefore, the cowshed is a logical place for the potentially dangerous situation of the new mother!

The five young health workers, who all come from remote villages themselves but whose home areas abandoned these customs at least a generation ago, were appalled. They refused to conduct deliveries in the cowshed, and amazingly, the villagers seemed to value their services enough to comply and find a spot under the awning or in a storage room for the actual time of childbirth.

But our health workers knew that as soon as they left the house of the new mother, the family would move her and the baby into the cowshed again, and they were very concerned about the risk of infection this poses to both mother and child, particularly as the vaccination rates for tetanus are quite low.

THE PLAN

The health workers held discussions among themselves, and with the FVHWs, the local teachers, and the men and women in the village, to discover options for encouraging change. It soon became clear that a number of opinion leaders felt that change was possible but that some sort of incentive was needed.

Incentives for behavior change are being used more and more all over the world, often within health systems (Marteau, Ashcroft, & Oliver, 2009). In Nepal, a scheme to increase the number of institutional deliveries is being supported by the UK Department of International Development (DFID). Women are given a cash incentive if they go to a hospital or primary care center to have their babies (Ministry of Health and Population, n.d.).

Our health workers and the community wanted to give an incentive that was meaningful to the very poor families they were dealing with, but that would

CHAPTER 5 Behavior Change Initiative

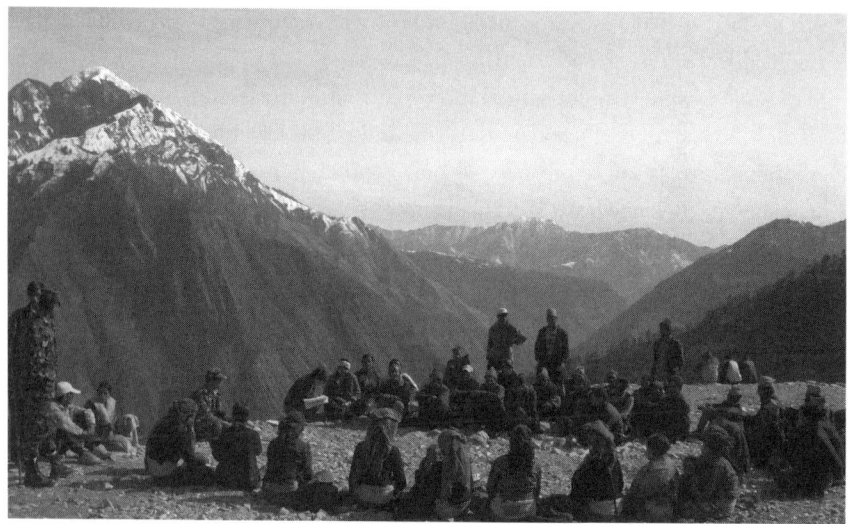

Figure 5-1   Community meeting in Maila.
Source: Courtesy of PHASE Nepal. Photo taken by Jiban Karki.

definitely benefit the mother and the baby and couldn't be diverted for other uses. They were worried that a cash payment might be used to buy nonessential luxury items, such as alcohol or sweets, and they wanted the gift to be substantial enough to justify change.

They believed that the resistance to change would not be very strong because many families already knew that this tradition was not kept up in other parts of the country. It was more the worry about being the first to be different, and the stigma this might carry, that kept families from making the change by themselves.

After many discussions, sometimes in groups of women, the health workers suggested to the PHASE central office that we should consider offering a set of new clothes to the mother and child. If they were bought in Kathmandu, one set of clothes would cost about 350 Nepalese rupees (~US$4.00), including transportation costs. But in terms of value to the family, they would be worth much more because similar-quality clothes would usually not be available locally at all.

Because the cost of the clothes was not included in the annual budget of the project, a private donor was found to finance 50 sets of clothes—traditional Nepali-style sets of trousers, jacket, and hat for the babies and sarees for the mothers.

THE SOLUTION

Starting in October 2008, PHASE health workers started distributing clothes to new mothers and babies. They had long discussions with the communities to decide where mothers would be able to spend the first month after childbirth because few families were prepared to ignore the tradition of untouchability completely.

Different areas of the community came up with different solutions. In one place, the neighborhood built a small house specifically for this purpose; it could be used by any family who had contributed to the construction. Elsewhere, families prepared for the birth by building a lean-to near the main living area. Some families decided to just give one of the rooms in the house over to the new mother, and some relaxed the rule so far as to let her stay in the general living area as long as she didn't get near the cooking area or sleep on the beds.

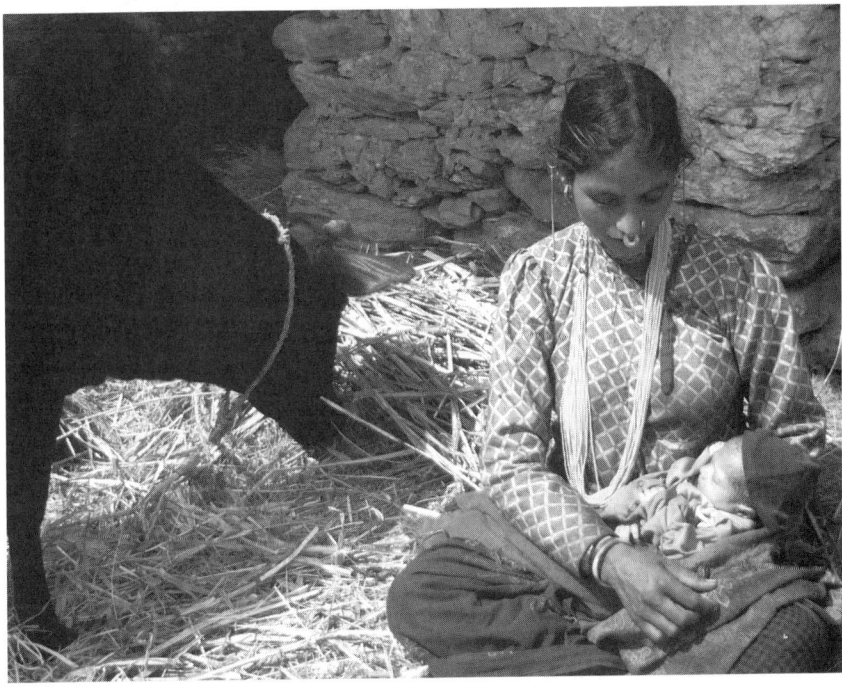

Figure 5-2 Mother with her newborn baby before the PHASE program.
Source: Courtesy of PHASE Nepal. Photo taken by Sr Urmila Adhikari.

CHAPTER 5 Behavior Change Initiative

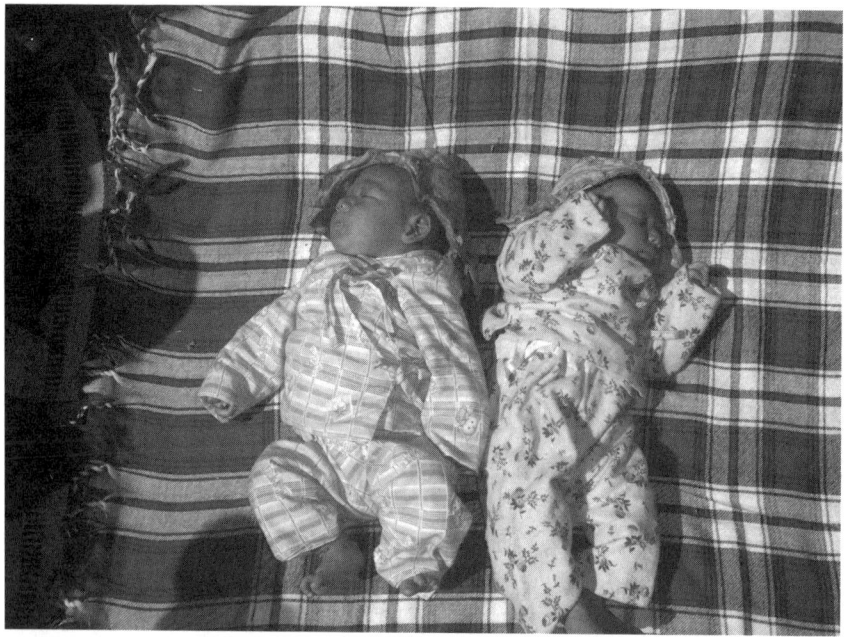

Figure 5-3   Two babies in new clothes.
Source: Courtesy of PHASE Nepal. Photo taken by Sr Urmila Adhikari.

   Whichever solution was chosen, the family had to make a small contract with the PHASE health workers to document that they agreed to not use the cowshed as living quarters for the new mother and her child. If any family violated the contract, it would be a matter for the whole community to decide how they should be penalized.
   Within six months, about 30 sets of new clothes have been distributed, and no violations of the contract have occurred, as far as our health workers know. They almost always revisit the house within a week of a delivery so they can get an impression of how the young mother is housed, and they are very confident that things have improved. In many cases, the mothers are now staying indoors, which makes a big difference to their comfort, especially in the more extreme seasons when it is very hot or very cold. It also seems to already have made a difference to infections in newborns, although of course the numbers are too small to be sure.

One mother explained the change like this: "Before, everyone just thought that this is how it has always been—life is hard for young mothers, and it is normal for babies to die in their first year. Then, PHASE nurses came along, and told us that it is not so in other parts of Nepal. They gave us nice new clothes, and they gave us a chance to stay in a clean, safe place with our babies. Now, everyone has seen that it is OK to stay indoors, and fewer babies are dying."

OUTCOMES

Before the initiative, no births were attended by a local skilled health worker. More than 90% of mothers in childbed were forced to stay in cowsheds or goat sheds for a month after delivery. Although it is not possible to get exact numbers, anecdotally the incidence of newborn sepsis and puerperal infections was high.

After implementation of the initiative, more than 50% of births are now attended by a skilled health worker, and among those that are attended, almost 100% agree to the conditional gift of clothes and to house the mother and baby in a clean, safe environment.

LESSONS LEARNED

Many organizations working in very remote areas find it difficult to change the health behaviors of potential clients. People often do not seek preventive health care, like vaccinations or antenatal care, and they often do not seek help for a serious illness at all or until it is very advanced.

Health workers often ascribe this behavior to inherent resistance to change in the population, and they blame the older generation for preventing younger people to effect change. PHASE health workers in Humla have demonstrated conclusively that an incentive scheme to change behavior can work, if certain conditions are met. In this particular case, trusted health professionals promoted the change with rational explanations and through enlisting the help of community members (FVHWs). They also offered acceptable alternatives to the traditional behavior and were nonjudgmental about local customs. Furthermore, they enlisted the help of the whole community in promoting the change and agreed on sanctions if the family did not stick to the agreement. The most important factor is probably that the health workers themselves, who are closely involved with the community, were strongly convinced of the idea.

CHAPTER 5 Behavior Change Initiative

> **Discussion Questions**
>
> 1. What factors determine if individuals, families, or communities abandon a long tradition in favor of new behavior?
> 2. What strategies were used to change traditional behaviors surrounding childbirth and delivery?
> 3. What were some of the possible impacts of the door-to-door outreach and data collection?
> 4. Given the remoteness of the area, how successful would the DFID-funded program be if it had been implemented?
> 5. Discuss the decision to give the families an incentive of clothing instead of cash. What were the impacts to the program, the women, and their families?

REFERENCES

Marteau, T. M., Ashcroft, R. E., & Oliver, A. (2009). Using financial incentives to achieve healthy behavior. *British Medical Journal, 338*, b1415.

Ministry of Health and Population, Government of Nepal. (n.d.). Nepal health sector programme implementation plan II (NHSP-IP 2) 2010–2015.

Ministry of Health and Population, Government of Nepal. (2006). Nepal demographic and health survey. Retrieved from http://www.measuredhs.com/pubs/pdf/fr191/fr191.pdf.

Ministry of Health and Population, Government of Nepal. (2011). Nepal demographic and health survey. Retrieved from http://measuredhs.com/pubs/pdf/FR257/FR257[13April2012].pdf.

United Nations Development Programme. (2011). International human development indicators. Retrieved from http://hdrstats.undp.org/en/countries/profiles/NPL.html.

World Health Organization. (2007). Maternal mortality in 2005. Estimates developed by WHO, UNICEF, UNFPA, and The World Bank. Geneva, Switzerland: Author.

PART III

The Impact of War

War creates a challenging environment in which to be healthy and to promote health. The outcome of armed conflict is death, disability, and conditions that often serve to spread disease, such as poor sanitation and lack of clean water. In the presence of conflict, people focus on their safety, and in order to preserve life and limb they often have to migrate quickly. War also destroys the institutional structures and supply chains that preserve and promote health. Healthcare workers may want to stay in conflict zones but have to leave to preserve their own lives. In the melee and confusion that precede and follow conflict, the health of local populations is greatly affected. With few human resources and destroyed physical resources, the health care of the most vulnerable populations suffers the most; among these are women, infants, and children.

Médecins Sans Frontiérs have won awards for providing health services to refugees from war as well as in areas of armed conflict. The United Nations also provides services under similar conditions. There are also local responses to armed conflict that provide essential services to people affected by war, by local people in their local languages. The instability that follows war makes it an environment where not many foreign agencies want to provide services due to safety risks to staff and the impact of conflict on supply chains and infrastructure.

With regard to maternal, newborn, and child health, pregnant women find it hard to leave areas of conflict, and leaving with young children is particularly challenging to moving quickly or providing for their care while on the run, in a refugee camp, or in a foreign country. Women may have to deliver under highly unsanitary conditions with no skilled attendant and their newborns may be at risk. Pregnant and parenting women in areas of conflict are highly unlikely to have prenatal care or to be able to access whatever limited health services may be available. Conflict can also cause mental illness and this can have a negative impact on the ability of mothers to care for their children.

The cases presented here are about a local response to conflict that is a shining example of what local people can do using their own resources. One case in particular features a collaboration between local foreign organizations. Different models with different strategies but with a similar goal of improving the health of women and children.

It should be noted that the case of rape as a weapon of war in the Congo is particularly intense and discretion is recommended when using this case in a classroom setting. However, it is particularly because of this women-centered strategy of combat and its horrendous impacts on reproductive, social, and cultural life, as well as on maternal and child health, that this story was included in this book.

CHAPTER 6

Integrating Child Spacing with Maternal Care in Postconflict Timor-Leste

Susan Thompson, MPH
Mary Anne Mercer, DrPH, MPH

Location: Timor-Leste

Sponsoring Organizations: Health Alliance International, funded by the U.S. Agency for International Development (USAID) and the Australian Agency for International Development (AusAID)

Target Population: Women of childbearing age and their families in the six districts of the central region of Timor-Leste

Project Goal: Assist the Timor-Leste Ministry of Health (MOH) to improve the quality of child spacing services and integrate activities for community promotion of child spacing into the national maternal and child health program

Project Objectives: (1) Better understand the perspective of Timorese families in relation to fertility regulation; (2) Assure access to quality contraceptive methods by Timorese families; and (3) Develop materials and approaches through which the MOH staff can motivate communities to adopt child spacing methods

CHAPTER 6   Integrating Child Spacing with Maternal Care

BACKGROUND

Timor-Leste, formerly East Timor, is a new democratic nation of great natural beauty with a tragic past. As a backwater colony of Portugal for several hundred years, East Timor was released to independence in 1975 (along with all of Portugal's other foreign colonies). The Revolutionary Front for an Independent East Timor (FRETILIN) declared the country independent on November 28, 1975. Nine days later the territory was invaded and occupied by Indonesian troops, leading to the integration of East Timor as the 27th "province" of Indonesia. However, Indonesian sovereignty was never recognized by the majority of Timorese or by the United Nations (Alonso & Brugha, 2006). The Timorese people suffered 24 years of brutal and illegal occupation by Indonesia; few Timorese families were without horrific stories of the torture, rape, disappearances, assassinations, and other forms of abuse that they had endured during this period. An estimated 200,000 Timorese died (25% of the population), either from direct warfare, starvation, or disease (Amnesty International, 1994). However, even when they were virtually ignored by the outside world, the Timorese people continued to organize a clandestine resistance against the Indonesian occupation based in the remote central mountains of the island.

In 1998, a change of government in Indonesia led to the promise of a "popular consultation," or referendum, on the choice of full Timorese independence from Indonesia or special autonomy as an Indonesian province. The announcement of the vote was followed by a bloody campaign of intimidation by the military and Timorese militias that they supported. Regardless of the threats, however, 98% of the registered voters turned out to express their wishes, with 78% voting for full independence from Indonesia. The announcement of the result of the vote was immediately followed by a systematic scorched-earth orgy of burning and violence by the military and their militias, destroying or seriously damaging an estimated 70% of the infrastructure and resulting in more deaths of Timorese citizens and the displacement of two-thirds of the population (Alonso & Brugha, 2006). In late September 1999, after 3 weeks of unrestrained destruction, troops sanctioned by the United Nations (UN) arrived and East Timor became a "non-self governing territory" of the UN. The devastation of the country was almost complete, including public services, banking, and commercial outlets, and there was a scarcity of trained Timorese personnel.

Following full independence in 2002, the newly formed government of what is now called Timor-Leste was faced with many competing challenges. The

Ministry of Health (MOH), in particular, had to cope with the destruction of more than a third of the health facilities. Virtually all equipment and supplies were damaged or looted, and a very small number of physicians and midlevel managers were available to address the health needs of a traumatized population. Additionally, the MOH was responsible for developing an entirely new healthcare system (National Research Council, 2003). This chapter reviews how Health Alliance International (HAI), a U.S.-based nongovernmental organization (NGO), worked in full partnership with the MOH from this early stage to help develop an integrated maternal/newborn health and family planning program in six rural districts in the central region of Timor-Leste. It describes the challenges addressed, results achieved, and lessons learned along the way.

HEALTH IN THE DEMOCRATIC REPUBLIC OF TIMOR-LESTE

Timor-Leste has a population of just over 1 million people, occupying the eastern half of the island of Timor in the Indonesian archipelago. It has a beautiful natural landscape that stands in stark contrast to the marginal conditions in which many Timorese live (**Figure 6-1**). There is widespread poverty, low literacy, and some of the worst maternal and child health statistics in the Southeast Asian region. After independence, maternal mortality was estimated at 660 per 100,000 live births (*Maternal mortality*, 2004), infant mortality was 80–90/1,000 live births, and 120 children per 1,000 died before reaching age 5 years. The utilization of health services was also very low. At that time only about half of women received any antenatal care during pregnancy, the use of a skilled birth attendant was less than 20%, and fewer than 10% of births occurred at a health facility (Ministry of Health and National Statistics, 2004).

Contributing to high maternal mortality was a fertility rate of 7.8, the highest recorded in the world. Only 10% of women were current users of a contraceptive method, which is common for families that aim to increase their numbers during an immediate postconflict period (Ministry of Health and National Statistics, 2004). However, 2003 survey data also pointed to very little community knowledge about how to go about spacing pregnancies if it was desired. Only 18% of ever-married women and 22% of ever-married men could recognize a contraceptive method, and they similarly had very little knowledge about where to obtain family planning methods or information (Ministry of Health and National Statistics, 2004). Other factors that may have influenced high fertility were a

CHAPTER 6 Integrating Child Spacing with Maternal Care

bride-price system (*barlake*), where new wives felt obligated to provide children for their husband's family, the dominant Catholic religion in the country, and cultural tradition that placed a high value on having many children. Clearly, a responsive and proactive healthcare system that would address the reproductive health needs of Timorese families was badly needed.

HAI is a U.S.-based international NGO with health programs in several countries and is closely affiliated with the Department of Global Health at the University of Washington in Seattle. HAI began operations in East Timor in early 1999 with support for maternity services in Dili, the capital. In response to the suggestion of the Minister of Health, HAI subsequently used a small foundation grant to develop an outreach component of a rural health program run by the Salesian Catholic Sisters. In 2004, USAID awarded HAI a health grant to support the new Timor-Leste MOH to strengthen maternal and newborn care in six districts of the central region of the country (**Figure 6-2**), followed in 2006 by a family planning grant, also from USAID. The central region comprises a large portion of the country and contains about 36% of the population. According to 2000 census data there were an estimated 244,930 women of reproductive age in the region (*Timor-Leste census*, 2006).

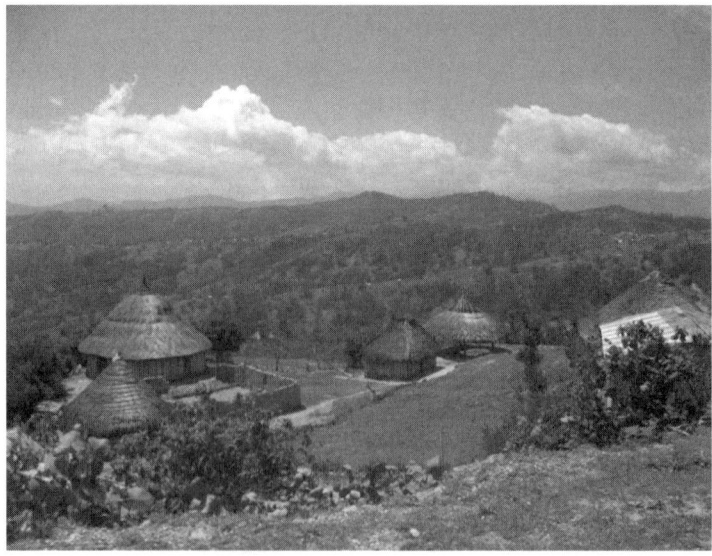

Figure 6-1   Rural Timor-Leste village of Maumete.
Source: Courtesy of Health Alliance International.

Health in the Democratic Republic of Timor-Leste

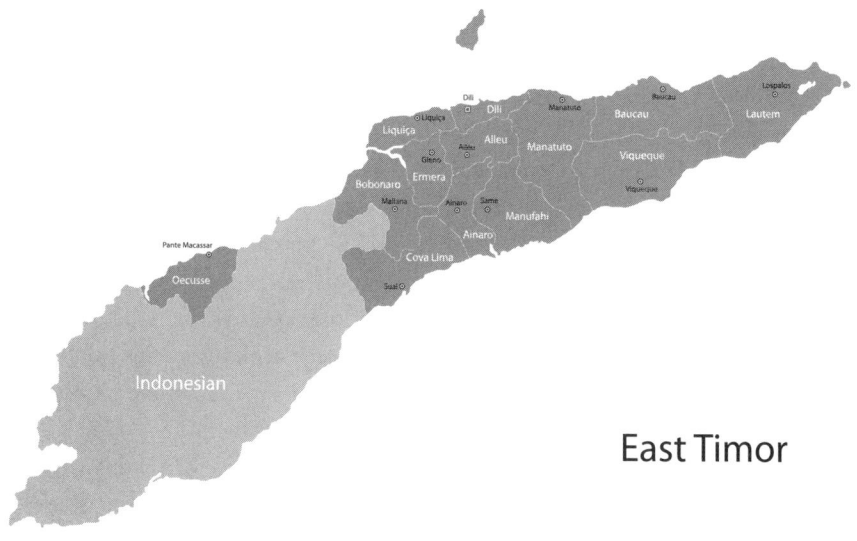

Figure 6-2 A map of Timor-Leste. HAI program districts in the central part of the country are highlighted in dark gray.
Source: © Volina/ShutterStock, Inc.

HAI's primary mission is to promote policies and support programs that strengthen government primary healthcare systems and promote decision making by national MOH staff. This contrasts with the common development model whereby an external organization, usually from the North, develops a short-term project and is understood to control the project budget and hold the balance of power in decision making (Girgis, 2007). The main operating principle in HAI programs is to participate in MOH initiatives in whatever ways are most helpful and to work with MOH staff in developing and pilot testing new activities or approaches. During the more than 10 years that HAI has been active in Timor-Leste it has built strong relationships with MOH counterparts at the central, district, and subdistrict levels and implemented programs in consultation with the MOH at every stage. With these and subsequent awards, HAI became a key partner in the development and deployment of Timor-Leste's maternal, newborn, reproductive health, and family planning policies. HAI is typically one of only a few NGOs included as a responsible

CHAPTER 6 Integrating Child Spacing with Maternal Care

party in national planning meetings and documents and is cited, for example, as a provider of technical assistance for maternal and child health and family planning in the 2007 Health Sector Strategic Plan (Timor-Leste Ministry of Health, 2007).

In 2006, HAI began the integration of family planning into their existing maternal and newborn care program in the central region. Several aspects of the situation in Timor-Leste indicated that a careful approach to promoting family planning would be important in implementing a successful program. The postconflict environment meant that many families felt the need to grow again, in some cases replacing lost family members. The population was almost entirely Catholic. "During Indonesian times," a phrase used to indicate the period of the Indonesian military occupation, there were well-documented human rights abuses, including numerous reports of coercive practices in connection with the occupying government's family planning program. These reports include allegations of contraceptive injections of school-aged Timorese girls under the guise of a vaccination program; the use of the Indonesian military to recruit contraceptive "accepters" in order to meet government targets; and requiring family planning as a prerequisite to receiving government licenses or permits (Sisson, 1997). The Indonesian family planning program known as *Keluarga Berencana*, or KB, focused on the slogan *Dua Anak Cukup* (Two Children Are Enough), a message that many Timorese found offensive and believed was an effort to control their population size.

Although survey data had documented low numbers of family planning use and understanding, little was known about the Timorese culturally based ideas, attitudes, and beliefs about fertility regulation. HAI's first activity was a qualitative community assessment to gather information regarding experiences, knowledge, beliefs, preferences, and practices about family planning, and then to share this information with the MOH and use it to inform and direct program activities. Assessment activities also served as a vehicle for an early introduction of HAI program staff to district MOH personnel and into the communities in which they would be working.

Program staff worried that many Timorese, particularly women, would be reticent to discuss family planning issues for the assessment. However, they were not only quite willing to share their knowledge, traditions, and experiences, but they were very eager to learn more about family planning. In general, families did not favor the notion of limiting family size, but they were open to the idea of healthy timing and spacing of pregnancy. Timorese parents expressed a desire to space their children in order to adequately provide for their children's needs, such as school fees and adequate food. Many also expressed a desire to know more about modern contraceptive methods so they could more dependably space their children. The ideal number of children varied based on geographic location, but the majority of parents stated that three, four, or five children would be ideal. Those living in remote areas were more likely to express a desire to have 7–10 children. While some parents felt their family size was something for God to decide, the majority of those interviewed did not express a conflict between using modern family planning methods and their Catholic faith.

Reflecting the same results as the quantitative data from the 2003 survey, there was very poor knowledge about modern methods of child spacing among the men and women interviewed. There were often fears, misinformation, and rumors about side effects, including infertility, of some methods. Respondents discussed traditional practices of consuming particular plants or drinking teas to either promote or limit fertility. Other practices were explained, such as burying the placenta following a birth either close to or far away from the family hearth to determine the timing of the next pregnancy (with a nearby site promising another pregnancy soon, and a farther-away burial leading to a longer interval until the next pregnancy) (Health Alliance International, 2006).

These early conversations within communities helped shape HAI's early program strategies. It was clear that messages that suggested limiting family size, which echoed the Indonesian program, would not be well received. However, since a focus on healthy timing and spacing of children seemed to be acceptable, the term adopted for the Timor-Leste family planning program was *Espaso Oan*, meaning "child spacing." It was also clear that there was lack of information, and misinformation, about contraceptive methods that would need to be addressed at all levels of the community. HAI staff were encouraged by not only the receptivity they encountered, but also the strong desire expressed by communities for more information about how they could successfully space their children.

INTEGRATING CHILD SPACING INTO A MATERNAL AND NEWBORN PROGRAM

HAI's health and development model emphasizes working with governments to strengthen public sector primary healthcare systems. A strong health system with government-provided services as its basis may be only a future aim in some places, but it should be fostered and supported. This is particularly true for a region emerging from conflict such as Timor-Leste, where there was extensive destruction of health factilites and a newly developing MOH. In the early planning stages of the Timor-Leste MOH, the decision was made to publicly fund and provide health care to the Timorese people. The high proportion of the population living on less than US$0.55 per day was a strong driver for Timorese authorities to support free universal access as the only acceptable option (Alonso & Brugha, 2006).

Although the main focus of the family planning project was to work at the community level to increase demand for services, a need emerged early in the project to also build the capacity of MOH midwives to improve the quality of family planning services. In the understanding that health workers benefit most from on-site, on-the-job training and follow-up coaching to ensure that new skills are understood and applied correctly, a key function of HAI's maternal and newborn care program was to provide supportive supervision visits to MOH midwives. In the family planning program, the staff found it necessary to focus on supporting family planning clinical skills as well. For example, although midwives had been trained in the use of most family planning methods, their training did not include follow-up skills assessments that would allow each midwife to be certified to conduct procedures such as intrauterine device (IUD) or contraceptive implant insertion. HAI midwifery staff became "master trainers" for the national family planning program, and as a result they were able to provide a posttraining skills check for midwives who had received training in methods such as hormonal implants and IUD insertion. Toward that goal, family planning activities were added to the supervision tool used for routine monitoring of quality maternal care.

The MOH standards called for outreach into communities, but because of a lack of training and appropriate materials, among other reasons, MOH midwives rarely took on this task. The population demonstrated a limited understanding of the benefits of maternal and child health practices, however, including the spacing of children, so the need for outreach activities was clear. To help the district staff undertake effective community outreach in both maternal–newborn care and family planning, HAI undertook the development of materials and training for activities that the MOH staff could conduct as a part of their routine work, emphasizing interesting and compelling audiovisual approaches.

Mai Ita Koko! (Come Let's Try!)

The Timor-Leste MOH began active implementation of a volunteer family health promoter program (Promotores Saude Familia, or PSFs) in 2006. Community members were selected to be PSFs by village leadership and were trained by the MOH staff to provide basic community health services, with a focus on teaching and motivation of families they visited. HAI provided additional training, materials, and supervision to PSFs in their house-to-house visits with pregnant mothers in a campaign called *Mai Ita Koko! (Come Let's Try!)*. The purpose of the home visit is to educate pregnant women and their families about healthy maternal and newborn behaviors and to encourage the adoption of a child spacing method in the postpartum period. Ten photo cards that depict relevant Timorese images and portray recommended maternal behaviors were developed. The images and messages on the cards are simple, clear, culturally relevant, and action oriented.

PSFs have been trained to use the cards as an educational tool during home visits and to encourage women and families to adopt one or more behaviors, such as having a skilled birth attendant or selecting a family planning method after delivery. The chosen behavior(s) is checked off on a colorful poster that contains each of the photos and is left with the family to remind them of their choice. The PSF follows up with families throughout the mother's pregnancy to monitor progress toward their goals.

The home visits have been well received by mothers who appreciate the support provided by the PSFs. Some district health staff members note that they see increased utilization of safe motherhood and family planning services that they credit to the Mai Ita Koko! program (Frey, 2009).

Film as a Health Promotion Tool

Where community understanding of safe maternal practices is poor and access to services is a challenge, it is important to provide believable evidence of its importance to the health and well-being of women and their children. Modern film technologies can make that aim feasible even in very resource-poor settings. In collaboration with the MOH and as part of the efforts to increase community knowledge of appropriate care-seeking behavior during pregnancy and delivery, HAI produced a film called *Feto Nia Funu* (A Woman's War). The film title reflected the idea that although the dangers of the war they had lived through for 24 years was fought heavily by men, women were regularly at risk of death every time they became pregnant. Directed by an internationally known filmmaker and filmed on location in Timor-Leste, the film portrays powerful scenes of pregnancy, birth, and the postpartum period, including actual scenes of newborn and maternal complications and the successful resuscitation of a newborn with asphyxia. The film has been shown widely to rural audiences to provide women and families with visual evidence of the dangers of delivery without a skilled attendant, and it promotes healthy maternal and newborn behavior change.

CHAPTER 6   Integrating Child Spacing with Maternal Care

With community audiences primed and the response to *Feto Nia Funu* so positive, HAI contracted with the same filmmaker to direct a two-part film, called *Espaso Oan*, about child spacing. The first part describes the benefits of child spacing for the health of the mother, children, and family; the second part provides detailed information about modern contraceptive methods, including natural methods. During film production HAI gathered broad support for *Espaso Oan* within the MOH, among community leaders, and even within the Catholic church leadership. The Vice Minister of Health gives an introduction to the film, and a prominent Timorese Catholic bishop is onscreen asserting that responsible parents need to adequately space their children. A nun explains natural methods. These onscreen appearances lend a great deal of credibility for Timorese audiences.

A local community-based organization was trained to use the film for health promotion in HAI program districts. They load up four-wheel-drive vehicles with generators, televisions, and DVD players and set out to tour small rural villages, district by district, to conduct screenings of *Espaso Oan*. They work with the district health staff to gather community audiences and lead lively community discussions following the film to answer lingering questions or clear up confusion. One of the highlights for participants in the after-film discussion groups is when midwives don an anatomical apron that illustrates the anatomy of both female and male reproductive systems (see **Figure 6-3**). The apron is used to show how and where specific contraceptive methods, such as the IUD, work. Audience responses to the film have been overwhelmingly positive. In late 2010, the film was shown on national television to an estimated audience of 150,000 people.

KEY FINDINGS

HAI and MOH staff members have regular discussions about the best ways to evaluate the integrated maternal care and family planning activities and make use of both qualitative and quantitative approaches to assess effects.

Findings from Community Discussions

Mindful of potential sensitivities in rolling out the *Espaso Oan* film in remote and rural Timorese villages, HAI decided to get an early sense of audience reaction through focus group discussions with men and women who watched the film and who participated in the guided disccusion groups. The responses were extremely enthusiastic; there appeared to be a real thirst for general and detailed knowledge of family planning methods. The majority of people stayed for the discussion

Key Findings

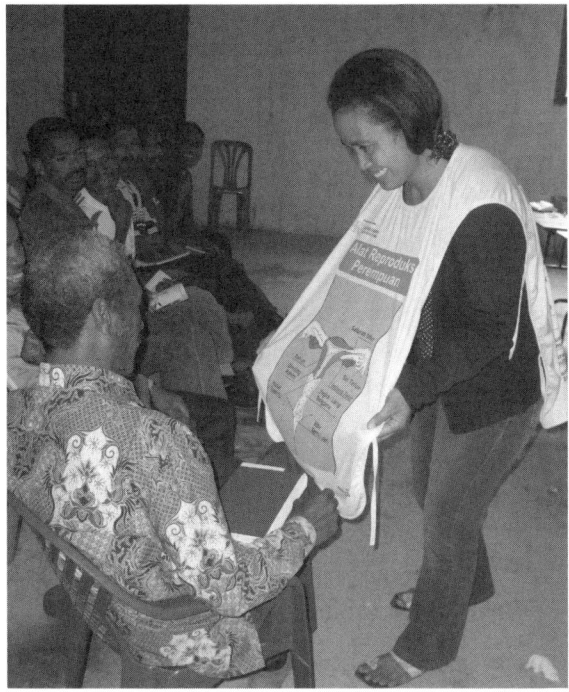

Figure 6-3 Midwife leading a post-film discussion on family planning methods.
Source: Courtesy of Health Alliance International.

following the film, even when the setting was hot and crowded or they were looking after restless babies. Most people in these rural locations had not heard about any methods except injectable contraception and, occasionally, the pill.

What knowledge was observed in communities about contraceptive methods appeared to be restricted to people who would have been of childbearing age during Indonesian times and thus had greater exposure to family planning messages and commodities. There was an apparent lack of knowledge among the younger generation (less than 35 years of age) about any form of family planning—this is understandable because in the early years after independence, family planning and the availability of commodities in the country was not a first priority of the Timorese MOH, which was overwhelmed with building an entirely new health system, essentially from the ground up.

Several women and some men in the audience voiced concern that methods that rely on abstinence, such as the Standard Days Cycle Beads and the calendar

113

method, would not work well when a man comes home after drinking. Women mentioned a lack of power to refuse their husbands, and both men and women talked about an obligation for wives to "serve" men due to a bride price paid as part of the marriage custom.

In 2009, HAI conducted another set of focus group discussions with men and women to evaluate the impact of the *Espaso Oan* film. The audience response remained universally favorable. The message that spacing children at least 3 years apart is better for the health of the mother, for the children, and for the economic future of the family resonated with the families we spoke to. Parents expressed appreciation in learning how to adequately and dependably space their children, and they continued to be eager to learn about specific contraceptive methods. One focus group participant commented, "After we saw the film, we [felt] better because in the past we had too many children; some died because there was not enough food and they didn't have healthy bodies . . . The film shows us what child spacing is [and] how to choose our own child spacing methods." Many of the participants asserted that they had been exposed to family planning during Indonesian times but had not heard of several of the methods presented in the film. They were appreciative of the new information: "Before the film came, I thought I had to have lots of children . . . We learned that child spacing gives health value for children [and] after three to five years [we] can have another child" (Hohl, Mercer, Thompson, Elson, & Harrison, 2010).

Survey Results

In 2003, an Australian university conducted a Demographic and Health Survey (DHS) across the entire country to assess the status of health indicators, including maternal and child health and family planning. Using the same methods, a second DHS was conducted in 2009, and the health changes that occurred over that 6-year period were impressive (**Figure 6-4**). The rates of facility deliveries and contraceptive prevalence more than doubled, with substantial increases in other indicators. In the 6 years between the 2003 and 2009 survey, the total fertility rate decreased from 7.9 to 5.7.

CHALLENGES

Working in a Postconflict Setting

In any resource-poor setting, and particularly in a postconflict situation such as that of Timor-Leste, a range of challenges are to be expected. HAI found that

Challenges

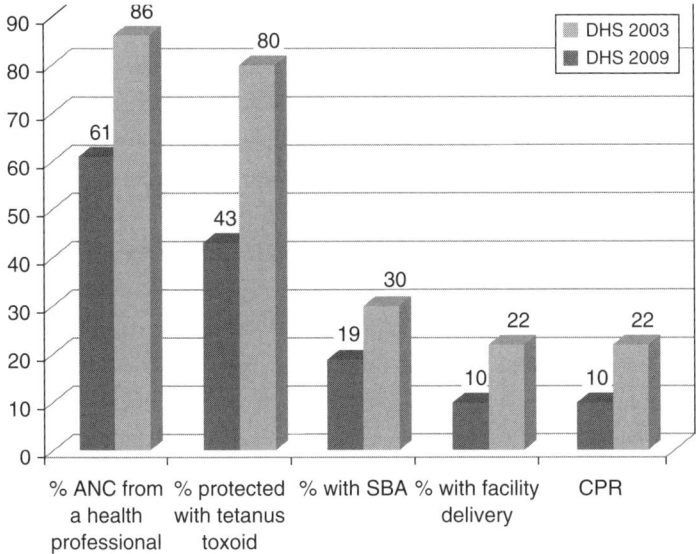

ANC : Antenatal care
CPR: Cardiopulmonary Resuscitation
SBA: Skilled Birth Attendant

Figure 6-4 National maternal health indicators for 2003 and 2009.

Source: Data from Ministry of Health and National Statistics Office, Timor-Leste, University of Newcastle, The Australian National University, ACIL Australia Pty Ltd. Timor-Leste 2003 Demographic and Health Survey. Newcastle, Australia: University of Newcastle; 200, and National Statistics Directorate (NSD) Timor-Leste, Ministry of Finance and ICF Macro. (2010). Timor-Leste Demographic and Health Survey 2009–2010. Dili, Timor-Leste: NSD and ICF Macro.

staff members of the fledgling MOH were often overwhelmed with a wide range of new undertakings and demands from multiple donors, making it sometimes difficult to assure their active involvement in new activities or initiatives. Formal MOH review and approval of the family planning film, for example, took several months after its completion due to the many competing priorities of MOH staff members. There was also a need to develop program approaches that would respond to an ever-changing situation, approaches not necessarily included in initial project plans. HAI was fortunate to have flexible support and collaboration both from the MOH and from their funders, USAID and AusAID, that allowed them to respond to new information and observe needs with fresh approaches during the course of the project.

CHAPTER 6 Integrating Child Spacing with Maternal Care

Civil Unrest

Working in a postconflict setting comes with the possibility of a return of the conflict. The political stability of Timor-Leste was threatened in 2006 with several months of violent civil unrest, particularly in the capital city, that sent large numbers of Timorese to internal displacement camps for extended periods—including some of HAI's counterpart staff from MOH. The unrest made travel to the districts difficult or impossible for several months and delayed important project activities. The expatriate staff of most NGOs and bilateral or multilateral organizations were evacuated out of concern for possibly increasing violence. However, the HAI staff continued to work throughout this time, despite the trauma of the period and the dislocation that several local staff members experienced. The Timorese staff expressed heartfelt gratitude to the expatriate HAI staff members who chose to remain in the country throughout the "situation" of 2006.

Cultural and Religious Barriers

Despite support from some in the Catholic hierarchy, there was ongoing sensitivity to possible cultural or religious objections to the discussion of specific family planning methods with the general public. Because the film was in two parts, HAI agreed to show the first film on family planning motivation to the public at large, and the second half of the film, where specific methods are explained, only to adults. This compromise was deemed important, even though it is clear that information about contraception would be useful for adolescents as well.

Information Systems

Assuring a strong health information system (HIS) is a major challenge to governments in transition. The Timor-Leste HIS underwent many changes during its first few years of development, and updates to improve accuracy and use of data continued. Efforts to provide accurate reports on family planning use were hindered by a lack of common definitions for standard indicators, such as a "new user" of contraception. Incomplete data submission by peripheral health units required the direct collection of health utilization data from the health units, a practice that was expected to be unnecessary when the system was fully developed. Reliable information about stocks of family planning commodities was similarly difficult to obtain, despite extensive inputs into the system by the United Nations Population Fund (UNFPA).

LESSONS LEARNED

The lessons learned from this project include the following:

- An integrated approach to support the government health system is crucial to effective and sustainable work with health systems and with communities. HAI programs in Timor-Leste (and elsewhere) are embedded within the MOH system. However, assuring access and use of quality family planning services at MOH facilities is tied to successful community-level health promotion to increase the demand for care—the two strategies need to go hand in hand. HAI's approach to working with district-level MOH midwives thus includes supporting both their clinical roles and their community outreach and motivational skills and resources.
- An integrated approach that weaves family planning activities into a maternal and newborn care project resulted in a program that was accepted by the community and providers alike. MOH midwives were initially hesitant to initiate family planning discussions with their clients because of its negative associations with the Indonesian period, lack of competency discussing the topic, and fear of disapproval by the church. Family planning activities that emphasized the health and social benefits of child spacing, however, were seen positively by midwives as an essential aspect of their role of caring for women and infants, and by communities as a believeable approach to promoting the welfare of their families. Family planning messages were integrated into all of the materials produced for the maternal and newborn care project, providing the midwives and health volunteers with easy transitions from more familiar information, such as assuring a safe delivery, to the newer topic of child spacing.
- Rural communities, even very traditional ones, may be open to learning how to dependably space their children. Learning about traditional methods of child spacing opened a discussion about other ways to accomplish that end. Simple information delivered with visual aids and ample opportunity for questions proved remarkably effective in stimulating discussions in even the most rural communities. Both men and women gave ample evidence of their openness to the use of modern family planning methods after basic information was provided and common myths were dispelled.
- The Catholic church can be a very effective ally. We found that many influential Catholic priests and nuns, and even one of the bishops of the

CHAPTER 6 Integrating Child Spacing with Maternal Care

country, were very open to supporting the need for child spacing when the extremely high fertility levels were made known. The appearance of both the bishop and nuns in the child spacing film added to its credibility.
- Film is an entertaining way to engage audiences in health promotion and is possible even in the most remote and rural locations. With the need for near-total rebuilding of the health infrastructure after 1999, modern audiovisual equipment was provided for many health facilties. Even where electricity is not available, small portable generators provide adequate power for showing films, which can be shown with LCD projectors or on laptop computers or televisons to small groups. The novelty of film in most of rural Timor-Leste has made it an in-demand addition to the materials available for rural health promotion.

CONCLUSION

HAI's experience in Timor-Leste has shown that close collaboration with the MOH to support both improved clinical services and active community promotion of family planning can be successful even in difficult postconflict situations. Anticipated barriers can be overcome by awareness about past traumas, sensitivity to local norms, programmatic flexibility, and integration into existing valued programs. Audiovisual materials that speak to local realities can go far to promote understanding and acceptance of unfamiliar ideas when the benefits to mothers, families, and the communities in which they live are made clear.

Discussion Questions

1. What rationale was given by HAI for closely linking with MOH? What do you think of this strategy?
2. What are the benefits and drawbacks of linking so closely with a MOH? Consider this question from the perspectives of HAI, MOH, and service recipients.
3. What were some of the challenges to creating a family planning program? How did MOH and HAI address each of them?
4. If you were to implement a film-based outreach or education program, what are some of the issues you would have to consider?

REFERENCES

Alonso, A., & Brugha, R. (2006). Rehabilitating the health system after conflict in East Timor: A shift from NGO to government leadership. *Health Policy Plan, 21*(3), 206–216.

Amnesty International. (1994). *Power and impunity: Human rights under the new order.* London, England: Author.

Frey, M. (2009). The use of photo cards in the PSF program in two districts of Timor-Leste: An implementation evaluation. Unpublished report.

Girgis, M. (2007). The capacity-building paradox: Using friendship to build capacity in the South. *Development in Practice, 17*(3).

Health Alliance International. (2006). *Qualitative community assessment: Aileu and Manatuto districts.* Seattle, WA: Author.

Hohl, S., Mercer, M., Thompson, S., Elson, E., & Harrison, M. (2010). *Espaso Oan: Evaluating a reproductive health film in post-conflict Timor-Leste.* Seattle, WA: University of Washington.

Ministry of Health and National Statistics, Timor-Leste; ACIL Australia Pty Ltd., University of Newcastle; & Australian National University, Australia. (2004). Timor-Leste 2003. Demographic and health survey: Key findings. Dili, Timor-Leste: Ministry of Health.

National Research Council. (2003). Tulloch, J., Saadah, F., Araujo, R., de Jesus, R., Lobo, S., Hemming, I., . . . Morris, I. *Initial steps in rebuilding the health sector in East Timor.* Washington, DC: The National Academies Press.

Sisson, M. (1997). *From one day to another: Violations of women's reproductive and sexual rights in East Timor.* Fitzroy, Australia: East Timor Human Rights Center.

Timor-Leste census 2004 overview. (2006). Dili, Timor-Leste: Pradet Timor Lorosa'e.

Timor-Leste Ministry of Health. (2007). Health sector strategic plan 2008–2012. Dili, Timor-Leste: Author.

World Health Organization & Dept. of Reproductive Health and Research. (2004). Maternal mortality in 2000: Estimates developed by WHO, UNICEF, and UNFPA. Geneva, Switzerland: World Health Organization.

CHAPTER 7

LifeLine Community Healthcare Program: Reducing Maternal and Infant Mortality in Liberia

Lucy November, MPH

Location: New Georgia Area, Monrovia, Liberia, West Africa

Name of Project: LifeLine Community Healthcare Program

Target Population: 10,000–15,000

Project Goal: Help reduce high rates of maternal and infant mortality in Liberia

Project Objectives: (1) Encourage and promote healthy living in the community with appropriate and effective health promotion activities; (2) Provide a comprehensive community health service, including laboratory service, diagnosis and treatment of common diseases, and maternity and child health activities; (3) Reach out to the less fortunate in the community with relief and humanitarian assistance; (4) Train traditional birth attendants (TBAs), using a recognized national program, to the level of Trained Traditional Midwife (TTM); and Demonstrate God's love by treating people with a high level of care and respect

This case study was compiled by Lucy November, with Ruth Swallie, Tage Swallie, Ezekiel Swallie, and Henry Powoe, in September 2009.

CHAPTER 7   LifeLine Community Healthcare Program

BACKGROUND

After being plagued by civil war for 14 long years, Liberia published new figures for maternal and infant mortality (Liberia Institute of Statistics and Geo-Information Services, 2008). They are horrific statistics, with maternal mortality at 994 of every 100,000 births in 2007, compared with 578 of every 100,000 births in 1987. Infant mortality decreased from 139 per 1,000 live births in 1992 to 71 per 1,000 live births from 2002–2006. Many thousands of women live with birth injuries, the threat of sexually transmitted infections (STIs) and unwanted pregnancies, and the dread of their babies succumbing to malaria, pneumonia, or diarrhea. With an unemployment rate of 85%, most people survive by petty market trading and live a hand-to-mouth existence. Health provision is scanty, with the majority of the 325 health centers in Liberia totally or partially destroyed, and the number of trained staff members is severely depleted by death and emigration. There are now 50 qualified doctors in Liberia for a population of 3.5 million; in 1989, prior to the war, there were 250.

Regarding midwives, Liberian Health Minister Walter Gwenigale stated that the country needs 1,400 midwives and there are only 300 currently working. A strong dependence prevails after years of handouts from international humanitarian organizations' efforts to relieve the worst of people's suffering; international nongovernmental organizations (NGOs) are exploring exit strategies in light of an ingrained belief that Liberia is incapable of ever providing for its own ("Life after the NGOs," 2009).

THE PLAYERS

Ruth Swallie, her husband, Tage Swallie, and their team are Liberians with a different mentality. Both born in 1962 in a Swedish mission compound, Ruth and Tage were childhood friends and sweethearts. She was small in stature, so Ruth was denied the opportunity to start school with her peers because she did not pass the entry test for the mission's infant school—the ability to reach over her head and touch her ear. At the time, this was the missionaries' way of judging if a child was aged 5 years or older. (The fact that Ruth was born at the mission hospital did not seem to be proof enough of her age!) Despite this faltering start, Ruth did very well in school and was quickly promoted the following year to rejoin her peers. Her own experience of hospitals started early when, at age 12, she was blinded in her left eye by a stone flung from her brother's sling as the two children were on scarecrow duty during the rice harvest.

In order to graduate from school, the children had to travel to the county's capital, and they met a man who would have a strong influence on both of their lives—the late Richard Cole, who dedicated his life to rescuing boy soldiers during Sierra Leone's long years of diamond-fueled rebel war. At this time, he was a young Christian evangelist who believed strongly that young people could change their destiny and that of their country if they could see themselves as the solutions to their country's problems and not victims. Throughout the 1980s, Tage joined Richard in building communities in provincial Liberia based around a farm, a clinic, and a school, enabling people to work together to be productive and improve their own health and education.

BECOMING A MIDWIFE

Ruth was keen to get into business too, and planned to go to college to study accounting. However, her mother, a trained traditional midwife, encouraged her to do midwifery training first. "You should always listen to your mother," said Ruth with a smile. She managed to get a place at Phebe—a prestigious nursing and midwifery school in Monrovia—and made the long journey to the city to study. With little money, she was unable to travel either back to her mother's home or to see Tage, and she stayed for 2 years in the students' dormitory. Ruth thinks she gained a wealth of extra experience at this time because, since she could not afford to go out on the weekends as her friends were doing, she spent most weekends and evenings with the midwives on the labor ward, learning to deliver breech babies and twins, learning how to deal with emergencies, and learning how to suture and other advanced skills. Graduation came, and with the lack of trained staff in the country, these newly qualified midwives were not given the luxury of a junior role working under more senior colleagues. Ruth returned to her home town and was put in charge of the maternity ward of a busy mission hospital.

With fighting breaking out indiscriminately across the region at that time, women would come not simply from the area of Foya where the hospital was situated, but from Guinea and Sierra Leone, in this area of Liberia where the three borders meet. Ruth recalls with amusement that her mother also worked in the hospital, with Ruth as her boss! Ruth and Tage faced huge criticism at this time for not marrying and having children earlier, which was the cultural norm,

CHAPTER 7   LifeLine Community Healthcare Program

instead of pursuing their individual callings—some said that Ruth had so many abortions that she could no longer conceive; others said that she was infertile and that was why she had pursued her training. Reflecting on it 20 years later, Ruth was not bitter—she recognized that many girls did not have the support that she had from her mother and Tage, and they were jealous of her success. When three baby girls came along in quick succession soon after their marriage in 1988, many people congratulated her and expressed their shamed apologies.

CHILDBIRTH IN LIBERIA

In Liberia, as elsewhere in Africa, most babies were (and still are in the provinces) delivered in their villages by untrained traditional birth attendants (TBAs). During those years in the province of Foya, Ruth witnessed the horrific effects of some very dangerous practices on women and their babies. She was able to save many women's lives through prompt action and treatment, but for others, by the time they reached the hospital, after having been in labor for several days or having a retained placenta or heavy bleeding, it was too late. One practice Ruth described is when a woman is taken to a clearing in the bush and is made to run around for hours while in labor and then is told to push (in the absence of an urge to push or any visible signs of the second stage of labor), with the TBA pushing on or sitting on her abdomen. Following this, many babies were stillborn, and many women died from a ruptured uterus or severe bleeding; many women in Liberia have had more stillbirths and neonatal deaths than live births. Blame is usually apportioned to the woman, who is accused of unfaithfulness or of being a witch, which "causes the child to die."

TRAINING TRADITIONAL BIRTH ATTENDANTS

When Ruth received an invitation to be part of a national plan for training TBAs to become Trained Traditional Midwives (TTMs), she was delighted and knew this would make a big difference for women's health in her country. Leaving baby Cecilia with her mother and Tage, she made the journey to Monrovia and did the 2-week training course. Armed with her new knowledge, a curriculum, and some resources, she started the local training program. TBAs were selected by village elders—one per village—and attended the 6-month program. They learned which women to refer to the hospital; which could be safely delivered at home; how to conduct a clean delivery; hand washing;

how to deal with common emergencies, such as bleeding; and other issues of general health, such as the importance of immunizations and family planning. Upon graduation, they were presented with delivery kits containing basic equipment that they had learned how to use—gloves, a nailbrush, clamps and scissors, a large bowl, local cord tie and alcohol for sterilizing—all provided by the Ministry of Health.

Ruth taught the students to ask a literate person to make records, and she visited their villages to supervise their practice and to immunize children. During these visits, Ruth experienced overwhelming gratitude from the people whose very lives had been saved by the improved skills of the TTMs; it was not uncommon for her to return home with a chicken, a bag of rice, and a gallon of oil. The jealousy of others had been replaced with a high level of respect and recognition. Women were now sent to the hospital as soon as a problem arose because of the trusting relationship that the TTMs had with Ruth. All women who were having their first baby were sent to the hospital, and overall there was a noticeable difference in the local rate of maternal and infant mortality. Ruth recalls one woman who had had six stillbirths prior to the TTM training, all at the hands of the untrained TBAs. Sent by the trained TTMs, she went on to have six live babies! These TTMs were not paid salaries, but in many villages, community elders would ensure that families would make small contributions, or other community members would help on their farms when the TTMs were busy caring for a laboring woman.

WAR

In 1993, the war in Liberia intensified. As rebel soldiers raided villages all over Foya, looting, raping, and killing indiscriminately, Tage and Ruth had no choice but to flee for their lives to Guinea. With their three little girls—aged 4, 3, and 1 year old—they literally ran all night through the forest and bushland until they reached the river that is the border between Liberia and Guinea. Not knowing what was ahead, but being sure that she would need them, Ruth had grabbed her two clamps, her scissors, and her bulb syringe, and wrapped them in one of baby Annette's nappies. Only women and children were allowed to cross the river to the refugee camps on the other side, because the Guinean authorities feared that they would unknowingly allow rebels into the country, so Ruth crossed alone with the girls. Tage managed to follow later, crossing quietly one night by canoe farther up the river.

CHAPTER 7 LifeLine Community Healthcare Program

Life in the camp was very tough, and Ruth made a living by going into the forest to chop wood that she carried on her head back to the camp to sell. In this way, she managed to feed the family and used a little money to buy some essential drugs to treat some of the common illnesses that were rife in the cramped conditions of the refugee camp. Ironically, children who had escaped the rebels in Liberia were now dying of malaria, pneumonia, diarrhea, and malnutrition in the refugee camp in Guinea. Gradually, Liberian families who had previously known Ruth and Tage sought them out in the nearest town, at the small house that was loaned to them by a local church pastor, and Ruth started to deliver babies in their one room. Tage would get out of bed, go outside with the children, and pray, while Ruth cared for the woman.

The refugee hospitals in this area of Guinea were being run by Médecins Sans Frontières, and when Ruth heard that they were recruiting for local midwives, she eagerly applied and scored first in the selection exam. Once again, she was put in charge of a busy maternity clinic, with one TTM (an ex-student from Foya) working alongside her. The clinic was very busy, serving not only the Liberian women from the camps, but also local Guinean women who came into the camp just to access the health care. Ruth recalls one night when a Guinean woman was brought to the clinic after delivering her baby out in the bush. She was bleeding heavily because part of her placenta was retained, and she was surrounded by distraught family members who were wailing as they could see the life literally draining out of her. Ruth sent the relatives out, prayed hard, and did her first manual removal of a placenta. She gave the woman IV oxytocin and antibiotics and called her relatives back to care for her. Her life was saved, the word spread, and more and more people came with emergency cases to the refugee clinic.

GOING HOME

When the college where Tage had been studying reopened, Ruth and Tage decided to move to Monrovia so that he could finish his studies. Life in Monrovia was desperate at that time, flooded with displaced people from the provinces and refugees. Finding accommodation was difficult, and Ruth was not able to find work as a midwife because jobs were only available in hospitals further afield. To make ends meet, Ruth and her children had to resort to filling small plastic bags with drinking water, chilling them overnight with ice blocks, and walking around Monrovia selling them. After her years of managing maternity units and gaining a huge amount of respect, this was not an easy time. However, with the money they made, Ruth managed to save enough to take a short course as a pastry cook. They bought a small coal oven so that Ruth could get up early in the morning and make doughnuts, which they would then sell along with the water. Because they always reinvested their money, however small, Tage and Ruth eventually managed to send the girls back to school and find themselves a one-room house to call home in an area of Monrovia called Chicken Soup Factory, named after the stock cube processing plant that had been a big employer before the war.

BUILDING A CLINIC

Ruth noticed an old shop that had been empty for years after being ransacked by rebel soldiers; it was locked up and dilapidated. Tage and Ruth sought the owner and made arrangements to renovate the shop and use it free of charge. Here Ruth started a small pharmacy, getting to know local people who would come to the store with sick children at all hours of the day or night needing common but lifesaving treatments for malaria, pneumonia, diarrhea, and other diseases. Inevitably, one night a woman came to Ruth in strong labor. Ruth closed the shop and delivered the baby there, where she had a makeshift bed and her essential delivery instruments. Government hospitals were in a serious state of disrepair, there were very few health professionals, and the pervasive corruption made a hospital stay a very expensive exercise, so when word got out that Ruth was a midwife, women started to regularly ask her to take on their care.

During the years at Chicken Soup Factory, Ruth recalls referring only two women to the main hospital. One woman came alone to the house; she was in labor and had no antenatal care, then developed eclampsia. Tage remembers running around the community desperately asking where her husband lived. Finding a car to transport the woman to the hospital was almost impossible, so Tage and the woman's husband carried her to the nearest military checkpoint where armed police persuaded a local taxi driver to make the hour-long journey to the hospital. Amazingly, the woman and her baby survived and returned to thank Tage and Ruth. Ruth charged these families a small set fee for delivery and drugs, and in this way she managed to help support the family while improving the health outcomes for the women and children in the local community of Chicken Soup Factory.

CHAPTER 7 LifeLine Community Healthcare Program

Ruth was again called on to train TBAs, and many went on to work alongside certified midwives in government health posts and clinics. Using hands-on methods, storyboards, drama, and song, many women without proper schooling were trained by Ruth to be very safe practitioners. Ruth and Tage had an idea to expand the service and build a bigger community clinic that would be a local supplement to the big, impersonal government hospital. It would be a place where local people would be treated with care and respect, bringing their children for immunization and treatment; a place that could become a hub, a gathering point for the community that was suffering so badly from fragmentation and family breakup.

They discussed the idea with Ruth's brother and his wife, who owned a plot of land in the New Georgia area of Monrovia. They decided to use some of the land to build a clinic, and they set to work making bricks at the end of every month, as money allowed. After several months, they had sufficient bricks to start the project, and Ruth's elderly father, who had been a mason, laid the foundation in 2001. This process of making bricks until there were enough to build the next stage continued until finally, in July 2003, The Healthline Medical Clinic was ready for operation. On the same plot, they also put up a covered structure to use as a church for the local Christian community. Tage describes the clinic as a Christian medical institution and a medical arm of the church ministry.

From the beginning, the financial accounting was very transparent. Ruth and Tage were determined to work on a different basis than other healthcare providers. Though they had to charge people for the service, they were clear that there would be no under-the-table charges, only an established charge for drugs, delivery, and laboratory tests. Even within the family, to avoid future misunderstandings, Ruth and Tage started to pay monthly rent to Ruth's brother for the land in return for continued use of the land—an arrangement that was legally binding. Right from the beginning, after paying salaries and buying basic drugs, all profits went toward developing the building and the service offerings.

The clinic has a large covered waiting and registration area where immunizations are done and babies are weighed. Here mothers can talk through general health concerns, such as feeding, weaning, etc. There is a small dispensary; a consultation room where sick people are seen by the physician's assistant, Henry Powoe; an antenatal room where pregnant women are seen for their regular checkups with Ruth and her staff; a labor room; and a four-bed women's room for postnatal women and women in early labor. There is also a laboratory room where simple blood tests for malaria, stool tests for worms, and urinalysis tests are carried out while patients wait. In a three-bed day room, patients who are ill can rest while commencing treatment or waiting for test results.

The clinic is fully registered with the Ministry of Health, with whom the clinic team has a very good relationship. They are kept fully informed of any new government initiatives, are invited to attend training alongside government health staff, and are part of the national Expanded Program on Immunization (EPI). Student nurses in national training programs are regularly sent to the clinic for clinical experience, and statistics are sent monthly to the Ministry of Health as part of national health data.

JOINING LIFELINE

In 2008, Tage was invited to take part in a business enterprise conference in the United Kingdom base of LifeLine Network (www.lifelinenetwork.org). LifeLine Network is a coalition of grassroots development organizations in 15 nations whose aim is to equip its members with the skills and resources to build sustainable models of community development through income-generating projects and to foster regional networks to enable sharing of skills and ideas. This conference confirmed in Tage's mind the vision he and Ruth always had of reinvestment and sustainability.

One outcome of becoming part of the LifeLine Network was being given a loan to start an Internet cafe in downtown Monrovia, where no such facility existed, to raise funds to expand the clinic and its services. As of September 2009, this project was going ahead and was managed by Tage's brother Ezekiel Swallie. The team (Tage, Ruth, Ezekiel, and Henry) was also working on other ideas for expansion to other needy areas of the city and developing their health promotion activities with parents. This focused on prevention of sickness by teaching about issues such as sexual health, diet for children, hygiene, and treatment of common illnesses at home, as well as ways to help women start small businesses to provide for their children. In response to a desperate need in their locality where parents could not afford to send their children to school, the church started a small school, as members asserted their belief that local problems can often be solved by local people.

Until its involvement with LifeLine Network, Healthline Clinic had no external sources of funding or support, and yet this team achieved such a high

CHAPTER 7 LifeLine Community Healthcare Program

level of success. Families sought out the clinic as its reputation spread. It was not free at the point of delivery because this is not sustainable, but it did reduce charges for particularly impoverished families. They also charged less for a delivery if the woman has attended for antenatal care, thus providing an incentive for women to access care throughout their pregnancy—an important factor in reducing maternal mortality. In a country where the annual per capita expenditure on health was US$2, this smaller, more flexible, locally managed model of healthcare provision was a realistic, viable addition to government provision. As Ezekiel summarized: "It is evident that the solution to the health problems in Liberia cannot be met by yesterday's answers. It calls for new answers from the minds of flexible visionary people."

Responding to the question, "What lessons have you learned from the experience setting up and running this project?," members of the team made the following statements:

- "As Liberians, we are able to make a big difference to Liberia."
- "Don't sit and wait for money to come to you. Whatever small resources you have available can be effective if used wisely."
- "Our attitude of love and respect goes a long way in building people's self-esteem. Health care is not just about giving out medicine. It is about kindness and respect."
- "By serving you learn. By learning you grow."

Discussion Questions

1. Explore mechanisms for financially sustainable healthcare services for poor people.
2. What are the implications of using volunteers for the provision of a primary healthcare service?
3. What were some of the health impacts of the war on Ruth, her family, her community, and her country?
4. How do you think that external sources of funding would change the operation of the clinic?
5. What were some of the differences between a hospital birth and a community birth?

REFERENCES

Liberia Institute of Statistics and Geo-Information Services. (2008). Liberia demographic and health survey 2007. Retrieved from http://www.measuredhs.com/pubs/pdf/fr201/fr201.pdf

Life after the NGOs. (2009, September 16). *New Democrat* (Monrovia, Liberia).

CHAPTER 8

Rape as a Weapon of War: Stories from the Democratic Republic of Congo

Elaine Dietsch, PhD
Luc Mulimbalimba-Masururu, MD

Location: MHCD is a not-for-profit, African nongovernmental organization (NGO). It has two bases, one in Kenya on the Kenyan–Ugandan border and the other in the Democratic Republic of Congo (DRC). North and South Kivu are the easternmost provinces of DRC and border Rwanda and Burundi, and they are the area of focus for MHCD: MCH programs.

Name of Project: Mission in Health Care and Development (MHCD): Maternal and Child Health (MCH) program

Sponsoring Organization: MHCD has no funding or sponsoring organization as such. Individuals in Australia, America, Switzerland, Kenya, DRC, and New Zealand provide financial support. One

Note: Warning: Many readers will find the contents of this chapter very distressing. It has been written with the expressed permission and plea of the women to share their stories as widely as possible, so that the world learns what is happening to them. Their stories are told to honor their request.

CHAPTER 8 Rape as a Weapon of War

company provides ongoing support to enable equipping and maintenance of a school for street children, orphans, rescued child soldiers, and internally displaced children. Community groups and clubs, various churches, and a number of schools in Australia are very generous with their financial support. Birth Kits Foundation Australia (BKFA) sponsors traditional midwifery and maternal and child health nurse education, and it supplies many thousands of birth kits through AusAID for traditional midwives associated with MHCD.

Target Population: Women and children in Eastern Congo.

"In eastern Congo, there is a war on women. There is such a pattern of rape and sexual violence that the world has never before seen its equivalent" (Lewis, 2008, p. 309). Women, especially those with infants and young children, are the most adversely affected by war (Almedom et al., 2003), and in DRC that impact is more damaging than any ever experienced at any time or in any place before (Lewis, 2008). MHCD: MCH programs serve the women and their children who have been traumatized, tortured, and often displaced as a result of rebel and militia action perpetrated against them. Many of the women seen in antenatal clinics and cared for by the traditional midwives associated with MHCD have conceived when they were raped; they were often raped on multiple occasions and over long periods of time. These women and their children usually have no means of support, having been banished by their communities and families following rape(s). Although a refugee is usually defined as a person who has sought refuge in another country, and an internally displaced person is someone forced to leave their home and community to seek refuge elsewhere in their own community (United Nations High Commissioner for Refugees, 1999), in this chapter the term "refugee" refers to any person forced to leave their home and community to seek refuge due to war or conflict, whether or not they have left their country of origin.

In the Kivu provinces, malnutrition is endemic and evident in the majority of women and, after they are weaned, the children who attend MHCD: MCH clinics. Women commonly seek diagnosis and treatment for chronic illnesses, including the increasing prevalence of HIV/AIDS (61% of those living with AIDS are women and girls, and in DRC this is estimated to be much higher; UNAIDS, 2008), gonorrhea, syphilis, malaria, cholera, and typhoid. Acute illnesses such as diarrhea and acute respiratory infections have the biggest burden on very young children (Kandala, Emina, Nzita, & Cappuccio, 2009) and are also commonly seen in the infants and young children brought to MCH services. Not all children are brought to MHCD clinics by their biological mothers because many are orphans and street children, who are also the priority for MHCD schooling. This is not surprising because there are more than 4 million orphans in DRC, a land where nearly half the school-age population receives no education (UNICEF, 2008). On an almost daily basis, women with their daughters seek assistance for injuries including rectovaginal and vesico-urethral-vaginal fistulae caused by sharp objects rammed into their vaginas during or following rape. Other injuries are caused by physical assault and include fractured limbs that have never been fixed. Severe back pain, headaches, deafness caused by beating, scarring caused by mutilation, and blindness from having their eyes gouged out by rebels or militia groups, intent on causing as much pain and long-lasting and visible reminders of their attack as possible, are common. Poverty, inadequate basic health services, and disruption of civil society are all exacerbated by a war that has created a humanitarian crisis that has no equal (Lewis, 2008). Emotional distress, fear (more akin to terror than fear), depression, and anxiety from being the victim or witness of war crimes is immeasurable and adds to the burden of injury and illness in the women and children attending MCH clinics facilitated by MHCD. Lewis (2008, 2009) describes DRC as the worst place in the world for women.

Government and systematic approaches to maternal and child health improvements have been impossible to sustain in this area of DRC due to huge numbers of refugees, high HIV prevalence, malaria and comorbidities, lack of basic healthcare facilities and medications, and the most destructive force of all, the continued violence perpetrated by armed militia and rebel groups. The MHCD: MCH programs seek to provide a service in these most disadvantaged areas of DRC where the war has had its most catastrophic effect on human security and sustainable development (Kandala et al., 2009).

CHAPTER 8 Rape as a Weapon of War

> **Project Goal (DRC):** Fight poverty using sustainable strategies, and in so doing improve the health of the women and children who have been traumatized by war in the North and South Kivu provinces of DRC
>
> **Project Objectives:** The MHCD goals and objectives mirror and are, in fact, a microcosm of the United Nations (UN) Millennium Development Goals (see Table 8-1; United Nations, 2000)

BACKGROUND

They are the nameless, faceless bandits, rebels, military; They abuse our bodies, take our souls, empty our guts, then throw us away. We are the trash they leave behind in their wars. We are the silent ones you see by the side of the road, the ones once called Mama, sister, wife, daughter. We are the ones discarded by husbands. We are used up, defiled by other men, dirty, unwanted, unseen, unheard, undone. We are the battleground, the ammunition in a war. (United Nations Integrated Regional Information Networks, 2004, p. 1)

Following the Rwandan genocide in April 1994, a million Hutus, including the Interahamwe soldiers (extremist youth wing of the Hutu militia and responsible for the majority of murders in the Rwandan genocide), escaped into what was then Zaire but is now known as DRC (Lewis, 2008; McGreal, 2008, May 15). War was officially declared against the Congolese people in 1996. However, militant Hutus are not the only Rwandan group to wage war on DRC civilians. In more recent years, Laurent Nkunda, a Tutsi warlord, and his soldiers, allegedly fearing that Hutu extremists might once again threaten Tutsis in Rwanda, waged war against the Interahamwe rebels and Congolese citizens in the North Kivu province of DRC. Reprisal attacks are common in the Kivu provinces, from multiple Congolese militia and rebel groups, including the infamous Mai Mai, and the Congolese Government Army is unable to significantly reduce the murders and torture against their citizens. Men from every known military group, and even some members of the UN peacekeeping forces, are implicated by women attending MCH clinics as perpetrators of sexual assault.

Table 8-1 MHCD: MCH objectives articulated with the UN Millennium Development Goals

The MHCD: MCH project objective is to provide women and their children with	UN Millennium Development Goal
Holistic support of those who have survived sexual assault in DRC. This includes financial and emotional support and essential primary health care.	Eradicate extreme poverty and hunger. Promote gender equality and empower women. Reduce child mortality. Improve maternal health. Combat HIV/AIDS, malaria, and other diseases.
Microfinancing of interest-free loans for small businesses for Congolese women (individual and community microfinancing projects)	Eradicate extreme poverty and hunger. Promote gender equality and empower women. Improve maternal health. Ensure environmental sustainability.
Mobile and outreach health clinics (medical and naturopathic) to fight chronic and infectious diseases, including HIV/AIDS	Reduce child mortality. Improve maternal health. Combat HIV/AIDS, malaria, and other diseases.
Antenatal, labor and birthing, postnatal and newborn, and MCH care through traditional midwives and community health workers who are equipped with birth kits and basic health and midwifery education	Promote gender equality and empower women. Reduce child mortality. Improve maternal health. Combat HIV/AIDS, malaria, and other diseases.
Education, medical care, and one meal per day for the street children, orphans, rescued child soldiers, and those displaced from their communities through war and ongoing violence	Achieve universal primary education. Promote gender equality and empower women. Reduce child mortality. Combat HIV/AIDS, malaria, and other diseases.
Mercy ministries that involve emergency support for sick and malnourished women and their children, orphans, street children, and rescued child soldiers	Eradicate extreme poverty and hunger. Reduce child mortality. Improve maternal health. Combat HIV/AIDS, malaria, and other diseases.
A strategy that enables women, at their request, to discuss their experiences with each other or a counselor in the knowledge that the counselor will share their stories with people and the media outside Africa to increase awareness of the horror that persists in DRC	Promote gender equality and empower women. Develop a global partnership for development.

Sources: Data from United Nations (2012). United Nations Millennium Development Goals. http://www.un.org/millenniumgoals/. Accessed July 24, 2012; and Mulimbalimba Masururu, Medical Director of Mission in Health Care and Development. Personal communication, 25th July, 2012.

CHAPTER 8 Rape as a Weapon of War

More people have died in the DRC war than in any war since World War II, and sadly the final number of fatalities in DRC is yet to be tallied. In the 10 year period from 1998 to 2008, it was conservatively estimated by the UN, World Health Organization (WHO), and Human Rights Watch (HRW) that at least 5.4 million Congolese men, women, and children were killed as a direct or indirect result of the war (Luu, 2008). The war may have been declared officially over in 2003, but carnage continues and the negative peace that persists is becoming increasingly more deadly. In 2005, in the North and South Kivu provinces, it was estimated that 30,000 people a month were murdered, and in 2008 the number of murders had increased to 45,000 people a month, half of them small children (McGreal, 2008, January 22). The UN and HRW estimated that between January and September 2008, a further 1.3 million people were displaced from their homes in the North Kivu province, and more than 50% of those were secondary displacements. As stated, sexual violence continues to escalate, and there has been renewed and increasing recruitment of child soldiers since 2008 (Luu, 2008; McGreal, 2008, January 22). Another ceasefire was called in November 2008, but it too was broken (Amnesty International, 2008).

Vinck, Pham, Baldo, and Shigekane (2008) attended a population-based survey of 2,620 adults, selected through systematic random sampling in the North and South Kivu provinces of DRC. It paints a detailed picture of how this forgotten war (forgotten by everyone but the Congolese people themselves), has impacted the lives of so many. Congolese adults who participated in the study were adversely affected by lack of income, homelessness, and experiences of abduction, rape, rejection, fear, and having loved ones disappear or be killed. Surprisingly, their sense of optimism remains strong with almost all participants (90%) believing that peace can be achieved in DRC. The Vinck et al. (2008) study found that 93% of participants earned less than US$2 a day, and more than 20% had no income at all. Only 4% of participants believed the UN peacekeeping force (MONUC) provided them with any protection. A large majority (85%) of participants had been displaced from their homes due to conflict, and on average, most had been made homeless more than three times. More than 33% of participants had been abducted for at least a week, and well over 50% had been interrogated or persecuted by armed guards. Nearly 66% of participants had one or more household members who had disappeared permanently. More than 66% had a family member or close friend who had met a violent death, and almost 50% had been threatened with death themselves. Sexual assault reports are known to be extremely conservative due to intense stigma and fear of rejection, but approximately 66% of all women have been sexually assaulted, with 20% of participants reporting multiple rapes and nearly 33% having witnessed sexual assault. Women fear rejection by their partners, families, and communities if they admit to having been sexually assaulted. This fear is validated when 33% of participants admitted they would not accept a victim of rape back into their family or community, especially if she had conceived through rape, but 66% said they were willing to forgive war criminals and perpetrators and reintegrate them back into their communities. A perpetrator is more than twice as likely to be welcomed back into the community than a woman who had conceived through rape!

Given the impact of war, it is not surprising that few nations in the world, if any, have worse maternal and child health outcomes than DRC. It is 1 of only 10 nations in the world where more than 20% of children die before the age of 5 years (United Nations Children's Fund, 2009). Furthermore, there has been no improvement and some worsening in life expectancy and maternal and child mortality rates between 1994 and 2004 (United Nations Children's Fund, 2009; Vinck et al., 2008). Sexual violence in DRC ranks at the top in the world and is increasing (Human Rights Watch, 2008). Many women attending MHCD maternal and child health clinics have outlined their understanding of why the rebels and militia groups continue to rape and torture women and girls. They argue it is a deliberate strategy to transmit HIV to DRC; to infect communities with sexually transmissible infections, such as syphilis and gonorrhea; to dehumanize the women and girls and the men who love them; to murder and kill; to destroy the Congolese identity through the conception of foreigner-fathered babies; to destroy marriages and families; to save bullets; to take advantage of the fact that the law and justice were destroyed during the war in DRC; and to commit genocide and make the most of the blackout that blankets DRC.

THE STORY

What the rebels do to the women is another form of genocide—to destroy women, to destroy mamas, is to destroy the whole nation! (Dietsch & Mulimbalimba-Masururu, 2006, p. 468)

This story is not about health professionals or systems. It is not about an African NGO, MHCD, nor its Australian connections. It is not a war story. This story is not even just a maternal and child healthcare case study! This story belongs to the women and girls of the North and South Kivu provinces of DRC; women

CHAPTER 8 Rape as a Weapon of War

and girls who attend MCH clinics and have survived innumerable attempts to destroy them. They have been mutilated, watched their children and partners be killed, and have seen guns inserted into their little girls' vaginas and shot. They have been slashed with knives and forced to eat and drink their own urine and feces and those of their rapists. These women are so strong and courageous that they can survive unspeakable horror and continue to not only live, but love, dance, sing, and even laugh. The lives of the mamas and children who access MHCD maternal and child health services are not cheap! They are priceless, absolutely invaluable, and all the more precious because of the fragility and unpredictability of the very air they breathe.

The statistics previously cited from the Vinck et al. (2008) study demonstrate the severity of the war, but it is not until you sit down and listen to the women themselves, watch their body language, and look into their haunted eyes that you realize the hellish impact war continues to have on maternal and child health. We have the privilege of working with and regularly listening to the women who have suffered in the North and South Kivu provinces of DRC. The women who attend mobile, outreach, and fixed MHCD facilities have pleaded with us to share their stories with the world. We do this now in honor of these strong, courageous women and out of respect for them and at their request. In doing so we hope to demonstrate that these war statistics, often referred to as collateral damage, have human beings behind them, often mothers and children. All names and identifying information have been changed to protect each woman's confidentiality. The stories were told to us, the authors, between December 2004 and June 2008; where appropriate, the women's translated words are used verbatim. Only a small number of the hundreds of stories that could be told in this case study are shared here.

Silaha attended an antenatal clinic near Goma. She was 35 years old and very tall, but she weighed only 45 kilograms. She was about 5 months pregnant and shared the following:

> The men found me in the house and they took me to the forest. There they beat me and raped me. I was raped by so many men, I have no idea of the number. They would not give me water to drink for many days. I was crying and so thirsty; they forced me to drink my own strong urine while they stood around me and laughed. I was in the forest for about two months, I was so worried for my children. One day some government soldiers came close by and I ran and ran until I caught up with them and they brought me home. I have had no medical attention since I was raped and I smell very bad. That is why I have come to see you today.

As part of Silaha's examination, a vaginal examination was attended, and when I removed my fingers there were feces on them, indicating she had a rectovaginal fistula. This is a very common injury for women following rape and torture in DRC. Silaha, a widow, is the mother of eight children, and she is now pregnant again after the rapes. She and her children are destitute, and repair surgery is not possible for this Goma woman. Such is the horror that is Goma, that many women who have been admitted to hospitals for injuries such as fistulae they suffered when they were raped, have died of starvation in the hospital. There is no one to bring them food. Silaha told me, "If people have mercy on me, they feed me and my children, otherwise we have nothing to eat."

Silaha's story has common threads with others that we have heard. Sometimes the husband's family keeps the children after a woman has been raped and refuses the mother any contact. Rape and torture of women and girls is a deliberate strategy used in DRC. One of the purposes is to conceive children fathered by foreigners, non-Congolese men. Mele, whose story follows, was 18 years old. Mele and her young husband were using condoms for contraception so they could delay having a family. Mele was raped and conceived a child who, at the time when she came to the MCH clinic, was about 4 months old. Mele said:

> Our family says, "take this child to her father!" They say very bad things. But this is impossible because I was raped by about 6–10 men. How do I know who is the father? My husband will accept me but not the child. He says, "take this child out of my house!"

On a barren hill on the outskirts of a town, on the shores of Lake Tanganyika, a thousand or more displaced women and children have made their makeshift homes, and MHCD provides an outreach MCH service on the hill. There are no roads, only rocky tracks. We walked up the hill to visit Mwabijangala and her baby. Her home is closest to the top of the hill and would be the first one accessed by rebels or soldiers if they come over the hill. Mwabijangala, like so many other women, has no door on her home. Her story was unusual because Mwabijangala shared how both her and her husband had been raped. The fact that her husband was raped does not make her experience unique; rather, her willingness to disclose what happened sets it apart.

Homosexuality is not tolerated as a lifestyle choice in DRC, and given that almost all perpetrators are male, an extra level of stigma is added when a man is raped. Linos (2009) argues that this inevitably leads to underreporting and reduced health service seeking behavior. Affleck (2009) also reports that in this

CHAPTER 8   Rape as a Weapon of War

area, both genders are raped by Democratic Forces for the Liberation of Rwanda (FDLR) militia members, but females continue to outnumber males. Mwabijangala shared how her husband, as a sexual assault survivor, suffers even greater shame and stigma than she does. Their two sons, aged 10 and 14 years, were placed in care with the family of the MHCD director to protect them from violence and malnutrition, which had already killed three of Mwabijangala's children. At the time of our visit, Mwabijangala's husband had gone back to their village to search for food. His need to feed his family overcame his fear of violence, and Mwabijangala reports that he said, "If they kill me, they kill me, but I have to feed my family, otherwise I am dead already."

Mwabijangala mentioned the doctor's family where her two sons were living. This family home served as an MHCD orphanage, medical center, naturopathy clinic, antenatal clinic, maternal and child health clinic, and sexual assault counseling service until 2008, when the health facilities moved; now the home serves mainly as an orphanage and family home in Bukavu.

Around one cluster of villages outside Bukavu, the Interahamwe had set up mobile camps and had been hidden in the area for a number of years. Those villagers that could flee to the town to live had done so. Those who were left had come together to offer a small degree of protection and support for one another. The women in the village had been tested for HIV, and 70% were HIV positive. The only antiretrovirals available in this area are supplied by Médecins Sans Frontières (MSF), as prophylaxis, when a person is able to reach the MSF base (18 kilometers away from these villages) within 72 hours of the assault and they are screened as HIV negative. On the day we visited this cluster of villages, there were approximately 400 women, 6 men, and innumerable children. The antenatal and MCH clinics were attended. Pauline was one of the many women attending the clinic, who asked to share her experience:

> I have been pregnant eight times. I have had seven children but three of them have died. Two died because I could not get enough food for them to eat and one of my children was killed. I was pregnant last year when three rebels came into my home. They took our chair outside. They pushed me down on the ground and one man started to rape me while the other men were laughing and cheering. I think they were high on drugs . . . I cried and I screamed until my husband who was working in a nearby field heard me. He came running in and tried to pull the rebel off me but another rebel pushed him back and shot him dead. The rapist still did not stop even though my husband's body was lying there beside me. I tried but I could not stop screaming . . . Another rebel started to rape me. I think it was the one who shot my

husband. My neighbor's husband came and tried to stop them but the rebels shot him too . . . That evening I was raped by three rebels while my little children stood watching and sobbing. The rebels told me I had to shut them up or we would all be killed. I honestly don't know what happened next because I think I lost consciousness when they beat me. When I woke up, it was dawn. The rebels had gone but the bodies of my husband and neighbor were still lying there. My children were sleeping. I tried to drag out my husband's body before the children woke up but I couldn't do it. I tried to drag out my neighbor's body but he was too heavy. I went to our village leader and asked for help to please bury the bodies. He refused to allow anyone to help me because she said it was my fault that two men had been killed. He said that if I hadn't screamed when I was being raped that these two men would still be alive . . . I took my children to the forest and we lived there for nearly a month before my neighbors came and found me. My neighbors, some of the women you saw here today, helped me to move my husband and his friend's body and bury them.

The small selection of stories shared demonstrate the hell and horror for so many women and children attending MHCD: MCH programs in the Kivu provinces of DRC. Their terror is incomprehensible, but so is their hope! How can women like Pauline not only survive but laugh and love and have hope for her own children's future, and that of their children?

Pauline was one of a group of women who had received a community microfinancing loan from MHCD. The women had planted amaranth, a crop with multiple uses that is also an excellent source of iron. The crop is distributed to all women of childbearing age and their children in the village. The remainder is taken into town and sold, and the women share the profits. There is another advantage. The women who grow the amaranth previously had no choice but to carry loads of wood, up to 50 kilograms, to town every day. They would walk more than 18 kilometers to town with these huge loads, then back 18 kilometers to the village, and they would be paid between 5 cents and 30 cents per load. Pregnant and nonpregnant women between the ages of 12 and 70 years completed this task every day and were treated as beasts of burden by the landowners. Now the women who grow the amaranth have to travel to town only infrequently to sell their crop. The amaranth is much lighter than wood and is far more valuable; and importantly, all of the money earned is shared among the women in this particular community development project and does not go to some exploitative landowner. After harvest, the inedible roots are used as fish food.

In turn, the women who have a microfinancing loan for the fish farms give the women with the amaranth free fish. There are currently five fish ponds dug out and filled with fingerling fish that grow and are caught to meet the protein needs of the women and their children. Any surplus fish are dried, smoked, and sold at the markets in town. The secondary advantage of fish farms is that the fish eat the mosquito larvae, thereby reducing the risk of malaria for the nearby villagers.

Other microfinanced community development projects around this area include rabbit and guinea pig farms. The animals breed quickly and can be used as a source of protein. Pigs, which are good breeders and have six to eight piglets per litter, are also a great source of protein and fertilizer for the women with the amaranth.

About 150 kilometers away from the area with the fish ponds and amaranth is another village on the edge of a swamp. This village is accessible only by small boat. Most of the men in this South Kivu village were either murdered or fled when rebels from Burundi attacked and then occupied the village for a number of years until late 2007 or early 2008. Twenty women, who have infants and small children and who conceived when they were raped by the occupying rebels, received a microfinancing loan for a ground nut project. The loan for US$120 provided the women with hoes, ground nut seeds, and basic food, so the hungry women would not be tempted to eat the seeds. The first crop had just been harvested, and from the proceeds these women paid back the interest-free loan; gave a US$50 gift and 5 kilograms of ground nuts to MHCD to help feed other vulnerable women and children; bought seeds for the next season's crop; stored ground nuts for all the families in the project to meet their future protein needs until the next harvest; sold the remaining ground nuts to a neighboring village co-op (another microfinanced community project); and shared the remaining US$680 profit among the 20 women involved in the project.

DRC has been and continues to be a literal hell for millions of men, women, and children. The women in the MCH clinics believed that no one outside DRC knew what was happening to them, and that is why they pleaded with us to share their stories. However, the women's own courage, strength, and resilience, coupled with the MHCD maternal and child health strategies outlined in this case study, are giving them hope—hope that the future for them and their children will be peaceful, safe, healthy, and with a standard of living that enables them to meet their daily needs.

LESSONS LEARNED

It is not possible to provide statistical evidence of improved health outcomes for women and children as a result of the strategies outlined in this case study. DRC is a nation where births and deaths often go unrecorded. Few people know their date of birth or even their age. Verifiable statistics relating to health outcomes and improvements in health outcomes since the projects commenced are not available, nor are they likely to become available in the near future. It would be difficult, if not immoral, to justify the time, energy, and financial costs that would be devoted to verifiable research at the expense of fighting poverty and providing life-saving primary health care.

On a number of occasions, MHCD has tried to transport goods, such as birth kits supplied by AusAID, donated blankets, clothes, exercise books, pencils, crayons, medications, medical supplies, etc., across Rwandan borders to DRC. Each time, border officials from Rwanda have demanded money (US$1,200–$2,500) to allow the donated goods to cross their border and transit Rwanda to DRC. This is not sustainable, and new strategies must be developed to enable the most vulnerable of the world's citizens—women and children in DRC—to receive the gifts that have been given to them without unfair interference.

It would be wonderful to report that all microfinanced projects have been successful. This would not be accurate. One village received seven pigs to breed and use to meet their protein needs. Sadly, the villagers (and MHCD volunteers) did not realize the need for the pigs to be vaccinated, and six of the pigs died. This was a difficult but invaluable lesson, and it will not be repeated.

The power of partnerships built on reciprocal trust, respect, and cultural humility can never be underestimated. Partnerships among women themselves in community microfinancing projects; partnerships between women and the MHCD volunteers; partnerships between MHCD and its international supporters; and partnerships among the MHCD volunteers themselves optimize health outcomes for mothers and children and the sense of reward and satisfaction for the volunteers. More than anything else, we've come to appreciate the strength, courage, and resilience of women and children in the Kivu provinces of DRC.

ABOUT THE AUTHORS

MHCD commenced in 2004 when two Congolese brothers, Dr. Freddy Nguliro and Dr. Luc Mulimbalimba-Masururu, both medical practitioners and naturopaths from the South Kivu province, identified the link between poor maternal and child health outcomes and war-induced poverty. They identified the need for sustainable community development and individual projects that would enable women to break out of the poverty that trapped them and their children in a cycle of ill health, which killed one in five of their children before they reached age 5 years (United Nations Children's Fund, 2009). Elaine Dietsch and Luc met at the end of 2004 when Elaine, a midwifery academic from Charles Sturt University (CSU), Wagga Wagga campus in Australia, attended midwifery faculty practice in Africa. Luc shared the MHCD vision and objectives with Elaine and invited her and her husband, John, to work in partnership with MHCD to improve maternal and child health outcomes. Elaine and John have worked with MHCD on a 4–6 week voluntary basis each year since 2004. Luc, Freddy, MHCD community health workers, traditional midwives, and teachers work tirelessly in DRC in an endeavor to meet the MHCD Maternal and Child Health goals previously cited. The School of Nursing and Midwifery at CSU is committed to social justice and promoting primary health care. As an extension of that philosophical framework, they provide in-principle support of MHCD and the work that Elaine does in Africa.

Discussion Questions

1. What does "rape as a weapon of war" mean?
2. What are the social, cultural, and health impacts of the mass rape of women in DRC?
3. Discuss the role of patriarchy in the vulnerability of women to sexual violence and its consequences in DRC?
4. What are some of the direct and indirect impacts of the microfinanced projects? What are the particular strengths of the models described?
5. In the "Lessons Learned" section, the authors suggest that it would be immoral to conduct research at the expense of fighting poverty and providing life-saving care. Discuss the implications of this statement for research conducted in resource-poor environments.

ACKNOWLEDGMENTS

First and foremost, we acknowledge the incredible Congolese women who shared their experiences with us so that more people might know the reality that is maternal and child health in the Democratic Republic of Congo. We also acknowledge the support of Charles Sturt University, Centre for Inland Health and the School of Nursing, Midwifery, and Indigenous Health for their continued support.

REFERENCES

Affleck, B. (2009, February 23). Glimmer of hope in Africa. *Time*, 22–27.

Almedom, A., Tesfamichael, B., Yacob, A., Debretsion, Z., Teklehaimanot, K., Beyone, T., . . . Alemu, Z. (2003). Maternal psycho-social well-being in Eritrea: Application of participatory methods and tools of investigation and analysis in complex emergency settings. *Bulletin of the World Health Organization, 81*(5), 360–366.

Amnesty International. (2008). Renewed fighting in DRC breaks precarious ceasefire. Retrieved from http://www.amnesty.org.au/news/comments/19696/

Dietsch, E., & Mulimbalimba-Masururu, L. (2006). We ask the world please hear us . . . women from the Democratic Republic of Congo (DRC) share their stories of survival. *MIDIRS Midwifery Digest, 16*(4), 467–469.

Human Rights Watch. (2008). Submission to the Committee on the Rights of the Child For the Periodic Review of the Democratic Republic of Congo. Retrieved from http://www.hrw.org/sites/default/files/related_material/hrw.drc.crc.0808.pdf

Kandala, N., Emina, J., Nzita, P., & Cappuccio, F. (2009). Diarrhoea, acute respiratory infection, and fever among children in the Democratic Republic of Congo. *Social Science and Medicine*, xxx, 1–9. doi:10.1016/j.socscimed.2009.02..004

Lewis, S. (2008). Building global alliances in a world of health care inequities. *Policy, Politics and Nursing Practice, 9*(4), 307–312. doi: 10.1177/1527154408329312

Lewis, S. (2009, May). *Portraits of war: The Democratic Republic of Congo*. Remarks at the photo exhibit of AIDS-Free World, Washington, DC.

Linos, N. (2009). Rethinking gender-based violence during war: Is violence against civilian men a problem worth addressing? *Social Science and Medicine 68*(8), 1548–1551.

Luu, K. (2008). *Democratic Republic of Congo—complex emergency*. Washington, DC: Office of US Foreign Disaster Assistance. Retrieved from http://transition.usaid.gov/our_work/humanitarian_assistance/disaster_assistance/countries/drc/template/fs_sr/fy2008/drc_ce_sr02_10-15-2008.pdf

McGreal, C. (2008, January 22). War in Congo kills 45,000 people each month. *The Guardian*. Retrieved from http://www.guardian.co.uk/world/2008/jan/23/congo.international

McGreal, C. (2008, May 15). We have to kill Tutsis wherever they are. *The Guardian*. Retrieved from http://www.guardian.co.uk/world/2008/may/16/congo.rwanda

CHAPTER 8 Rape as a Weapon of War

UNAIDS. (2008). *Sub Saharan Africa AIDS epidemic update regional summary.* Retrieved from http://data.unaids.org/pub/Report/2008/jc1526_epibriefs_ssafrica_en.pdf

UNICEF. (2008). *The state of the world's children.* Retrieved from http://www.unicef.org/publications/files/The_State_of_the_Worlds_Children_2008.pdf.

United Nations. (2000). *United Nations millennium declaration.* Retrieved from http://www.un.org/millenniumgoals/

United Nations Children's Fund. (2009). *State of the world's children.* New York, NY: UNICEF.

United Nations High Commissioner for Refugees. (1999). *Reproductive health in refugee situations: An international field manual.* Geneva, Switzerland: Author.

United Nations Integrated Regional Informational Networks. (2004). *Our bodies . . . their battleground: Gender-based violence during conflict.* Retrieved from http://www.plusnews.org/Report.aspx?ReportId=60995

Vinck, P., Pham, P., Baldo, S., & Shigekane, R. (2008). *Living with fear: A population based survey on attitudes about peace, justice and social reconstruction in Eastern Democratic Republic of Congo.* New York, NY: International Center for Transitional Justice.

PART IV

Support Groups

Support groups are a model of intervention used throughout the world to address different issues that impact human beings. From substance abuse to cancer, from pregnancy to divorce, people get together in groups to provide emotional support to each other around a common issue or problem. Sometimes these groups are run independently of professionals such as Alcoholics Anonymous, while other times a professional facilitates the meeting and provides additional links to resources that may be of benefit to participants.

The case presented here is about a group of women who have many challenges that put their pregnancies at high-risk. Through sharing and professional support, the impacts of their difficulties are reduced not only through the psychological support gained from the process but also by gleaning information that becomes useful to them in their daily lives.

CHAPTER 9

Enhancing Outcomes for At-Risk Moms: The Moms Mentoring Moms Program

Blythe Shepard, PhD
Meg Kapil, MA, CCC
Lara Shepard, BA

Location: Victoria, British Columbia, Canada

Name of Project: Moms Mentoring Moms

Sponsoring Organizations: Fetal Alcohol Spectrum Disorder Community Circle and Prostitutes Empowerment Education and Recovery Society (PEERS)

Target Population: Women with substance abuse problems who may have given birth or are at risk of giving birth to a child with fetal alcohol spectrum disorder

Project Objectives: (1) Healthcare education; (2) Reduction of alcohol intake during pregnancy; (3) Empowerment of families; (4) Reduced involvement with the foster care system; (5) Creation of positive community relationships; and (6) Building of mentoring capacity

CHAPTER 9 Enhancing Outcomes for At-Risk Moms

INTRODUCTION

Stigma is a heavy burden for substance-using women (Howell, Herser, & Harrington, 1999) and in particular for pregnant women and mothers (Poole, 2003b; Rutman, Callahan, Lundquist, Jackson, & Field, 2000; Tait, 2000). Stigma hinders a mother's access to services due to feelings of shame, fear of losing custody of her children if she requests help, and anticipation of being treated poorly and judged because she has a substance use problem (Poole & Isaac, 2001). Certain policies cause additional barriers to accessing care for women of childbearing years, including the refusal of many transition houses to accept women with substance use concerns because abstinence is often a requirement for admission to treatment (Poole, 2003b). Inadequate protocols for supporting pregnant women through withdrawal management in detoxification services (Poole, 2003b) and lack of immediate support and therapeutic interventions have also been cited (Leslie & DeMarchi, 2004). Poole warns against an overly narrow and simplistic prevention focus that may imply that women are ignorant of risks when, in fact, they are unable to stop using alcohol during pregnancy. Health, social, and economic concerns also play a role in women's alcohol use, as identified in the report released by the United Nations Office on Drugs and Crime (2004), which noted that women who use alcohol

> hav[e] fewer resources (education, employment, income) than men, are more likely to be living with a partner with a substance use problem, have care of dependent children and have more severe problems at the beginning of treatment . . . [They] also have higher rates than men of trauma related to physical and sexual abuse and concurrent psychiatric disorders, particularly post-traumatic stress disorder and anxiety disorders. (p. 1)

Therefore, a comprehensive approach is needed to address the issues faced by pregnant women and mothers who have given birth to prenatally exposed children.

In Canada, a number of programs are now providing holistic, community-wide interventions to mothers at risk. The Moms Mentoring Moms program in Victoria, British Columbia, is targeted to moms who are pregnant and those who have already given birth to children with fetal alcohol spectrum disorder (FASD). The goal of the program is to provide support for high-risk women in whom addiction has been identified as a barrier in their ability to parent. The overall intent of the program is to connect with moms to provide support whether or not their children are in foster care; to develop appropriate parenting strategies; and to determine the women's needs and to help them make informed, healthy life choices. In accordance with the Centre of Excellence for Women's Health recommendations (Johnson, Greaves, & Repta, 2007), the program addresses broad health determinants using a multipronged, holistic approach.

In this chapter, a women-centered program built on a mentorship model is described. The program focuses on mothers or mothers-to-be who have substance use problems. An overview of FASD and its effects is presented, followed by a detailed description of the Moms Mentoring Moms program and its participants. Outcomes of the program are evaluated with regard to their impact on participants and in meeting program objectives. The chapter concludes with a discussion of lessons learned for future programming.

FETAL ALCOHOL SPECTRUM DISORDER

Fetal alcohol spectrum disorder (FASD) is a nondiagnostic term that depicts various physical and developmental problems associated with prenatal alcohol exposure. A continuum of birth defects and developmental disabilities are associated with the consumption of alcohol during pregnancy. For a diagnosis of full fetal alcohol syndrome (FAS), three criteria are used (Chudley et al., 2005): (1) a pattern of facial abnormalities, (2) growth deficiencies, and (3) central nervous system impairment. Related conditions include partial FAS (pFAS), alcohol-related birth defects (ARBD), and alcohol-related neurodevelopmental disorder (ARND). With FASD it is paramount to focus on prevention because the effects of FASD are irreversible and permanent, and they represent the most common form of brain damage to infants in the Western world (Poole, 2003a).

Alcohol use and other drug use during pregnancy varies considerably, but the incidence has been reported as high as 46% in Vancouver's Downtown Eastside (Poole, 2003b). According to Health Canada (2004), FASD has a prevalence rate of approximately 9 out of every 1,000 babies born in Canada, and the 2002–2003 annual report from the Ministry of Children and Family Development (MCFD, 2003) regarding early childhood development activities estimates a prevalence rate of 3.5 per 1,000. Accurate estimates of FASD and related concerns are a challenge due to the paucity of accessible and evidence-based diagnostic measures. Informal labeling without confirmation of maternal alcohol use or professional assessment has been common and can be a barrier to accessing services for those affected by FASD (Greaves, Cormier, & Poole, 2002).

Prenatal alcohol exposure has been linked to more than 60 disease conditions, birth defects, and disabilities (World Health Organization, 2004). The damage encompasses a diverse continuum, from mild intellectual and behavioral issues to profound disabilities or premature death. Prenatal alcohol damage varies due to volume ingested, timing during pregnancy, peak blood alcohol levels, genetics, and environmental factors (Chudley et al., 2005). As children become adults, FASD does not disappear, but rather the issues translate into ongoing problems in family relationships, employment, mental health, and justice conflicts. The cost to the individuals affected, their families, and society are enormous.

Poole (2003b) recommends an FASD prevention strategy that focuses on improving women's health, in general, and addressing the multiple determinants of FASD and addiction in a manner that is coordinated and compassionate. This multifaceted prevention strategy also includes public awareness, health promotion, and community development on one level; a coordinated infrastructure of services that is directed to all women of childbearing age at another level; and the coordination of a comprehensive range of health and social supports to encompass pregnant women, mothers, and their children at yet another level. In their 10-year plan for addressing FASD in British Columbia, the MCFD also highlights the importance of working together to support women to have healthy pregnancies and to improve the lives of those living with FASD (Ministry of Children and Family Development [MCFD], 2008). The Moms Mentoring Moms program aimed to address all levels as identified by Poole (2003b).

THE MOMS MENTORING MOMS PROGRAM

The Moms Mentoring Moms program was funded collaboratively by FASD Community Circle and Prostitutes Empowerment Education and Recovery Society (PEERS). FASD Community Circle is dedicated to the prevention of birth defects caused by alcohol during pregnancy and the provision of quality education, support, and services for affected individuals and families. PEERS provides support and resources for past and current sex trade workers.

The overarching goal of the mentoring program was to develop a model of support for high-risk women that would encourage participants to have healthy pregnancies and to prevent or minimize the impact of FASD. Funding to evaluate the effectiveness of the program was provided by Victoria Foundation.

Facilitators, Mentors, and Assistants

The two facilitators, through their involvement with PEERS, had extensive experience in working with women who have addiction issues. As highly respected workers they formed strong relationships with the participants, who tended to be very isolated, difficult to reach, and understandably apprehensive about accessing community support. The program leader, a birth mother to a child with FASD, has been in addiction recovery for the past 15 years. She was assisted by an art therapist with more than 10 years of experience. The primary activities of the facilitators included organizing weekly group meetings and guest speakers, providing lunch for the group meetings, advocating for and supporting group members, fostering community connections and referrals, and offering individual counseling.

Two mentors from PEERS performed outreach activities and provided members with support while attending weekly group meetings. The majority of time spent by the mentors involved working with the women in the following areas: (1) support, (2) tangible needs, (3) advocacy, and (4) information. Their personal experience with substance use enhanced their credibility with participants and increased the likelihood of being viewed as role models for the women who were at different stages of recovery.

Additional assistance was provided by a nursing practicum student to establish a bridge between participants and hospital outpatient clinics. By meeting individually with participants, the student determined which women would benefit from additional support during pregnancy. The relevant information about fostering healthy pregnancies was based on their specific needs.

A fourth-year medical student provided health information, including navigation of the healthcare system. In addition, she accompanied participants to meetings with social workers, lawyers, physicians, and others. The wide range of topics addressed during the one-on-one meetings with participants included appropriate use of antidepressants; joint pain; access to medication; nicotine replacement therapy; asthma pathophysiology and treatment; methadone withdrawal; fibromyalgia; healthy weight loss; neonatal abstinence syndrome and the perinatal effects of in utero drug exposure; adult FASD; hypothyroidism; migraines; coagulopathies; neurodevelopment; pediatric developmental milestones; and colic.

Participants

The participants were recruited through a number of agencies. The program's contact information was posted on bulletin boards, and fliers were distributed at local agencies. Twenty-six intakes were completed, with continuing inquiries made throughout the evaluation year. The participants ranged in age from 16 to 50 years, with 75% between the ages of 21 and 37 years. In terms of ethnicity,

CHAPTER 9   Enhancing Outcomes for At-Risk Moms

the majority self-identified as white, and 15% self-identified as aboriginal. Of the women who attended the Moms Mentoring Moms group, more than half had been in foster care as children, two were adopted, and only two were still in touch with their birth families. Most women had two or three children (aged newborn to adult), with 50 children in total born to the participants. The living situations of the children varied. Of the 50 children, 10 lived with their grandparents, 10 were adopted, 12 were either apprehended or in care, and 18 lived at least part time with their mothers. At the time of intake, four women were pregnant, and they were immediately connected with either a midwife or with some form of prenatal care. The number of children with FASD was difficult to assess because most children had not been evaluated.

The majority of participants (46%) received income assistance. Of the remaining participants, 30% received disability assistance, 8% identified a need for support to apply for income assistance, and 8% identified a need for support to apply for disability. Only 8% of the participants indicated that they were financially stable. In regards to housing, only one participant indicated that her housing situation was acceptable. The remaining participants either needed stable housing or larger accommodations. In Victoria, finding affordable housing was challenging and presented a large barrier for most participants. The Canada Mortgage and Housing Corporation speculated that at the time of this evaluation, the vacancy rate for Victoria was at 0.8%, with an average rental cost of US$579 for a bachelor unit, US$709 for a one-bedroom unit, US$892 for a two-bedroom unit, and US$1,115 for a three-bedroom unit. Social assistance provided about US$520 per month for housing. The participants' capacity to retain affordable housing was challenging due to cuts to child care subsidies, women's centers, advocacy groups, employment training, and shelters and day centers for women leaving abusive relationships (Canada Mortgage and Housing Corporation, 2007).

On intake, participants indicated a need for assistance in the following areas: recovery from drug and/or alcohol use, parenting and child support, housing, financial assistance, negotiating the return of an apprehended child, nutrition, counseling, employment, medical issues, advocacy with government agencies, support with MCFD interactions, and assistance with the disability application. According to the staff, the women most in need of support were those who were homeless; individuals new to recovery; women who had their children apprehended; individuals who were affected by FASD; and those at risk for self-harm. Long wait lists and the necessity of leaving Vancouver Island for treatment were additional barriers. Language and technology *literacy* were also barriers to *accessing government services*.

Of the 26 participants, about 10 members attended the weekly group meeting, with different members attending each week. Two to three days per week were needed to address ongoing crises such as court attendance, dispute resolution, school issues, and child apprehension.

Sources of Data

A range of data collection approaches was taken, including qualitative semi-structured interviews at trimonthly intervals with facilitators, mentors, and assistants, as well as interviews with community partners. Participant feedback was obtained through case notes, group feedback, art assessments, and pre- and post-questionnaires.

OVERALL EFFECT OF PROGRAM ON PARTICIPANTS

I think of what we do as a patch work quilt, if you make one, some [of] the squares get a bit of tension but if you look at the next square it is fitting nicely so it ebbs and flows but it all works together that whole connectivity is what is really a key piece to it, we are a team.

—Art therapist

Through their involvement in the program, participants reported a variety of positive changes in their lives. Some noted that attending group meetings and coming out of isolation were important components in staying clean and sober. "I named my baby Miracle. The group helped me stay clean and sober throughout my pregnancy." Others credited the program with greatly improving relationships with their children and, for some, reuniting with them. "My son is coming home at long last." Participants attributed their involvement in the program with their increased ability to connect with community resources and to develop a support and advocacy network for themselves and their children. "This program has given me the ongoing support and courage to carry out a successful life today . . . I am a better and stronger advocate for myself." Some spoke of their sense of resiliency. "I am much more vocal about me and my family's needs and not willing to be bullied into accepting 'bad' situations . . . I am more resilient and have a very positive perspective." One outcome described by a number of participants was the ability to articulate ideas and to take responsibility for their lives. A spin-off was an increased sense of hope and optimism. "I had a positive experience at the hospital. Unlike my previous deliveries where the hospital staff treated me like the scrap off the bottom of their shoe because I'm a drug addict, this time they treated me with respect." All participants mentioned an increase in health knowledge. "I now know so much more about FASD and prenatal exposure to alcohol. I've learned how to have a better diet even though I don't have lots of money to buy food. I am definitely healthier. Most of all, I am much more aware of how substance misuse and how I live can impact my baby."

In response to the question "Has this group been helpful or useful to you?" all participants rated the Moms Mentoring Moms program as a 10 (with 1 being the least helpful and 10 the most helpful). When asked what changes they would like to see, participants indicated a need for more mentors, an additional group meeting during the week, and continuation of the group beyond the year.

Their confidence in their ability to parent rose from 5.6 at the beginning of the program to 8 at the end of the year (on a Likert scale with 1 = not confident, 10 = very confident). Similarly, their confidence in dealing with agencies increased from 4.8 to 8.9 on the same scale. Their comfort levels in seeking out support from community agencies also increased from 6.1 to 8.8. The overall effectiveness of the Moms Mentoring Moms program was rated at 9.8, indicating a very high level of satisfaction from the participants of the group.

Art activities were reported to be valuable for group members as a way to explore their life experiences and their sense of hope. In particular, participants found that art allowed them to discover new things about themselves (e.g., their inner creativity), to be able to express and release feelings, and to share a process with other people. Engaging in art activities helped them to relax and to connect with childhood issues. Upon reflection, one participant noticed a gradual progression in the projects she worked on in terms of depth of expression. Additionally, participants indicated that art definitely helped them to reflect some of the recent positive changes in their life.

MEETING PROGRAM OBJECTIVES

Six specific program objectives were identified: (1) educate participants about the healthcare system and their health, (2) support women to reduce their intake during pregnancy, (3) empower families by teaching them parenting strategies and life skills, (4) reduce unnecessary involvement with the foster care system, (5) build positive working relationships within the community, and (6) build the capacity of women to mentor other women.

Educate Participants about the Healthcare System and Their Health

Participants completed a questionnaire about their experiences with the healthcare system and information about their bodies and their health. Participants, for example, were asked to identify the most important qualities of a doctor. Honesty was indicated to be the most important attribute, followed by being nonjudgmental. Other qualities identified included being compassionate, having intelligence, being empathic, having specific knowledge, being friendly and showing respect, having a sense of humor, being professional, and demonstrating integrity.

When reviewing the pre- and post-questionnaires it was evident that the women had gained a better understanding of physicians' roles and developed a greater sense of empowerment within the physician–patient relationship. For example, the participants' agreement with the statement "Doctors have their patients' best interests at heart" improved from the intake to the exit questionnaire, as did their agreement with the statement "Doctors are trustworthy." There was improvement between the pre- and post-questionnaires in the level of agreement with the statement "I leave my doctors' appointments with a better understanding of my own health," perhaps suggesting that the women were feeling more empowered to advocate for themselves in the clinical setting and to effectively request explanations related to their health concerns.

Interestingly, the participants' agreement with the statements "I feel healthy" and "I know my body best" both decreased between the intake and exit surveys. This trend perhaps reflected the reality of health-related events that transpired between the two questionnaires, or it could imply that these women need more tools to improve their own health. It could also suggest that the participants were becoming more informed, and this greater awareness indicated recognition of the complexities of their own health (e.g., awareness of the true health implications of smoking, or awareness of the dangers of obesity). One statement with which all respondents remained emphatically in agreement was "I would like to understand my health better," indicating an ongoing need for health education and advocacy.

There were anecdotal indications that participants were able to more effectively navigate the healthcare system and to advocate for themselves. For example, one mother who had suffered long-term chronic pain due to lack of funding for medication was supported to communicate with a pharmaceutical company and to advocate for medication. She now works with this company to advocate for more funding for others who suffer from chronic pain.

Support Women to Reduce Intake During Pregnancy

Facilitators and mentors provided information and support in a nonjudgmental manner regarding substance use during pregnancy. The facilitators and mentors reported that for several women, substance use either reduced or stopped. As a FASD key worker whose role it was to provide information, advocacy, and support to families with children and youth (aged 0–18 years) where FASD is suspected or where there is a confirmed diagnosis, the program leader also provided assistance throughout an FASD assessment. This holistic approach helped to improve the outcomes for the children and met goals outlined in the provincial plan for British Columbia from 2008–2018 (MCFD, 2008), which suggest that prevention of FASD requires a comprehensive approach that includes "specialized holistic support of pregnant women with alcohol problems" (p. 3) and recommends "postpartum support for birth mothers directed at improving their health and social networks, as well as the health of their present and future children" (p. 3).

By liaising with hospitals, nurses were able to connect with the mothers during labor and delivery as well as during the postpartum period. Nurses reported shifting their perception of participants as "bad mothers" to people who needed help. These informal alliances had a direct positive impact on the women. Improved hospital care and better understanding from the nurses increased the likelihood of more receptive and helpful engagement with each person. Although there were direct benefits from these informal alliances, no new formal support or systemic changes occurred during the evaluation. High-risk women continue to stay under the radar as they worry about their baby being apprehended. Preventive versus punitive thinking toward these women would go a long way to help reduce prevalence rates, with the snowball effect resulting in children who have parents who are better supported.

Empower Families

A number of guest speakers attended the weekly group meetings to educate participants on a variety of topics in addition to the parenting strategies and life skills taught by facilitators. Mentors provided assistance with nutrition information, grocery shopping, finding bargains, coping with daily stressors, helping people move, becoming familiar with the community, organizing the house, or planning the day. Information about schools and child care and how to clearly define goals as concrete, realistic, and manageable steps was also provided. Participants connected with services in the community and learned how to advocate for the return of their children, and they learned to navigate important processes such as income assistance and housing.

Reduce Unnecessary Involvement with the Foster Care System

The facilitators advocated for the women by communicating with social workers, attending meetings with MCFD regarding the apprehension of children, and empowering the women through support and education to better care for their children. Workshops conducted by social workers educated group participants on how to communicate and build positive relationships with government workers. Interviews with MCFD indicated an increase in the number of referrals from social workers to the Moms Mentoring Moms group. In their roles as advocates, the facilitators and the mentors were able to communicate recovery successes and positive wellness steps made by group participants to relevant community workers and agencies. In this way, the women were more likely to be recognized for any positive steps they had made toward a healthy pregnancy or toward reduced involvement with substances. Modeling healthy relationships and communication with different systems was integral to the success of this program as the women learned to navigate various systems effectively.

Five mothers gave birth during the program. One mother's baby was apprehended, one mother and her baby entered a collaborative care project, and three mothers went home with their babies and have had success as parents. In addition, four children were returned from the British Columbia Ministry of Child and Family Development (MCFD) care due, in part, to the support they received from the program that bridged the gap between the women and the social workers. One mother was supported in putting her child, who had significant behavioral challenges, into voluntary care in order to protect another child in the home. For some participants, their children would not be returned from care; however, the group encouraged them to stay connected to their child in a productive manner.

Build Positive Working Relationships within the Community

Involvement with the Moms Mentoring Moms group was viewed by MCFD as a strong asset in working toward effective parenting. Facilitators helped group members to communicate wellness steps taken as a result of attending the group and to advocate for their needs and the needs of their children with the MCFD. In the group, women were empowered to articulate their needs in a nonadversarial and confident manner. This is especially important for women who have themselves been in care and often lack close family connections and stable relationships in their lives. In this case, the mentors and facilitators modeled healthy and effective communication and relationships that the women were able to transfer to other contexts. The participants were assisted with completing forms, making phone calls, arranging rides to agencies, and obtaining information about bus routes. Frequently a mentor would accompany a woman to a meeting, particularly when there was a previous relationship with an agency and assistance was needed to obtain fair treatment. Through workshops, group members developed a tool kit of skills that could be used to manage conflict and strategies to navigate different systems effectively.

In turn, the staff helped other professionals to communicate appropriately with group participants. For example, when one woman was diagnosed with FAS, the facilitators and mentors educated the involved lawyers to use concrete, specific language with their client. The facilitators fostered strong connections with midwives and social workers at the hospital and with drug and alcohol services that encouraged women to access the healthcare system at an early stage in pregnancy. Through fostering liaisons and providing referrals to many community agencies, positive working relationships between the community and the mothers were encouraged. The shame was taken out of addiction and pregnancy, and a bridge was built between the hospital and detox centers. Although the facilitators continually advocated for housing, the lack of affordable and suitable housing remained a key issue.

Build Mentoring Capacity

Mentorship was central to the functioning and outcome of the program and was the means by which knowledge acquisition and transfer, wellness, and the mutual sharing of resources and information occurred. The mentors, who had personal experiences with substance misuse, were able to share their experiences with group members and to serve as role models. Although participants had experienced shame, disrespect, and stigma as a result of their involvement with substance use and their challenges with parenting, here they were accepted while they were in their recovery process. The principle of mentorship set the tone for the collaborative and respectful nature of the groups and for the cascading effect of positive mentoring relationships that followed. At the end of the first year, several participants were identified as potential mentors.

LESSONS LEARNED AND RECOMMENDATIONS

With recognition that shame, guilt and mistrust of the systems scrutinizing women who use alcohol during pregnancy have been identified as barriers in accessing care, programs have shifted toward an empowering, strengths-based and women-centered approach. Central to this approach is an openness for allowing women to set goals for improving their health that may not give immediate priority to substance use issues, and when they do, accommodating goals of reduced use rather than immediate abstinence. (Dell & Roberts, 2005, p. 62)

FASD and the use of alcohol by pregnant women are both significant health considerations. While addiction during pregnancy clearly has detrimental effects on both the mother and the child, the path to recovery is far from clear (McIntosh & McKeganey, 2000). People who misuse substances have much to tell us about their lives, and social and life experiences have the potential to shape current wellness and the path to recovery.

Societal narratives typically portray drug misusers as people with negative personal and psychological characteristics, without consideration for life experiences or the social, political, and economic conditions that form the context of a person's life and the path to addiction (Etherington, 2006). Women's health has been inextricably linked to the context and circumstances of their lives (Benoit & Nuernberger, 2006). Through respectful listening in an appropriate forum, the women's shared accounts of resilience and resistance, which may otherwise be overlooked, can be witnessed (Etherington, 2006).

Many programs focus only on individual wellness strategies. The benefit of the Moms Mentoring Moms program was the systemic perspective, which included building healthy relationships as a sustainable strategy for individual and community wellness. The navigation of multiple systems and relationships was central to the success of the program. For example, the staff learned to navigate the social systems of participants, and the participants learned to navigate various social support systems in order to address their many barriers to wellness. A variety of relationships evolved and became important conduits in knowledge transfer.

An important contribution of mentorship is the formation of a particular type of learning climate that includes autonomy and agency, accountability, communication, education and training, mentoring opportunities, and safety (Davis,

2001). *Autonomy and agency* developed as all individuals involved became collaborative partners by creating spaces where all voices were heard. Mothers connected with other community resources and were supported until they were able to access resources on their own. Participants were encouraged to make informed decisions regarding their health and their lifestyle as they received nutritional and financial education and were supported by advocacy actions in areas of social assistance, legal aid, and independent housing.

Defining the roles and responsibilities of participants, mentors, and facilitators contributed to *accountability*. Group participants were encouraged to take charge of their own recovery and wellness, including relapse prevention strategies, nutrition, and health. Participants were also supported to regain custody of their children and to problem solve existing parenting challenges. Open *communication* supported *education and training*, which involved candid feedback, sharing of resources and experiences, the opportunity to test out ideas and take risks, and mutual support. The group participants provided input on which speakers to invite to the meetings, and staff members presented relevant material to the group, thus transferring their experience and knowledge regarding wellness and substance misuse to the group. The sharing of knowledge and information among facilitators, mentors, and participants provided *mentoring opportunities* for all involved. The collaborative and respectful climates characteristic of this mentorship approach fostered *safety* for participants, an important factor in building individual capacity. The modeling of respect and nonjudgment demonstrated to members that everyone was valued as part of the supportive community. In addition, psychosocial support was a key component of safety for the group and included affirmation, encouragement, counseling, and friendship.

As Poole (2003b) notes, little effort has been made to understand women's substance use during pregnancy and to develop interventions to prevent or reduce the impact of having a child diagnosed with FASD. The focus has typically been on the child, and less attention has been paid to women's health and to the nature of women's substance use during pregnancy (Poole, 2003b). For example, often overlooked is the fact that young mothers who have been in care, like many participants of the Moms Mentoring Moms group, are often stigmatized by social workers, which perpetuates the cycle of youth in care who have children that end up in care (Rutman, Strega, Callahan, & Dominelli, 2002). When compared to mainstream youth in British Columbia, youths from care are more likely to be on income assistance, engage in higher levels of alcohol and substance misuse, have tenuous ties to family, and have a more fragile social support network (Rutman,

Hubberstey, Barlow, & Brown, 2005). A stable relationship with a caring adult and strong social supports are protective factors for individuals who have aged out of care (Rutman et al., 2005). A significant function of the Moms Mentoring Moms program was to provide the social support needed by participants and to provide the stable and caring relationships listed as protective factors for women who have been part of the foster care system.

SUMMARY

The Moms Mentoring Moms program endeavored to address women's health, substance misuse and pregnancy, and issues related to FASD in a respectful, integrated, multifaceted, and flexible way. The multipronged approach included attending to health promotion and community development, the provision of an interface of services, and the development of comprehensive support systems for the mothers and their children. The benefits of the Moms Mentoring Moms program reached beyond the four walls of the group room; participants learned about their personal assets, strengths, and skills, and for the most part they were able to transfer this knowledge to other situations in their lives.

Moms Mentoring Moms Closing Prayer

May today there be peace within
May today we trust our highest power that we are exactly where we are meant to be
May we not forget the infinite possibilities that are born of faith
May we use those gifts that we have received, and pass on the love that has been given us
May we be content knowing we are children of the Universe
Let this presence settle into our bones and allow our souls the freedom to sing, dance, praise, and love. It is there for each and every one of us.

Discussion Questions

1. In general, what are some of the advantages and disadvantages of using a support group? What about for this population?
2. What are some of the ethical issues related to working with mothers who are also addicts?

CHAPTER 9 Enhancing Outcomes for At-Risk Moms

3. Do you think that facilitation of this group requires a leader who has overcome the same issues as the women in the program?
4. Considering that most of the children were not residing with their mothers, and considering the involvement the mothers had with the child welfare system, suggest some prevention strategies for this problem in this population.
5. List at least five strategies that were used with the participants, and evaluate the success of the strategies.

REFERENCES

Benoit, C., & Nuernberger, K. (2006). *Health determinants and women's health.* Victoria, British Columbia: Women's Health Research Network, University of Victoria.

Canada Mortgage and Housing Corporation. (2007, second quarter). *Housing market outlook.* Victoria, British Columbia: Author. Retrieved from www.cmhc.ca/housingmarketinformation

Chudley, A., Conry, J., Cook, J., Loock, C., Rosales, T., & LeBlanc, N. (2005). Fetal alcohol spectrum disorders: Canadian guidelines for diagnosis. *Canadian Medical Association Journal, 172*(Suppl. 5), 1–21. doi:10.1503/cmaj.1040302

Davis, K. S. (2001). "Peripheral and subversive": Women making connections and challenging the boundaries of the science community. *Science Education, 85,* 368–409.

Dell, C. A., & Roberts, G. (2005). *Alcohol use and pregnancy: An important Canadian public health and social issue.* Ottawa, Ontario: FASD Team, Public Health Agency of Canada.

Etherington, K. (2006). Understanding drug misuse and changing identities: A life story approach. *Drugs: Education, Prevention, and Policy, 13,* 233–245.

Greaves, L., Cormier, R., & Poole, N. (2002). *Fetal alcohol syndrome and women's health: Setting a women-centered research agenda.* Vancouver, British Columbia: Centre for Excellence for Women's Health. Retrieved from http://www.bccewh.bc.ca/publications-resources/documents/fasworkshop.pdf

Health Canada. (2004). *Fetal alcohol spectrum disorder. Knowledge and attitudes of health professionals about fetal alcohol syndrome: Results of a national survey.* Ottawa, Ontario: Author. Retrieved from http://www.phac-aspc.gc.ca/about_apropos/reports/2008-09/fasd-etcap/findings3.1-eng.php.

Howell, E. M., Heiser, N., & Harrington, M. (1999). A review of recent findings on substance abuse treatment for pregnant women. *Journal of Substance Abuse Treatment, 16,* 195–219. doi: 10.1016/S0740–5472(98)00032–4

Johnson, J., Greaves, L., & Repta, R. (2007). *Better science with sex and gender. A primer for health research.* Vancouver, British Columbia: Women's Health Research Network.

Leslie, M., & DeMarchi, G. (2004, Spring). Engaging pregnant women using substances: A review of the Breaking the Cycle Pregnancy Outreach program. *IMPrint: Newsletter of the*

References

Infant Mental Health Promotion Project (IMP), 39. Retrieved from http://www.mothercraft.ca/resource-library/publications/Engaging_Pregnant_Women.pdf

McIntosh, J., & McKeganey, N. (2000). Addicts' narratives of recovery from drug use: Constructing a non-addict identity. *Social Science and Medicine, 50,* 1501–1510.

Ministry of Children and Family Development. (2003). *British Columbia's annual report on early childhood development activities—2002/2003.* Victoria, British Columbia: Author.

Ministry of Children and Family Development. (2008). *Fetal alcohol spectrum disorder: Building on strengths together—a provincial plan for British Columbia 2008–2018.* Victoria, British Columbia: Author.

Poole, N. (2003a). *Fetal alcohol spectrum disorder: A strategic plan for British Columbia.* Victoria, British Columbia: Government of British Columbia, Ministry for Children and Family Development.

Poole, N. (2003b). *Mother and child reunion: Preventing fetal alcohol spectrum disorder by promoting women's health.* Vancouver, British Columbia: Centre for Women's Health, Policy Series. Retrieved from http://www.cewh-cesf.ca/PDF/bccewh/FASbrief.pdf

Poole, N., & Isaac, B. (2001). *Apprehensions: Barriers to treatment for substance-using mothers.* Vancouver, British Columbia: Centre of Excellence for Women's Health. Retrieved from http://www.bccewh.bc.ca/publications-resources/documents/apprehensions.pdf

Rutman, D., Callahan, M., Lundquist, A., Jackson, S., & Field, B. (2000). *Substance use and pregnancy: Conceiving women in the policy-making process.* Ottawa, Ontario: Status of Women Canada. Retrieved from http://publications.gc.ca/collections/Collection/SW21-47-2000E.pdf

Rutman, D., Hubberstey, C., Barlow, A., & Brown, E. (2005). *When youth age out of care: A report on baseline findings.* Victoria, British Columbia: School of Social Work, University of Victoria.

Rutman, D., Strega, S., Callahan, M., & Dominelli, L. (2002). "Undeserving" mothers? Practitioners' experiences working with young mothers in/from care. *Child and Family Social Work, 7*(3), 149–160.

Tait, C. L. (2000). *A study of the service needs of pregnant addicted women in Manitoba.* Winnipeg, Manitoba: Manitoba Health. Retrieved from http://www.gov.mb.ca/health/documents/PWHCE_June2000.pdf

United Nations Office on Drugs and Crime. (2004). *Substance abuse treatment and care for women: Case studies and lessons learned.* New York, NY: Author. Retrieved from http://www.unodc.org/pdf/report_2004-08-30_1.pdf

World Health Organization. (2004). *Global status report on alcohol.* Geneva, Switzerland: Department of Mental Health and Substance Abuse. Retrieved from http://www.faslink.org/WHO_global_alcohol_status_report_2004.pdf

PART V

Birthing Centers

Birthing centers are a low-tech alternative to a more industrialized hospital setting for giving birth. The natural process of birth is stressed and medical interventions are usually kept to a minimum. The centers can be staffed by midwives, doulas, nurse–midwives, or obstetricians. Because they are outside of a hospital setting, they are more home linked and provide options like food or drink during labor, music, presence of more family members, and other methods to make mothers more comfortable. They are usually for women who are expecting to have low-risk, uncomplicated births, but are still equipped for maternal and infant emergencies.

Birthing centers have grown in response to the medicalization and industrialization of labor and delivery, particularly in developed countries, where women were beginning to feel less in control of the birth process than they would prefer. Across the Organisation for Economic Cooperation and Development member countries, there is a wide range of birthing practices but the comparison point for these chapters is the privately insured, heavily interventionist, hospital-focused labor and delivery system of the United States. Therefore, in the United States birth centers support a woman's ability to give birth on her own and provide the support systems for her to do this including showers and bathtubs, freedom of movement, and lots of support from staff members and family and friends. Because they have fewer interventions, birth centers cost about one-third less than hospital births in the United States. The United States has an accrediting agency for birth centers called the American Association of Birth Centers.

In developing countries, when birthing centers are available, they are often the only option for a local birth because hospitals are often far away and inaccessible at the time of birth. Maison de Naissance is a nonprofit organization registered in the United States and has funding challenges—their website seeks donations from visitors to keep services going. In the two cases presented here, both communities were in need of maternity care that was close to the community and the birthing centers, and that focused on providing a home-like environment where the community could meet the sociocultural and psychological needs of the women they served with minimal technology. They also needed back-up care with a focus on midwifery provided by a medical doctor at a hospital outside of the community. MamaBaby Haiti, founded in 2004, is another birth center that started in 2010 with midwives and naturopaths that provide many of the same services as Maisson de Naissance. They are also a nonprofit organization that has expanded their maternity services to include a more holistic perspective to the health of the community. These cases serve as an interesting contrast to each other because of the differences

PART V   Birthing Centers

in the resources available, the sponsorship of the centers, and the provider of the services. The reader may want to compare these cases along those lines.

In New Zealand, there are other publicly funded birth centers that are funded through the Ministry of Health and local health authorities. Free services are provided by midwives, some of which include prenatal services, postnatal care and postnatal visits, water births, and referrals to specialists. Other birth centers like River Ridge Birth Center and Waterford Center are also publicly funded, privately operated, and staffed by midwives like the clinic in Warkworth. These birthing centers grew out of government health reforms in 1992 that facilitated new initiatives in the provision of health services.

Maison de Naissance: A Community Birthing Home in Haiti

Whitney A. Smith, BA
Natasha Massoudi, MPH
Stanley G. Shaffer, MD

Location: Torbeck Plain, Haiti, Caribbean

Project Goals: Reduce infant and mother morbidity and mortality; increase utilization of family planning, prenatal care, and skilled attendants at birth

Project Sponsor: The St. Luke's Hospital Center for Women and Infants (University of Missouri–Kansas City, School of Medicine)

CASE STUDY

Madeleine was 28 years old. She had three children and was pregnant with her fourth. She had experienced no problems during her pregnancy, and labor began as it had before. She planned to deliver at home with the assistance of neighbors, but labor became painful and she started to have heavy bleeding. Her sister became alarmed and sought help to take her to a hospital. It was nighttime, and no transportation was available. The bleeding continued. Madeleine lost consciousness. She was carried on a mattress for 2 hours until they reached a road, then she was taken on a truck for 1 hour to the hospital. Madeleine arrived in shock and died a short time later.

BACKGROUND

Haiti has the highest rate of maternal mortality in the Western Hemisphere. An estimated 670 maternal deaths occur for every 100,000 live births (World Health Organization [WHO], 2009), an order of magnitude greater than neighboring Latin American countries. Globally, the rate is higher only in Afghanistan, Nepal, and sub-Saharan Africa. Alongside the issue of maternal mortality lies the burden of child mortality. In Haiti, the child mortality rate is 76 deaths per 1,000 live births (WHO, 2009). Though the disparity of the child mortality rate is not quite as extreme as the maternal mortality rate, Haiti's rate is still an order of magnitude greater than the lowest-rate countries in the Western Hemisphere (Canada, Cuba, the United States, and Chile). The issues of maternity care and child health are intimately related, because more than one-third of child deaths occur in the newborn period. For both mothers and their children, birth is a critical time of vulnerability.

The disparity of health conditions that afflicts Haitian mothers and their children is magnified by social and economic disparities that exist within Haiti. These include geographic and accessibility factors, distribution of health professionals and services, availability of communication and transportation, and local attitudes toward available healthcare options. In combination, these factors influence health-seeking behavior, the success of healthcare delivery, and ultimately health outcomes. For example, child mortality is 30% higher in rural versus urban areas, 50% higher for low-income versus high-income families, and 100% higher if mothers are uneducated versus educated (WHO, 2006).

Disparities of maternal and child survival point to the need to understand local social conditions and restraints prior to determining remedies. The following describes a community-based maternity program that began with an attempt to define common barriers that limit healthcare access for a specific rural community. A combination of social and medical interventions led to improved pregnancy outcomes. The program has attempted to incorporate mechanisms that will allow it to continue to respond to community needs.

PURPOSE

In 2004, a healthcare team from the St. Luke's Hospital Center for Women and Infants (University of Missouri–Kansas City, School of Medicine) began an initiative to decrease maternal and neonatal mortality in a rural area of southern Haiti. The approach was threefold: address social barriers that limit access to health care, employ evidence-based interventions for pregnancy and newborn care, and institute systems for ongoing monitoring and evaluation of community impact.

FORMATIVE RESEARCH

A study population was selected based on preexisting knowledge of the region and upon a request from the community's leadership. Formative research was conducted to formally define the population and its demographics, health conditions, and health preferences.

The study population initially consisted of residents of 901 homes in the Torbeck Plain along Haiti's southern coast. This population was expanded, and subsequently a geographically defined zone of service was established that included the original study population among a total of 2,424 homes (Shaffer, Fryzelka, Obenhaus, & Wickstrom, 2007). The zone of service was approximately 100 square kilometers that were entirely rural. There was no electric service, pumped water, or sewage systems. There was no landline telephone service, but cellular networks have recently become available. The roads are dirt or gravel. Homes abut corporate agricultural fields, and most households have their own small gardens. Some houses are arranged in small clusters, but there are no formal villages, and a few public buses (*tap-taps*) cross the area on an irregular basis. A variety of traditional health workers (voodoo priests, leaf doctors, and traditional birth attendants) reside within the zone of service, but the area contains no hospitals or medical clinics. The closest hospitals are in the city of Les Cayes, a distance of 10–20 kilometers.

Methodology

Community health workers, who were indigenous to this area of Haiti, and foreign volunteers visited every household in the zone of service, recorded information about each home, registered all household members, surveyed all women of childbearing age, and conducted focus groups with community members. Home

CHAPTER 10 Maison de Naissance: A Community Birthing Home in Haiti

data included household size, construction materials, water sources, presence of a latrine, use of bed nets, and GPS location of each home. Health information included past pregnancy history, present vaccination status, and health-seeking practices. Survey and focus group data also included knowledge, attitudes, and desires regarding the availability of health services in the region. Data was entered into an online community health database. GPS data permitted the construction of a series of community health maps.

The original 901 homes included 5,496 residents. Histories of prior pregnancies were obtained from 764 women. These included a total of 1,951 pregnancies and 1,657 live births. Of these births, 1,460 children were still living. Of 197 childhood deaths, 66 occurred by 1 month of age, and 65 occurred between 1 and 5 years of age. The calculated neonatal mortality rate was 40 deaths per 1,000 live births (Shaffer et al., 2007).

Data

When asked details about their most recent pregnancies, 321 women reported that they had at least one prenatal visit, and the other 443 women reported that they had never visited a clinic or a hospital for care prior to delivery. Of the births, 101 occurred at a hospital, and 663 occurred at home with no assistance from skilled health staff. Eighty-one women were pregnant at the time of the survey, and only 30 had visited a prenatal clinic. Some women sought no health advice, and others sought health advice from a variety of sources, including traditional healers, leaf doctors, traditional birth attendants, voodoo priests, church clinics, and public clinics. When asked why they did not go to a hospital to deliver their babies, the women gave three common responses: the hospital is too expensive, the hospital is too far, and I don't trust the hospital (Barnes-Josiah, Myntti, & Augustin, 1998). (These responses are similar to what has been described as the "Three Delays" responsible for maternal mortality globally: delay in seeking health care, delay in reaching a healthcare provider, and delay in receiving appropriate care after reaching a healthcare provider.) Other specific reasons for not going to the hospital echoed this triad of concerns: not helpful to go to the hospital, no transportation to the hospital, fear of staff, rude staff, patients do not receive good care at the hospital ("women who go to the hospital die"), the cost is high, there are no supplies at the hospital, there is no food for the patients, and there is no one to care for my family at home. Basic prenatal clinic visits were also not popular. Women complained that they took time away from the responsibilities of family, home, and market work. Some women reported that their male partners objected to the time that would be spent at the clinic or to their receiving family planning (Shaffer et al., 2007).

In response to survey and group discussion questions regarding needed services, the community expressed a strong desire for pregnancy services located closer to home. The residents were specific in their requests for a convenient, clean, safe facility for birth and a good staff. The residents felt that health services should be free of charge (whereas most healthcare workers who were interviewed felt that payment was essential, otherwise treatments would be perceived as worthless). Other common desires were for better water, child health services, vaccinations, schools without fees, and food. Some women discussed the need for family planning services. Transportation to the city hospitals for routine care was not seen as a desirable option.

METHODS

The results of the formative research were used to guide the selection of interventions with the overall hope of improving reproductive health among women in the zone of service. The needs and desires of this community were clearly immense, and many desires did not relate directly to reproductive health. The investigators decided to focus resources narrowly on maternity care and actively seek development partnerships to address broader needs. Five strategic goals were selected to define outcome success:

1. Increase the prevalence of family planning
2. Increase the prevalence of prenatal care
3. Increase the prevalence of births supervised by a trained birth attendant
4. Increase neonatal survival
5. Increase maternal survival

Both medical and social realities were taken into consideration to establish specific program elements. Health surveys, discussions with medical personnel, and review of the available health statistics for this region suggested that the most common medical conditions associated with maternal mortality were peripartum hemorrhage, infections, and eclampsia. These are the same pathologies responsible for maternal mortality in most resource-poor areas of the world. Fortunately, global health research has defined the medical interventions most likely to reduce maternal and neonatal mortality from these causes (Darmstadt et al., 2005). These evidence-based interventions include maternal education, antenatal care packages, infection-related interventions, tetanus immunization, clean delivery practices, and providing trained and equipped birth attendant to supervise deliveries.

From a social perspective, the project's formative research had defined the specific barriers to healthcare access that were impairing health-seeking behaviors. These barriers and suggestions for their remediation were well described by the community. To eliminate the service fee barrier, all care needed to be free, regardless of where it was provided. To counteract the distance barrier, a plan was made to deliver most primary maternity services within the community. To remedy the barrier of mistrust, healthcare services needed to be delivered with compassion, courtesy, and consistency. These goals would be further enhanced by striving to maintain community engagement with patient involvement in health promotion, receiving feedback with positive health outcomes, planning community health events, attracting new development programs sponsored by other organizations, and creating new jobs for community members.

The Maison de Naissance Model
Facility-Based Services

Facility-based services were centered in a birthing home, or *Maison de Naissance* (MN). MN was designed as a home to highlight ideals of hospitality and to distinguish it from the negative attitudes associated with hospitals in the region. Nurse midwives were hired and trained, and they continue to operate and supervise the birthing home throughout the day and night. Standard protocols or clinical pathways guided most aspects of patient care. An emphasis is placed on patient education and continuity of care. There is no physician presence, but physician consultation is available by telephone and satellite Internet service. There is a laboratory, pharmacy, and obstetrical ultrasound. MN provides family planning, prenatal care, triage and referral of patients with significant pregnancy complications, vaginal delivery of uncomplicated patients, postpartum care for mothers and newborns, and HIV screening and treatment for the prevention of maternal-to-child transmission of HIV. When an obstetrical emergency situation arises, women are transferred to a regional hospital by ambulance. Supplies and service fees are provided for patients who are referred for care.

Community-Based Services

Community members warmly received home visits during the period of formative research. Home visits were therefore continued and have evolved into a robust system for patient education, distribution of community health interventions, data collection, outcome monitoring, and ongoing community engagement.

Community health workers initially conducted home visits. More recently, following suggestions from the community, neighborhood residents have taken on responsibility for routine home visits. The community and MN leadership now jointly select community members who are then trained as health promoters. Health promoters visit a defined set of 50 homes once each month to provide educational messaging, dispense medication for elimination of intestinal parasites, monitor compliance with prenatal care, organize vaccination posts, etc. The promoters provide a network for ongoing data collection and outcome monitoring. They also provide a neighborhood resource to respond to obstetrical emergencies and initiate patient transport. The institution of this new cadre of health providers both empowers local community members and gives other MN staff members additional time to pursue more complex activities in the community, such as home-based prenatal assessments and home-based family planning.

SUPPORTING TECHNOLOGY

MN has explored the use of technologies to enhance its services. Chief among these is an Internet-based electronic medical record system. Maintaining data in digital form permits transfer of information between clinical activities and expedites retrieval of data for review. Internet service, provided by satellite linkage, also permits frequent communication between MN in Haiti and consultants in the United States. Shared information and communication have been valuable for patient care, administration, and research.

MN's active community-based programs have presented special technical opportunities and challenges. A community health database includes the GPS location of all homes and many community services. Geographic information system (GIS) software is used to display health information in the form of maps. For example, it is possible to query a list of children who are eligible for deworming, vitamin A, or specific vaccines according to their age and history of prior treatments. The homes of these children are then displayed on a satellite image map (Google Earth), and outreach teams can plan targeted services. Community health teams have also explored methods of data collection in the field (laptop computers, personal digital assistants, and GPS devices). Recent availability of cell phone communication in the region promises further innovations with communication and data transfer.

Because MN is located in a remote area off the power grid, a generator was required to provide electricity. Until recently, diesel fuel was the largest operational cost for the birthing center. Fuel shortages due to economic embargoes or civil unrest sometimes disrupted power, communication, and data management. A solar power system has recently been installed. Operational costs have significantly decreased, and MN's power security has been enhanced.

MONITORING AND EVALUATION

Monitoring and evaluation is essential to providing quality care. Ongoing program assessments at MN include the community, the staff, and external advisors. Because patient records are Internet based, it is possible to employ many of the same quality assessment tools used in United States hospitals. Clinical volumes, compliance with protocols, and outcome data are compiled and reviewed both at MN and remotely.

To promote the goal of continuity of care, a specific quality assessment tool was developed to monitor major benchmarks that should occur with each pregnancy. The tool is called *TiPa TiPa*, which means step by step in Haitian Creole. Nurse midwives can review these steps with patients, and scorecards can be created for individuals or groups. Grouped data can reveal service delivery problems that require process changes. For example, an early assessment indicated that only 70% of women who delivered at MN had received a tetanus vaccination prior to delivery. An investigation revealed that the nurse midwives were following a protocol set forth by the Haitian government that said women should receive a tetanus vaccination before 32 weeks in their pregnancy. Thus, women who arrived for a first prenatal visit after 32 weeks were not being offered a tetanus vaccination. The protocol was misunderstood; it is best for women to receive the vaccination as early as possible in their pregnancy, but it is not detrimental for them to receive it after 32 weeks. After this misunderstanding was identified, it was easy to explain the purpose of the protocol and to increase vaccinations in women who had been pregnant for more than 32 weeks. As another example, *TiPa TiPa* monitors recently demonstrated an increasing number of mothers initiating prenatal care at MN but not delivering at MN. Further investigation revealed that many of these patients lived at a greater distance from MN or went into labor at night when travel would be more difficult. This finding has led to a search for new patient communication and transportation options, again with input from the community.

RESULTS

MN has been able to measure progress toward each of its five strategic goals. The prevalence of family planning has increased from 15–55% of women of childbearing age. Home births have decreased, and the percentage of births supervised by a skilled birth attendant (MN or referral hospitals) has increased from a baseline of 23% to 93% 3 years after the MN programs began. The most significant change has been a decline of neonatal mortality rate from 40 to 9 deaths per 1,000 live births. The number of births from this zone of service (300–500 per year) is too low to measure a statistically significant change in maternal mortality, which is measured in deaths per 100,000 live births. However, 17% of mothers in labor have been transported to a regional hospital because of pregnancy complications or obstetrical emergencies. It is likely that many of these women would have died without recognition and transport assistance (Shaffer et al., 2007).

In addition to measured success with its strategic goals, many community changes have been observed. Women of the community congregate at MN for conversation, education, and mutual support. New mothers encourage and educate prenatal patients. Some of these mothers have initiated formal mothers' clubs. Other mothers have volunteered to become health promoters for the neighborhoods. These are hopeful signs of community impact and empowerment.

Finally, MN continues to nurture partnerships with other organizations to seek complementary services and wide-based development. The Episcopal Church of Haiti is an administrative partner that provides programs for primary education, social development, pastoral care, and microfinance. Project Hope is a partner for pediatric referrals. USAID also serves as a partner that conducts an agriculture project to supply fruit trees and vegetables and teach agricultural skills to the families of HIV-positive mothers.

CHAPTER 10   Maison de Naissance: A Community Birthing Home in Haiti

DISCUSSION

Each year complications of childbirth result in countless deaths of mothers and newborns worldwide. Many more have lifelong disabilities due to birth complications. These grim statistics are particularly tragic when it is known that most deaths could be averted with straightforward medical interventions and that most deaths occur in poor communities where there are social barriers preventing access to care. For many women, childbirth continues to remain a time of fear and intense vulnerability.

The social context of childbirth in Haiti is similar to most resource-poor regions of the world: women struggle to get health care. For prenatal care, they walk for hours to reach the nearest hospital. They must wait in a queue and pay user fees when they already have too little money to pay for necessities such as food. They must forgo expensive tests and medications that were prescribed and often walk home feeling that they have received little for their efforts. For a birth at the hospital, the obstacles are even greater. Because hospitals are unable to provide basic supplies, families must purchase birth supplies from the hospital: sterile gloves, antibiotics, IV fluids, and even bandages. Mothers are deterred from seeking prenatal care and hospital delivery. Instead, they deliver at home, often with unsanitary conditions and untrained assistants.

The maternity program described in this chapter is relatively small, with a target population of 10,000 persons. Yet this small size has permitted a strong community focus and an environment where grassroots or bottom-up strategies could evolve and where social and medical solutions could be integrated closely.

Community engagement was a significant factor for improving pregnancy outcomes among women living on the Plain of Torbeck in Haiti. The MN program began with formative research in the community to learn women's concerns and their suggestions for solutions to structural social problems. This research approach eventually set a precedent for ongoing community listening so that medical interventions could be integrated with the problems identified by the community. Research yielded not only knowledge, but also a surprising degree of community engagement. The methods used (surveys and focus groups) were fairly standard, but the location of the discussions may have resulted in the unexpected positive consequences. Conducting conversations in nearly 1,000 homes initiated widespread trust and community involvement. Collaborative participation by local church and civic leaders, who already held the public trust, was also likely helpful.

Maison de Naissance elected to continue a rotation of home visits to, in part, sustain the community ties that had been established during the period of formative research. Also, home visits uniquely express the ideal of maximizing healthcare access by moving health care to the patient rather than vice versa. Important public health interventions can be distributed and health information can be discussed in the format of a home visit. Home visit data collection and conversations have been an integral part of ongoing program monitoring and evaluation. Furthermore, the community engagement encouraged by home visits has given birth to new leadership roles reflected in parent clubs and a new cadre of community health promoters. Mining of the community now includes positive deviance investigations. As intractable problems are discussed, there are inevitably a few community members who have overcome these obstacles. For example, within a focus group there is usually a mother who achieved success with family planning, prenatal care, or infant nutrition. The solutions to intractable problems sometimes emerge from the success of individual community members. Current research highlights how the lessons learned from positive deviation can be shared, taught, and applied more broadly.

No single strategy is likely to unknot the complex net of poverty, illiteracy, and injustice that restricts access to care for poor mothers and their children. There will be no magic pill or new vaccine to reverse this health crisis. Preventing death and serious morbidity for mothers and babies will depend on closely integrated social and medical solutions. The present model demonstrates that communities can employ local resources and opportunities to discover pathways to improved health and well-being. In this process, there is an important role for organizations that can work nimbly and effectively to facilitate change by embracing bottom-up solutions and assisting with strategic resources.

CASE STUDY REVIEW

Madeleine's story is tragic; but it includes a powerful seed of hope. Madeleine died, but only after her community did everything in their power to prevent her death. Her sister sought help, and her neighbors carried her for hours on a mattress to reach a hospital. Stories like this are, unfortunately, common. At Maison de Naissance, we listen to each story like Madeleine's to learn the specifics of the barriers that women face and to join in the hope of already engaged communities to bring health care within reach.

> ### Discussion Questions
>
> 1. What was the role of community engagement in the data collection process?
> 2. What are the advantages and disadvantages of providing free health services?
> 3. Many of the reasons given for not going to the hospital for care pertained to dissatisfaction with hospital services. How would you address these issues if you did not have the resources to build a birth facility like MN?
> 4. Could Madeleine's life be saved given the situation she was in? Why or why not?
> 5. "Women who go to the hospital die." What are some of the reasons that women would say this, and how would you address this statement given that women may have to be transferred to the hospital from MN?

REFERENCES

Barnes-Josiah, D., Myntti, C., & Augustin, A. (1998). The "three delays" as a framework for examining maternal mortality in Haiti. *Social Science & Medicine, 46*(8), 981–993.

Darmstadt, G. L., Bhutta, Z., Cousens, S., Adam, T., Walker N., & de Bernis, L., for the Lancet Neonatal Survival Steering Team. (2005). Evidence-based, cost-effective interventions: how many newborn babies can we save? *Lancet, 365*(9463), 977–988.

Shaffer, S., Fryzelka, D., Obenhaus, C., & Wickstrom, E. (2007). Improving maternal healthcare access and neonatal survival through a birthing home model in rural Haiti. *Social Medicine, 2*(4), 177–185.

World Health Organization. (2006). *Global Health Observatory Data Repository—Haiti*. Retrieved from http://apps.who.int/ghodata/?vid=10000&theme=country

World Health Organization. (2009). *World health statistics*. Geneva, Switzerland: Author.

CHAPTER 11

Providing a Safe Space for Birth in Warkworth, New Zealand

Liz Smythe, PhD, RM, RGON
Deborah Payne, PhD, RGON
Sally Wilson, RM, RN, ADN
Sue Wynyard, RM, RN

Location: Warkworth, New Zealand

Name of Project: Warkworth Birthing Centre

Sponsoring Organization: Government of New Zealan

Target Population: A rural community of 90,000 people

Project Goal: Provide maternity services to a small rural community where the local hospital was closing

---

INTRODUCTION

New Zealand, a small country known for its innovative approach to finding solutions, has developed a unique maternity system. In 1990 the law changed, making it possible for a pregnant woman to book directly with a midwife to provide maternity care from early in pregnancy until 6 weeks after birth (Clarke,

---

Parts of this chapter courtesy of *New Zealand College of Midwives Journal*.

CHAPTER 11   Providing a Safe Space for Birth in Warkworth, New Zealand

1990). This change had come about through consumer groups of women and midwives lobbying government together. They argued that midwives could offer a continuity of care model of practice and preserve confidence in natural birth (Pelvin, 1990).

Prior to 1990, women had to access maternity care through a medical practitioner or a hospital system of midwifery care that always had a doctor in charge. The difference in 1990 was that now midwives could set up as self-employed practitioners, taking on their own case load of women (usually between five and seven women per month). With the structural change to legislation came the cultural change of new possibilities (and restraints) of care (Burton & Ariss, 2009). It is important to note that through New Zealand's social welfare state, all women have access to free maternity care unless they choose to have a private obstetrician as their maternity provider (Lovell-Smith, 1966), which was maintained.

In the small rural community of Warkworth, located in the Rodney district, where once they were employed on a roster basis to staff the maternity unit in a small government-funded community hospital, the midwives embraced the opportunity to be self-employed and to practice continuity of care with a woman and her family. They chose to become self-employed practitioners with their own case load. The government deemed the community hospital, which had always been a funding challenge, impossible to run. The initial transition was to offer birthing facilities only. This meant that the self-employed midwives could go with the woman to the hospital for labor, but after the birth the woman and her baby would need to go straight home. There was an uproar in the Warkworth community. They believed the postnatal service they had come to value over the past 80 years was too precious to lose. Women, midwives, and indeed the Warkworth community wanted to regain the option of a unit where women could not just give birth, but also stay and receive live-in postnatal care.

In 1992, two community meetings were held, and each were attended by 500 people. After 5 years of lobbying the Warkworth Birthing Centre (referred to hereon as Warkworth or the Centre) became a reality. In 1998, a Community Trust Board was founded with the aim that there would always be a birthing facility in Warkworth. Three midwives set up a private company to manage the service, yet they still drew on government funding to ensure that maternity care remained, and continues to remain, free for the women. In addition, a purpose-built facility was adapted from an old nurses' home for nine women, and registered nurses were employed to provide 24-hour postnatal care. Today eight local and eight remote self-employed midwives now provide labor care for the women in their case load at this birthing center. They support each other professionally and provide cover for days off and annual leave.

The Warkworth Birthing Centre offers a unique case study of excellent maternity care because of the following:

- Its values, structure, and way of providing care have emerged from a midwife–community partnership.
- Although the Centre is supported by government funds, because it is managed by a private company (currently two midwives, Sally Wilson and Sue Wynyard, are codirectors), decisions on how money gets spent are made by the people who are intimately involved in providing service. They have a firsthand understanding of the needs.
- The Centre does not have immediate access to epidurals, forceps delivery, and Cesarean sections that, in first world countries, are increasingly shaping how birth happens (McAra Couper, 2009). Thus, for a woman to choose to give birth at Warkworth is to believe that she is capable of giving birth without such intervention.
- Because the Centre is approximately a 50-minute drive from the nearest base hospital, midwives using Warkworth are challenged to ensure that their everyday assessment and management of childbirth ensures either timely transfer or safe emergency care.

This case study is drawn from a collaborative research study between the Auckland University of Technology (AUT) Centre for Midwifery and Women's Health Research and the codirectors of the Centre (Smythe, Payne, Wilson, & Wynyard, 2008). Data from that study will be used to bring the voice of the various stakeholders to the argument. An analysis and discussion are combined in each section.

THE CASE

Table 11-1 shows the birth rates from 2005–2008 at Warkworth. Approximately 14 women give birth at the Centre each month (three or four per week). This would be a daily quota in a city hospital. There is a much lower working demand at Warkworth. But it is important to note that the number of postnatal women is inflated by those who transfer back to Warkworth after birthing in a base hospital. The significant aspect of this case is that 88% of women who book at Warkworth achieve a normal birth without technological intervention. It is

CHAPTER 11   Providing a Safe Space for Birth in Warkworth, New Zealand

Table 11-1   Birth rates at Warkworth from 2005–2008

Table One	2005	2006	2007	2008
Normal birth	178	154	161	162
Primigravida	59	43	45	58
Multigravida	119	111	116	104
Transfer in Labour	18	20	20	22
Postnatal only	180	234	268	281
% of booked women who gave birth normally	91%	89%	89%	88%

Source: Smythe, L., Payne, D., Wilson, S., and Wynyard, S. (2009). Warkworth birthing centre: exemplifying the future. *New Zealand College of Midwives Journal, 41*, 7–11.

difficult to make statistical comparisons because some women, through need or choice, will make their initial booking in a base hospital. Nevertheless, at New Zealand's largest obstetric hospital in 2008, only 55.6% of women experienced a normal birth (spontaneous vertex birth), and 52% of women had an epidural for pain relief in labor (National Women's Health, 2008). Such statistical evidence suggests that it is becoming more and more uncommon for women to birth without some kind of intervention. In the United States, in the decade from 1996 to 2006, the Cesarean section rate rose by 50%, so less than two out of three women (62.3%) now have an unassisted vaginal birth (Birthstats, 2009). What was once called "normal" birth is no longer normal. Young, writing from an international perspective, calls for greater "support for natural childbirth and, hopefully, a more normal 'normal childbirth'" (2009, p. 3).

A Commitment to Local Community

The community of Rodney, from which this case study is drawn, has a population of just fewer than 90,000 people, and it is 30 minutes north of the large city of Auckland. It is a rural community with a mix of families who have lived there for several generations and others who have moved into the area specifically for the relaxed country lifestyle close to many beaches.

What galvanized this community to fight for its own birthing center? One young mother described why it was important for her to be able to birth in her local community:

> I wanted to have my baby here because I was born up here. So was my dad. Sue was my brother's and my midwife, that's why my mum remembered her. I wanted Warkworth on my daughter's birth certificate.

This first-time mother belonged to a long-standing and prominent Warkworth family. She wanted to continue her family history of children being born in Warkworth and to stay connected to her family roots. Also, she wanted be cared for by a midwife who was known and trusted to her family.

Other women talked of the history of birth in this community:

> You hear all the stories of Sister Brown and the old hospital, and you see all the old photos.

There is a strong sense of remembering that birth has occurred in, and has been part of, the Warkworth community for generations. It is normal and expected that this is where birth happens. Accompanying the historical practice of birthing in Warkworth is the holding of living memory that parents and grandparents were born without any of the technology available today.

Sally, one of the codirectors of the Centre, describes how it feels for the Centre to be associated with the community:

> We are part of this community, but we are also private. We are tucked up on the top of a hill in amongst a reserve. We are separated from the community in that respect. But people feel a part of it because they are encouraged to come in and visit. They've heard good stories. Wherever I go I hear "Your Centre is fantastic." They've all got really good things to say about it. They love the centre but they are not necessarily very involved with it.

This birthing center exists because of community demand, and therefore a sense of ownership has developed. Local people are very proud their community has such a center. For example, there is a large box of baby clothes in the Centre's lounge that are free for new mothers to take. They have been donated by families who no longer need them. Such is the spirit that underpins this center.

The other codirector, Sue, who has been a midwife in the community for 36 years, shares her own passion for the Centre:

> I'm not a local but I moved here when I was five. I've been a midwife in this area since I was 23. The oldest baby I birthed is now 36 and they've had four children with me. I just feel it's so important to be able to have a facility in your own community.

There is a growing trend toward economies of scale, building large hospitals that are accessible to the majority, and therefore removed from local communities. We argue that before discounting the possibility of building a small, local community birthing center one must first recognize that somehow confidence is held by keeping birthing within known territory, where people are known and trusted, and where the stories of safe birth become the fabric of everyday life. A commitment to community yields a culture of birth that no technology can ever replicate (Barlow, Hunter, Conroy, & Lennon, 2004). Hunter (2000, 2003) coined the term "real midwifery," which she argued helped sustain a belief in normal birth that allowed it to stay within the community. Equally, the existence of trusted community birthing units create a space that upholds women's belief that they can give birth without high-tech intervention, thereby legitimizing the concept of technology-free birth. Skinner and Lennox (2006) argue that women need to be informed of the implications for birth outcomes inherent in their choice of place to birth; that the very choice of a birthing center increases the chance of birthing without intervention. We argue that shared identity and reciprocity (Adams & Hess, 2001) emerges when midwives and women share a birthing space in community.

A Commitment to Building Confidence

Confidence is born of trust. It is a feeling, a mood vulnerable to being undermined by a look, a seed of doubt, a thoughtless remark. One woman who was expecting her first baby described it like this:

> My midwife did a lot of explaining and gave me lots of books because I was really frightened. She made me feel confident. I thought it would be the worst thing in the world but she built my confidence up. She took really good care of me. She didn't say much, she didn't interfere much. She let me do it myself. Because she seemed really confident, it gave my husband confidence and that made me feel confident.

The midwife's own confidence exuded a calmness that rubbed off on this woman and her husband. She made sure they had information to equip them for what they needed to know. She encouraged them. She let this new mother experience for herself that she could rise up to all that was expected of her.

Another woman expressed it this way:

> Nothing was ever a problem. No question was ever silly or daft. Everything was answered, no matter how big or how little it was. You feel as though you are asking a stupid question but you don't actually feel like you are daft. It was just "wow." It was just fantastic.

In these words there is a real sense of feeling safe to ask. This woman gained the confidence from the midwives and nurses to ask anything because she was never made to feel foolish or that she should not have asked such a question.

The nursing staff, who were on rosters to provide postnatal care, showed how such a climate of trust is achieved:

> I think we are really good at making the women feel listened to and cared for. They feel nurtured in the time we spend with them. Even when we are really busy we let them know that we are available. We carry phones so that they can ring us whenever they need us. Yet . . . we are helping them to cope on their own, giving them the skills to cope by themselves.

The nurses know how important it is for women to feel listened to and cared for. Even when the nurses are busy, the women can still contact them easily by calling them on the phones they carry. Thus, women never have to wait for their call to be answered. They get an immediate response and know how soon the nurse will be able to come to their room. The nurses talked of nurturing, yet they balanced this with the recognition that their ultimate aim was to help each woman cope on her own.

This example shows the commitment to building confidence:

> We had a woman with inverted nipples. She had no milk. We managed to keep her chilled. It's just our attitude I think. I said to her: If I start to look worried then you start to worry, and I'm not worried. And she was just so relaxed and the milk came in. It's keeping positive.

Nurses and midwives have seen many situations where what seems like an impossible breastfeeding scenario becomes straightforward as long as trust and confidence remain. The most important skill in the learning period is to show no signs of worry. If the woman can catch the confidence of those who know, she is much more likely to succeed. Confidence matters (Halldorsdottir & Karlsdottir, 1996). Research on how midwives support women through labor talks of "an inner conviction within some midwives which communicated itself to women and incites them to call upon something inside themselves" (Vague, 2004, p. 25). Similarly, Berg talks of "an enormous intrinsic power which exists in motherhood" (2005, p. 17). When the message is "of course you can do it," the woman comes to believe that for herself. When she is trusted, she trusts both "herself and the childbearing process in itself" (Lundgren & Berg, 2007).

A Commitment to Making the Centre Feel Like Home

Places of birth in New Zealand were once called Maternity homes (Donley, 1986). With the rise of medicalization of birth (Arney, 1982) came words such as

CHAPTER 11 Providing a Safe Space for Birth in Warkworth, New Zealand

obstetric hospital, and along with that came sterile environments, clinical ambience, and proudly displayed technological equipment. The Warkworth Birthing Centre strives to return to the notion of home. One mother described it like this:

> It felt like having a baby at home. You had the security of having it in a birthing centre but not that sterile environment of having it in a hospital. There was no smell of hospital. It felt like being in my own bedroom.

In one's own bedroom one is relaxed, at home, with a sense that one is free to do whatever one likes. These women were not at home. They sought the security of the birthing center where they knew there was equipment and staff that would keep them safe, yet they were delighted that the Centre in no way resembled a hospital. Even the smell was noted for its familiarity of being just like home. But it was more than the physical environment:

> When I came back here it felt like I was home again. They actually remembered who I was.

Other women talked of their anticipation of going back to a place they knew:

> When I found out I was pregnant again I said to my husband "Oh great. I get to stay at the birthing unit again."

Instead of labor, birth, and the postnatal stay being seen as a time of stress and strain, the women eagerly looked forward to what was ahead of them: another opportunity to go to the place they called home. But the Centre is not exclusive to women:

> They let your husbands stay one night.

Part of the homeliness of this center is that each woman has her own room, and in it a double bed. For the first-time mothers, especially, having their husband stay through the night was a special gift. They reported feeling so comforted by their husband's presence, as often they had never been separated since being together. Some would have loved their husbands to stay longer. However, the staff were mindful that too many men on the premises could become problematic. They also recognized the importance of helping the mother to cope with her baby on her own. The staff had found they were able to spend more time with the mothers teaching, supporting, and ensuring everything was going well after the partner had gone. But we are aware that having the partner stay one night was a very un-hospital-like thing to do.

The homeliness of the Centre is no accident. Sally describes how important this is to their approach:

> I love the homeliness of this birthing centre; that it is women centered and family centered. It's the simple things like "normal" beds, that the rooms are as comfortable as possible.

Keeping the Centre homely, and recognizing what can still be normal, matters. Yet, it is more than that:

> The receptionist, she always smiles. She's always helpful; nothing is ever a problem. She's enthusiastic. She restocks so you know there's plenty of food when you come in on the weekend.

Whoever visits the Centre, for whatever reason, is greeted with a smile. This is a place where people are made to feel welcome. There is an attitude of wanting to help. It was a midwife who made the previous comment. She knows that whenever she arrives with a woman in labor, she will find everything she needs in its place. This is a place where everyone relaxes because there is a team of people committed to getting it right.

The paradox of a place like the Warkworth Birthing Centre is that while some would call it a hospital, it strives to be a home, a place where women can simply be themselves, a place where they can be nurtured and tend to their bodily needs in comfort and trust.

A Commitment to Upholding Natural Birth

When a woman knows she is likely to birth in her own community amidst people she knows and trusts, when she has built up her confidence that she can give birth without intervention, when she arrives at the Centre, is greeted warmly, and feels at home, she is poised to labor effectively. One woman offers the mantra of this birthing center:

> South of the harbour bridge they are all saying "go for the drugs" but up here the midwives say "you can do it, you won't need it."

The women pick up the confidence of the midwives that they will be able to give birth without all the drugs. From the very beginning they come to believe they can "do it." And they do:

> I wanted to labour without an epidural to see what it was like. Afterwards I was on a huge high, like superwoman. It was a good experience.

CHAPTER 11 Providing a Safe Space for Birth in Warkworth, New Zealand

Not only did this mother birth without an epidural, but she emerged from the experience feeling like superwoman. The confidence she exuded in her own ability to birth still shone from her months later. And their stories said something quite different than "there was nothing to help me":

> They are not saying "this is natural birth and there are no options." You have the gas, you can have the music you can have the oils, the rope ladder, or the tens machines. There are some things you can't have up here but they give you the options of what you can.

It was with a sense of pride that these women told of the variety of options they had available to them to assist them through labor. From their experience, such low-tech, low-cost, no-side-effect options worked. The midwives confirmed this:

> Most of our births here are amazing. You see people who are totally unstressed. It's not labour, they are relaxed and they enjoy it. Lots of women here, before their placentas are born, are talking about the next one. They feel really powerful afterwards like they have done something amazing.

When women enjoy their births, so do midwives. Everyone is relaxed. And after the birth there is a real sense of pride and exhilaration. Midwives see women empowered by their birth experience. It seems that again it is the simple things that make a difference:

> I think in labour they are not tied to one room, they can wander outside. They can wander round in the lounge in the night. They can be really, really mobile and have a sense of freedom. They can feel OK wandering about in their pyjamas. And the women can make a noise without it being a problem.

Being mobile in labor is known to promote a positive experience (Balaskas, 1992). For these women it is very easy to wander around, inside or outside, wearing anything they like. There is privacy in this Centre, tucked up on the hill overlooking the town with a backdrop of native bush. If they make a noise, the only people who might hear will understand. Women are free to labor with no sense of having to be a good patient. This is their place where they are able to stay completely focused on the labor itself and to stay in control. Such an empowered birth experience is not about any one thing. It is about everything coming together in a way that the woman has the confidence, freedom, and support to birth as generations of women before her have done. Sue describes how, as a rural midwife, she helps women understand the nature of birth:

> Education is important. It takes ages going through with the woman how the labour starts. I relate everything back to centuries ago: we are supposed to be born at night, it's safer, there are not so many predators around. They are usually more settled at night. And especially for primips, if they are not in established labour by the time the sun comes up it usually goes away again. And it starts again the next night when it gets dark. So we should keep in contact, and say "lie low, stay in bed, get peaceful." It's usually a long latent phase. And then they come in, 7cm dilated, about 10 pm at night because they have just slowly been doing something. And I guess coming from a farming background you are in tune with how it's really meant to be. The cat doesn't have her kittens in the middle of the lounge floor, she finds a quiet place. My husband has been involved in farming all his life. I've learnt a lot from him. It relates, it really does.

Sue knows labor happens best when the woman lies low, finds a quiet private place, and lets the long latent phase slowly progress. There is no sense of hurry or angst. Rather she coaches these first-time mothers to trust the instinctive process of birth. She almost expects that the contractions will go away in the harsh light of day, to return again in the safety of the dark night. Arriving at the Centre 7 cm dilated means the birth itself will not be that far away. In such a way birth just happens, just as it happens on the farm. Perhaps in a rural community there is more trust in nature, more confidence in the fruitfulness of simply waiting.

Why does it matter that there are pockets of natural birth expectancy within society? Is it important to keep the belief that women can have very satisfying birth experiences without technological help as a competing discourse in an era where in the Western world epidural and operative delivery rates continue to rise (Kennedy & Shannon, 2004)? Could it be that these women who talk of feeling empowered by their birth experiences have lower rates of postnatal depression, breastfeed for longer, and are less stressed by their mothering experience? Do children of such mothers get a better start in life? These are big bold questions, but as one talks with these women some months after their birth experiences, one senses that their account of a positive birth experience has influenced their ongoing experience of being new mothers within a community that offers ongoing support services. Lundgen and Berg (2007) reveal that in Sweden less than 10% of births can be defined as spontaneous childbirth without interventions, such as the births that happen at this Centre. To respond to Young's challenge that "perhaps it really is time for a rebirth of 'natural childbirth'" (2009, p. 2) is to reflect on the insights offered by the midwives and women in this case study.

CHAPTER 11 Providing a Safe Space for Birth in Warkworth, New Zealand

A Commitment to Mothering

The discourse of midwifery in New Zealand for the past two decades has been one where midwives and women work in partnership (Guilliland & Pairman, 1995), where midwives empower the women to make their own decisions. Yet, the word we heard these women use in relation to both the midwives and the nurses who provided care was "mother":

> They are like mothers. You trust them and feel safe. I don't like to be invaded like being asked to "flop it out." With the staff here I felt more comfortable. She was massaging my breasts and I didn't think anything of it. I wouldn't go to my doctor to do it and she's a woman.

There was something in the relationship that made this woman feel safe. She acknowledged her shyness about her body, yet with the staff in the Centre she felt no need to be. They were like mothers. The word "mother" to describe the midwives and nurses was used time and time again:

> After I had my baby there was something wrong with him—he ended up in Starship. My midwife was there with me all the way through that. She was like a Mum. She still keeps in contact too.

In a time of concern for her baby this woman experienced the motherly care of her midwife. She was alongside her through this time of worry, not doing anything but rather being there sharing the concern, just as a close family member would. Such closeness did not finish at the end of the 6-week postnatal period. The relationship continues.

Other women talked of the kind, tender gestures and practices that made such a difference:

> Just bringing you a Milo in the middle of the night. You are lying there and the nurse says: "Would you like a Milo?" I'm still trying to make the Milo like they do.

To be brought a mug of hot chocolate to drink in the middle of the night is to feel cosseted, pampered, made a fuss of. One woman describes a similar experience:

> I remember feeling sore in my stomach and they brought me a wheat bag and it was just so nice and I went straight to sleep.

While it is likely the nurse also brought her some medication for the pain, it is the hot wheat bag that this woman remembers. Someone took the trouble to bring her comfort. The nursing staff confirmed the language of mothering as being congruent with their approach to care:

> Mothering is what women need when they've just had babies. In the best of worlds they would have their mother helping them.

In earlier generations it is likely that the woman's mother would have been with her to care for her through her childbirth experience. These nurses believe it is very appropriate for them to take on a similar role. They know that the loving care of a mother is just what these new mothers need:

> It's pampering. The meals are taken in to them on trays. Nowhere in life do you get pampered like that. And at handover we always go around and introduce the oncoming staff to the mums.

The word "pampering" conveys thoughtfulness and flexibility on the part of the nurses to tailor their care to the woman's needs. Rather than women having to conform to the scheduled routines, the nurses and midwives allow the women to follow their own. They willingly go the extra mile to make these women feel personally cared for. They recognize that caring is a relational activity. They consider the little things:

> I always tell them that if they are hungry in the night that there is food, like toast and muffins because sometimes they are too embarrassed to tell you they are hungry.

In most maternity units the only food available during the night is likely to be through a coin (vending) machine. But at the Warkworth Birthing Centre, caring means making sure there is food available whenever the woman feels hungry, and making sure she is not shy to ask. There is a watchfulness about what the women need:

> We can see a roomful of visitors there and we can see the mothers beginning to wilt. And we'll ask the visitors to go.

On the one hand this Centre is very welcoming of visitors, yet on the other very protective of each woman's needs. If they see the new mother beginning to tire from exhaustion they do not hesitate to step in and ask the visitors to leave. This is not about rules; rather it is stepping into the gap and helping the woman regain the peace and quiet she most needs. Such an attitude is what the codirectors of the Centre seek to promote, as Sally describes:

> Nurturing is really important. We try and encourage the nurses to make sure the women get a good rest; that they don't get a meal thrust at them when they are not ready for it; we'll re-heat it if it's gone cold. If the Mum is really, really tired we will take her baby between a feed so she can get a good solid sleep. They often only

CHAPTER 11 Providing a Safe Space for Birth in Warkworth, New Zealand

> need it for one night and then they get back on the job again. The mother might be ready to throw her baby out the window. The nurse will wrap the baby up firmly and walk around with it for a bit and often it will go off to sleep. That's our conflict with the Baby friendly hospital policy. But we put our mothers ahead of any policy.

This is not a Centre that runs by the clock, or by any external policy that gets in the way of woman-centered care. The needs of each woman are watched over and responded to. She is given her hot meal when she is ready for it. Rather than insisting that the baby always stays with the mother, as baby-friendly policy dictates, there is an understanding that sometimes the thing that matters most is for the woman to know that someone else is watching over her baby. That frees her to have the sleep she is desperate for and equips her to face the next day. Common sense reigns, along with a responsive readiness to reach out to the mother who needs support:

> One day I heard a baby crying in the supermarket. I thought "oh that poor mother. If it's one of our babies then I'll go and rescue her." She was going through the checkout and so I asked her if she wanted me to take the baby for a minute. She said "thank you so much" and the next day a card arrived thanking me for helping her out.

In the local supermarket, off duty, the nurse shows she is always there to support these new mothers. While she may not have approached someone she didn't know, when she saw it was one of the mothers who had recently been in her own Centre she did not hesitate to offer to take the baby. This new mother clearly appreciated such support. When birth happens in the community, the support lives on.

The midwives and nurses mother new mothers, who in turn mother their newborn babies. One senses that a chain of care is infused with a regard for the other that goes beyond performance of tasks and recognizes vulnerability and responds proactively. The care goes beyond what might be expected and takes initiative for the sake of the other. Such attitudes, which are perhaps expected to be instinctual in mothering behaviors, are nurtured when mothers are cared for with love. To be mothered oneself empowers the new mother to respond lovingly to her own baby. Sally, the codirector, sees the importance of keeping the flow of care strong:

> We care for the midwives so they can care for the women. And we the midwives can leave our women in the care of the nurses because we know they will love and care for the women.

Heidegger (1995) talks of two modes of care. One is to leap ahead, as in a partnership relationship in which one equips and supports the other person to take care of herself. The other is to leap in, to take over care and help the other until she is strong and able to do for herself. The tension of midwifery practice is always to know when to leap ahead (the ideal) and when to leap in and take over (Smythe, 2003; Vague, 2004). The discourse of midwifery as a partnership (Guilliland & Pairman, 1995) perhaps silenced the very idea of mothering by staff. Perhaps the notion of mothering signals unequal power relationships. Yet it seemed the women in this study were expressing the love and care they experienced from those who looked after them "as a mother." We argue that there is a time when a new mother simply needs to be looked after, just as there is a time to encourage her to learn the skills of mothering her new baby and to step back as she takes charge and does it in her own way. To mother someone is not to patronize or undermine her. Rather it is to support her with care until she is ready to be independent; to be accessible, sensitive, and engaged but noninterventionist (Elvin-Nowak & Thomsson, 2001). The tension requires a skillful attunement on the part of the midwife, what van Manen refers to as tact:

> A tactful person has the sensitive ability to interpret inner thoughts, understandings feelings and desires from indirect clues such as gestures, demeanour, expression and body language . . . A tactful person is able, as it were, to read the inner life of the other person. (1991, p. 521)

To leap in and mother somebody who is perfectly capable of looking after herself is to misread the inner person and is likely to leave that woman feeling belittled. On the other hand, to leave a new mother alone who is feeling vulnerable, unsure, in pain, and emotionally fraught is to be negligent in one's care. Midwives and nurses need to learn how to tactfully read each situation, knowing that mothering moves to sistering (a more partnership approach), which moves again to a more professional distance as the woman reclaims her independence.

A Commitment to the Whole

The people involved with the Centre share a strong sense of what matters. In other words, there was a living philosophy of practice that ensured the core of what worked well stayed strong. One mother noticed the following:

> All the staff have been here for more than seven years and that tells you something about the place. I asked a few of the staff and they love their work. They love the contact with all the mums.

CHAPTER 11 Providing a Safe Space for Birth in Warkworth, New Zealand

This mother worked out for herself why this Centre works so well. All the staff love their work, and love working with the new mothers. Yes, it provided them with a job, but somehow working here was experienced as something more than a job. A midwife made the following comment:

> When I was up here once in the middle of the night the nurse who was on duty said "I really enjoy spoiling these women."

When the staff members love spoiling women, and the women love being spoiled, then it is hardly surprising that this place works well. The staff affirmed this:

> I think there is a feeling of love and respect for the women, wanting them to succeed and enjoy their experience. That infiltrates everybody who works here. I think we have a different attitude here. At the end of the day you feel like you are doing something worthwhile.

The word "infiltrates" shows how pervasive the attitude of caring is in this place. When everybody is trying to give these women the best experience possible, then any one person who brought a not-so-caring attitude would stand out. Caring is the only attitude that is acceptable in this place. Sally affirms that idea:

> I think the nurturing side is really important and it doesn't cost money. Because if you nurture them at this specific time then they become independent.

Caring or nurturing does not cost money, yet it is perhaps harder to ensure than a commodity that can be bought. The Centre cleaner talked of how she is able to care for the women:

> I like to meet people, I like talking to them. I like caring for them. I love to give them fresh towels and restock their nappies for their babies. I like everything.

In a less-personalized work environment, the cleaner could easily get caught up in the tedium of only doing the restocking and the cleaning, but this woman took real pride in her work. She had the privilege of giving these new mothers clean towels and diapers and to talk with them as she went about her work. That many of the women commented about the cleanliness of the Centre is testament to this woman's care. She knew she impacted their experience and was valued by the rest of the staff.

This service works because of the synergy of many components coming together. Each influences and shapes the other. One woman said the following:

> The whole experience is amazing, right from the time when I thought "Oh my God I'm pregnant" to the time when she actually came out.

This is a service where the enacted philosophy of care is congruent from the very beginning of pregnancy right through to the birth. For the women it mattered that everything happened at one place:

> I come from a long way away. I like having everything here. Antenatally I see my midwife here. I know this is where I come, this is where I have my baby. My family knows this is where I come. My children call this Sue's house. Just having everything here, it's great.

Everything is here. The whole family sees the Centre as the place where one goes for everything. It is not a hospital; it is "Sue's house," a safe place where even children feel at home and look forward to playing on the playground. And there is a sense that the care takes the woman on to the next step:

> They just don't give you a whole lot of information. They give you the right information and they make sure you understand it. Before I left they made sure I had all my contacts, like Plunket [baby care service] and Parent Port and coffee groups. They gave me a big information tree.

The staff made sure this woman knew exactly who could offer her support as a new mother in the community. They did more than just pass the information over. They helped her understand how to use such information and gave her the confidence to access the support she needed. This woman said the following:

> They look after you and do what's best for you but they want you to keep on coping when you go home. They not only want you to cope for the first days here but they want you to keep on coping when you go home.

As well as being concerned for the care needed in the current moment, it seems that the midwives and staff at the Centre also take seriously their responsibility to equip women for what comes next. There is a real sense of integrated community care.

The midwives and the staff who make this Centre work are special people, drawn to care, eager to give, willing to invest themselves in their commitment to one another and to the women in their care. In turn, they themselves are cared for. They laugh together and play together. There is a generosity of spirit that makes the Centre work. The women and families who come here sense that and in turn are generous in doing whatever they can to ensure this service is sustained within the local community.

Berg (2005) talks of a mode of midwifery practice where there is genuine caring. She suggests that such care comes from "the very nature of a midwife's way of

CHAPTER 11 Providing a Safe Space for Birth in Warkworth, New Zealand

being" (p. 16) and focuses on the woman with "absolute dignity" (p. 16) for who she is, with specific focus on her being a new mother. Within such a climate the women also come to trust the nurses and midwives, both as people and for their professional competence. Mutuality develops where each is willing to be open to the other. We found such a spirit of practice at the Warkworth Birthing Centre.

Inherent in such a spirit of care is the question of safety (Smythe, 2003).

And a Commitment to Being Safe

It is relatively easy to paint a rosy picture of a small birthing unit nestled against native bush, with caring staff, and a homely environment. Yet, at the end of the day the thing that matters most to women and their families is that they emerge from the experience having been kept safe (Smythe, 2003). If the health and well-being of the mother or baby is compromised, then none of the nice things matter. Safety is always paramount.

The midwives practicing at the Centre were very mindful that safety matters. They voiced a strong sense of feeling well supported to ensure safe practice:

> What keeps it safe is that you know it's well equipped, you know that there are always other people around to consult with if you are unsure. No-one is too far away.

First, there is confidence that everything is always in place for when a situation arises that needs equipment to be easily accessible. And second, there is a strong ethos of collegial support. There is always another midwife to ask or to come at a moment's notice to help. Sue gives an example:

> A woman came in, in strong labour. The foetal heart beat was dipping down, it was her second baby and she was about 7cm, so I ruptured her membranes to see if there was meconium liquor and found a cord at the side of the head. It was during the day. Sally was here. I kept the head up and she did all the organising. The baby was born by caesarean section 55 minutes after leaving here, and everything was fine.

There was no way this situation could have been predicted. It simply happened. But everything was in place to ensure the situation remained as safe as possible. The cohesive teamwork meant the woman was promptly on her way to the base hospital. They had the skills and processes to keep the woman safe and share in celebrating the positive outcome. Nevertheless, they do not take such success for granted:

> We have a good transfer policy. When we have our midwifery meetings on Fridays we go through cases and review how the transfer went.

Every case where something happens that requires a transfer to the base hospital is reviewed. The decision to transfer is based on a set of criteria that have been established by the midwifery directors with the local midwives and staff and have been refined over time and through experience. Questions are asked as to how practice could have been even better. Lessons are learned to ensure that women, babies, and staff are kept as safe as can be. Smith, Dixon, and Page (2009) researched the safety of the maternity service in England and concluded that safety was compromised by increasing complexity associated with the medicalization of birth, staff shortages, low staff morale, and poor management. The Warkworth Birth Centre is, perhaps in some ways, safer than a big city hospital because it stays focused on promoting natural birth and nurturing both women and the staff. Further, it embodies a spirit of safe practice (Smythe, 2003), which keeps the staff alert and attuned to possible unsafe situations so they can transfer the woman ahead of time and always be prepared to support each other in dealing with the unexpected.

Recognizing the paramount importance of physical safety, women can feel unsafe in other ways, especially from a cultural perspective when their ways of birth are frowned upon or not allowed (Ramsden, 2002). A Maori (indigenous culture of New Zealand) woman shared her experience:

> My experience was great. I'm a first time Mum. You are coming into an environment where you feel pretty vulnerable; hormones all over the place. My midwife was great: experienced, peaceful, calm. I found it really peaceful coming here. What I liked about it was with your birth plan everything was open. We did a karakia [prayer] when my daughter was born, and my husband did that. You could do whatever you liked and they were open to suggestions. I had all my family in when I had my baby, there were twenty of them and they were fine with that.

This woman expresses the cultural safety of her birth experience. Her husband clearly felt comfortable praying as their baby was born. Having 20 of her family members present, as is the custom for many Maori, was not a problem. What could have been an unsafe experience for this first-time mother on many different levels is described in very positive terms. Safety can be violated without the staff being aware that they have caused hurt and harm. An approach of openness to the behaviors and requests of women and their families, with the flexibility and space to allow things to happen without compromising the experience of other women, ensures cultural safety (Spence, 2001).

CHAPTER 11 Providing a Safe Space for Birth in Warkworth, New Zealand

SUMMARY

This case study reveals that there is no one thing that promotes a positive birth experience for women and their families, but rather an interconnected weaving of many things. Commitment is the common ingredient. When everybody, from the community to the cleaner, is committed to ensuring that each woman and her family has a safe and positive birth experience, then the chances of that being the reality are high. Commitment comes because people are clear about what they care about and who they care about. Commitment is nurtured by seeing deeply satisfied women and their families and receiving their thanks and acclaim. Commitment is tenacious when the rising intervention rates from obstetric hospitals continue to paint a very different picture of birth. This small community not only preserves a place where birth successfully happens in a cost-effective, low-tech manner similar to generations past, but perhaps it also preserves the possibilities that others may be challenged to reconsider how their own birthing services could be different.

The midwives at this birthing center say that most births are amazing. The women echoed this description. Something right is happening here.

Discussion Questions

1. How does the Warkworth Birthing Centre differ from a hospital setting in your country?
2. What are some of the advantages and disadvantages of birthing in a community?
3. Do you think the dynamics of the birth process would have changed if there had been a doctor on site? If so, how?
4. This case is possible because of New Zealand government funding arrangements, laws that allow self-employed midwifery practices, and cost-effective insurance arrangements for midwives. What barriers stand in the way of attaining a similar service in your country? Are there ways around such barriers?
5. How do you think the relationship between mothers and midwives influenced the birth process?

REFERENCES

Adams, D., & Hess, M. (2001). Community in public policy: Fad or foundation. *Australia Journal of Public Administration, 60*(2), 13–23.

Arney, W. R. (1982). *Power and the profession of obstetrics*. Chicago, IL: University of Chicago Press.

Balaskas, J. (1992). *Active birth: A new approach to giving birth naturally*. Boston, MA: Harvard Common Press.

Barlow, A., Hunter, M., Conroy, C., & Lennon, M. (2004). An evaluation of the midwifery services at a New Zealand community maternity unit (birth centre). *New Zealand College of Midwives Journal,* 7–12.

Berg, B. (2005). A midwifery model of care for childbearing women at high risk: Genuine caring in care for the genuine. *The Journal of Perinatal Education, 14*(1), 9–21.

Birthstats. (2009). Birthstats: Rates of Cesarean delivery, and unassisted and assisted vaginal delivery, United States, 1996, 2000, and 2006. *Birth, 36*(2), 167.

Burton, N., & Ariss, R. (2009). The critical social voice of midwifery: Midwives in Ontario. *Canadian Journal of Midwifery Research and Practice, 8*(1), 7–22.

Clark, H. (1990). Introduction of the Nurses Amendment Bill in Parliament, New Zealand. *College of Midwives Journal, 3,* 9–10.

Donley, J. (1986). *Save the midwife*. Auckland, New Zealand: New Women's Press.

Elvin-Nowak, Y., & Thomsson, H. (2001). Motherhood as idea and practice: A discursive understanding of employed mothers in Sweden. *Gender and Society, 15*(3), 407–428.

Guilliland, K., & Pairman, S. (1995). *The midwifery partnership: A model for practice* [Monograph series 95/1]. Department of Nursing and Midwifery, Victoria University of Wellington.

Halldorsdottir, S., & Karlsdottir, S. (1996). Journey through labour and delivery: Perceptions of women who have given birth. *Midwifery, 12,* 48–61.

Heidegger, M. (1995). *Being and time* (J. McQuarrie & E. Robinson, Trans.). Oxford, England: Basil Blackwell.

Hunter, M. (2000). *Autonomy, clinical freedom and responsibility: The paradoxes of providing intrapartum midwifery care in a small maternity unit as compared with a large obstetric hospital* (Unpublished master's thesis). Massey University, Palmerston North, New Zealand.

Hunter, M. (2003). Autonomy, clinical freedom and responsibility. In M. Kirkham (Ed.), *Birth centres, a social model for maternity care*. London, England: Books for Midwives.

Kennedy, H. P., & Shannon, M. T. (2004). Keeping birth normal: Research findings on midwifery care during childbirth. *Journal of Obstetric, Gynecologic, and Neonatal Nursing, 33*(5), 554–560.

Lovell-Smith, J. B. (1966). *The New Zealand doctor and the welfare state*. Auckland, New Zealand: Blackwood and Janet Paul.

Lundgren, I., & Berg, M. (2007). Central concepts in the midwife–woman relationship. *Scandinavian Journal of Caring Science, 21,* 220–228.

McAra Couper, J. (2009). *What is shaping the practice of health professionals and the understanding of the public in relation to increasing intervention in childbirth?* (Unpublished thesis). Auckland University of Technology, New Zealand.

National Women's Health. (2008). *Annual clinical report.* Retrieved from http://www.adhb.govt.nz/nwhealthinfo/

Pelvin, B. (1990). Nurses amendment bill—the implications for midwifery. *New Zealand College of Midwives Journal, 3,* 6–7.

Ramsden, I. (2002). *Cultural safety and nursing education in Aotearoa and Waipounamu* (Unpublished doctoral thesis). Victoria University, Wellington, New Zealand.

Skinner, J., & Lennox, S. (2006). Promoting normal birth: A case for birth centres. *New Zealand College of Midwives Journal, 34,* 15–18.

Smith, A. H. K., Dixon, A. L., & Page, L. A. (2009). Health-care professionals' views about safety in maternity services: A qualitative study. *Midwifery, 25,* 21–31.

Smythe, E. (2003). Uncovering the meaning of "being safe" in practice. *Contemporary Nurse, 14*(2), 196–204.

Smythe, L., Payne, D., Wilson, S., & Wynyard, S. (2008). *Warkworth Birthing Centre: An appreciative inquiry.* Retrieved from http://www.aut.ac.nz/__data/assets/pdf_file/0006/8556/warkworthbirthingcentre_finalreport.pdf

Spence, D. (2001). Prejudice, paradox and possibility: Nursing people from cultures other than ones own. *Journal of Transcultural Nursing, 12*(2), 100–106.

Vague, S. (2004). Midwives' experiences of working with women in labour: Interpreting the meaning of pain. *New Zealand College of Midwives Journal, 31,* 22–27.

van Manen, M. (1991). Reflectivity and the pedagogical moment: The normativity of pedagogical thinking and acting. *Journal of Curriculum Studies, 23*(6), 507–536.

Young, D. (2009). What is normal childbirth and do we need more statements about it? *Birth, 36*(36), 1–3.

PART VI

The Culture of Maternity

Like the way we think, speak, dress, eat, and interact, culture impacts the way we think and behave about the most primal of experiences: motherhood. We are not only influenced by the way we are mothered, but also by the way our societies perceive the role of motherhood, in particular, and gender roles, in general.

As a collection of stories from around the world, this book is explicitly about culture. However, the stories in this section focus generally on culture and not on specific cultural practices. Two of these cases are anthropological explorations of how maternity is experienced by different cultures in South America—one in Brazil and one in Argentina. In both cases, the stories fascinate us with difference. Though it is easy to think of these cultures as exotic, the lessons to be learned from the experiences of these scholars and those they studied can be generalized to populations with whom we work every day. Understanding how the indigenous peoples of South America have maintained and lost traditions related to health practices that were passed down through generations helps us understand how our own cultural practices may seem strange to others, and it challenges our own notions of what works and what does not.

Because of the ever-growing desire of students and professionals—from both North and South America—to work abroad as part of their studies or as professional development or as a career track, the issues raised regarding community partnership, sustainability, and study and service abroad are pertinent to the discussion of culture and maternity within the context of service delivery and community engagement. The ethics of cross-cultural interaction in a foreign context—often with a backdrop of colonialism or imperialism—and the inherent racial and economic factors inherent in these historical relationships are complex and sometimes ambiguous. Health practitioners who choose to work abroad must learn to live with the latent and explicit ethical challenges and contradictions in values that are common to the experience. The degree to which one engages with the communities in which they work can be a reflection of their comfort level with these contradictions and ethical challenges. While some people enjoy living in an environment that is very foreign to their own, others seek the comfort of other foreign workers. These choices influence practice through the strength of interpersonal relationships that connect people to the communities in which they work.

Though there is no way to eliminate the influence of culture on how we practice public health, there are ways to maximize the benefits and minimize the challenges of our differences, and the questions attached to each chapter in this section will help us explore how we can do this. Though it is not explicitly discussed in any of these chapters, the importance of linguistic ability cannot be overemphasized (this is particularly targeted to unilingual Anglophones). The expectation that there will be enough other people to speak English is itself an expression of power that shapes the helping relationship. So much of culture is reflected in language, so gaining fluency in the language of the culture in which you choose to practice should be as important to you as your public health training so you can maximize the effectiveness of your training toward your goal of working in partnership with populations other than your own.

CHAPTER 12

Maternal–Infant Care in the Brazilian Amazon

Reflections on the Well-Being of Indigenous and Peasant Communities

Louis C. Forline, PhD
Helena dos Santos, PhD

Location: Maranhão, Brazil, South America
Sponsoring Organization: Pan American Health Organization (PAHO)
Target Population: Guajá Indians
Project Goal: Attempt to problematize and identify some of the factors influencing maternal–infant health in the Brazilian Amazon, focusing on two ethnographic fieldwork and community surveys that examine local adaptations of peasant and indigenous communities

INTRODUCTION

Mother–infant health practices are of mounting importance in the developing world. The well-being of these actors is inextricably linked. Externalities bearing

CHAPTER 12 Maternal–Infant Care in the Brazilian Amazon

on mothers invariably affect the health of infants, while the cost of infant care increasingly puts demands on maternity. As international aid organizations gather an increasing ensemble of data to anticipate malnutrition, infant death, and maternal well-being, developing countries scramble to find solutions that would be compatible with local needs. Policies directed at these issues vary according to country, cultural beliefs and practices, and access to healthcare resources and information. In this chapter we attempt to problematize and identify some of the factors influencing maternal–infant health in the Brazilian Amazon, focusing on two separate studies. These studies comprise ethnographic fieldwork and community surveys that examine local adaptations of peasant and indigenous communities located in the Pará and Maranhão states of the eastern Amazon. This region has undergone rapid change in the past 40 years as a result of unbridled development, settlement patterns, changing cultural practices, and environmental degradation. Our study attempts to provide a common yet relativized thread of variables influencing maternal–infant health, placing an emphasis on breastfeeding and weaning practices. As we isolate variables influencing maternal–infant health, we also explore the discourse provided by community members and health workers in interpreting their well-being. Examined here are the Guajá Indians of Maranhão and a case study commissioned by the Pan American Health Organization (PAHO).

The first study comprises an ongoing investigation since 1990 by one of the authors (Forline) among the Guajá Indians of Maranhão state. This group came into permanent contact with Brazilian mainstream society in 1973 and has since been settled by Brazil's Indian service (FUNAI) into four separate communities. Before contact, the Guajá lived primarily by foraging and are now transitioning to a mixed subsistence strategy of hunting, gathering, fishing, and farming. Currently, the bulk of their diet stems from their agricultural products, accounting for nearly 60% of their caloric intake. While contact has opened up new resource options for the Guajá, it also exacted a heavy toll because a number of them succumbed to introduced illnesses and disease, primarily malaria and influenza. Because most indigenous peoples of the Americas have little resistance to Old World diseases, many of them perished during the first years of contact. One of the Guajá villages, for instance, was reduced to nearly one-fourth its original size. Additionally, because Guajá women bore the brunt of contact more than their male counterparts, this scenario has altered their social structure, subsistence patterns, and investment in women and children.

The second study was commissioned by PAHO in 1998 to examine feeding practices among mothers and infants. Five rural municípios (counties) of Pará state, a Tembé indigenous community, and the state capital of Belém were selected to explore factors influencing mother–infant feeding practices for purposes of elaborating national food guidelines and recommendations. In addition to recommending food guidelines and recommendations, this study also suggested elaborating alternative dietary parameters for the state of Pará to more accurately reflect local adaptations and needs. The first five of these communities are primarily rural agricultural and riverine communities, and the Tembé community represents an indigenous community that has been in contact with mainstream Brazilian society for more than 200 years. The sample selected for the state capital of Belém targeted a peripheral community of this city, a neighborhood initiated by a squatter settlement in the Guamá district.

The results of these studies will be discussed following a brief background on the Amazon region. This backdrop will better situate these communities within the context of health and nutrition as it pertains to mother–infant well-being. What follows, then, will contextualize mother–infant feeding practices within the scope of the Brazilian Amazon in light of ecology, history, and development.

THE BRAZILIAN AMAZON: REGIONAL ECOLOGY, HISTORY, AND DEVELOPMENT

The Amazon region contains the world's largest freshwater reserve and tropical forest area. The water volume flow of the Amazon River is 20% of the joint volume of all rivers on Earth. The Amazon River alone discharges 60 times more water per day than the Nile and 11 times more than the Mississippi. This river network is rich in biodiversity and is home to many peasant and indigenous communities, and it supplies a large gamut of resources for these dwellers. In addition to its abundant supply of fish, this hydrological basin supplies nutrients for the traditional farming methods utilized along its banks. Seasonal silt deposits provide the nutrient base for the soils upon which slash and burn horticulturalists use to clear land and plant and harvest crops. Similarly, riverine areas represent a very rich ecological zone for game animals that feed and breed in this area. As such, it draws together many resources that are managed and utilized by the inhabitants of the region. Even the interfluvial zones of the Amazon basin are cut by a series of seasonal streams that provide a multitude of resources for

CHAPTER 12 Maternal–Infant Care in the Brazilian Amazon

indigenous and peasant populations. Despite the massive road building projects that took to the wing since the 1970s, forests and rivers in this area provide its peoples with a natural transportation infrastructure and bounty of nature that sustain their livelihoods.

The landscapes of the region are also imbued with many myths regarding the origins of the earth's people and its creatures. Many indigenous legends persist to this day in various forms and, to some observers, a number of myths help safeguard natural resources from overpredation and exploitation. Thus, these myths serve as a "primitive Environmental Protection Agency" for these people (McDonald, 1977, p 734). For example, the concept of *panema* holds that greedy hunters would incur supernatural sanctions for overkilling animals and, in turn, would be cursed with bad luck. As such, observance of taboos and ritual protocols would keep hunters in favor with animal spirits and other animate forces of nature, maintaining a healthy balance between humans and their natural environment.

According to some accounts, most of the indigenous people in the Amazon region resided along its watercourses prior to the arrival of Europeans. As previously noted, it is not too startling that greater numbers of people would be drawn to rivers, streams, and lacustrine areas, given the bounty of resources that converge upon these ecological zones. Thus, even in times past it is speculated that these areas were disputed between pre-Columbian inhabitants. In this scenario, populations residing in interfluvial zones would have been residing there not necessarily as a matter of choice but because they were forced out of riverine areas as a result of competitive exclusion from stronger and more established groups (Sponsel, 1989). Later, during the time of conquest, European powers mapped over previously established indigenous communities and settled along river courses. In fact, a number of present-day cities of the Amazon region were formerly inhabited by large indigenous communities, such as Belém, Manaus, and Altamira.

In recent times, the Amazon region has been coveted for reasons of national security, geopolitical concerns, and, of course, its natural resources. Since the 1960s, the Brazilian government engineered projects aimed at settling the region to ensure its sovereignty over a resource-rich area that is still sparsely populated and larger than western Europe. During the heyday of Brazil's economic miracle of the 1970s, its government energetically jockeyed for position to establish land settlement projects for people from other areas of Brazil. The hallmark project of this era, Projeto de Integração Nacional (PIN, or Program for National

Integration), was touted as "land for men for men without land" (Velho, 1995). With this project and other ventures, Brazil's then military government hoped to accomplish two things. First, it would help diffuse civil unrest in other regions by siphoning off people to the Amazon and deeding out parcels of land. Second, as development planners pointed out, settlement in the region would occupy an area thought to be targeted by external powers. Official slogans such as *integrar para não entregar* (integrate the country lest we give it away) became popular mottos for this time period.

While the short-lived economic miracle fizzled out, settlement in the Amazon region proceeded at full steam, and the day and age of large-scale projects took to the wing. In addition to government and private colonization ventures, road building and massive mining projects were established. Along with these ventures a number of illegal activities surged in the wake of officially sponsored development, particularly gold mining, land grabbing, and logging. And given the large volume of water present year round in this region, developers saw in the Amazon a large potential for generating hydroelectric power.

All of these projects invariably affected Brazil's first inhabitants, its indigenous peoples. For one, the PIN project impacted approximately 96 different indigenous groups, or about 56% of the known Indian communities of the Brazilian Amazon (Ramos, 1984). The Carajás Mining Project (PGC) impacts, directly and indirectly, 40 indigenous communities along its 500 mile railway (Treece, 1987). For its part, the Balbina Dam forced the contact of a number of indigenous groups who had little or no contact with Brazilian mainstream society. As Davis pointed out (1978), many of these groups turned out to be victims of the Brazilian economic miracle of the 1970s. The rapid pace of development during the past 40 years also transformed the region's population profile and landscapes. Deforestation has been a major concern, removing the resource base for many peasant and indigenous communities. Many newcomers to the region introduced different management regimes and undermined the sustainability of local landscapes.

STUDY RESULTS, COMMUNITY FEEDBACK, AND REFLECTIONS

In light of this backdrop and brief introduction of our study communities, we discuss some of our results vis-à-vis mother–infant health and feeding practices. Although each of these studies varies in its principal focus, we attempt to analyze

CHAPTER 12   Maternal–Infant Care in the Brazilian Amazon

our results within the context of the Amazon's ecology, regional development, and history to establish common ground for discussing mother–infant well-being.

The Guajá

As previously noted, the Guajá are undergoing a rapid transition from foraging to farming. They have had an incipient introduction into the market economy, occasionally selling or bartering forest products and game with neighboring non-Indian communities. The demographic decline suffered by the Guajá in the wake of contact with Brazilian mainstream society left two of its communities with a large disparity in sex ratios. As a result, there were three men to one woman of reproductive age. One response to this was the formation of polyandrous marriages, a situation where one woman is married to two or more men. Some anthropologists speculate that polyandrous arrangements are one of the mechanisms used by indigenous groups of the Amazon to recover population losses and rebuild their communities (Laraia, 1974; Wagley, 1974).

Additionally, the betrothal of young girls is also thought to comprise a mechanism in recovering population losses and is a current practice among the Guajá. Polyandrous marriages, or associations, also correspond with a unique reproductive ideology that is commonly observed among indigenous groups throughout the Amazon region, partible paternity. Independent of language family, this complex is shared by many native Amazonians. Also termed multiple paternity, indigenous groups in Amazonia claim that if a woman has sex with more than one man that the sperm of each male is "mixed" and the child is, for all practical purposes, a "multi-paternity project." As such, the various fathers in this scenario would be imbued with a series of social obligations to the child and mother. In this light, Beckerman and Valentine (2002) posit that this complex may actually enhance the survivability of women and children. Thus, both the biological and putative fathers provide food and other goods and favors for the mother and her children. These provisions would primarily be offered during the *couvade* period, where parents would have to observe certain ritual protocols to protect the child and improve his or her chances for survival. These protocols include ritual behavior, food taboos, and, on some occasions, sexual abstinence.

In light of these cultural practices, Beckerman and Valentine (2002) also speculate that partible paternity may have been more common in the past, when humans lived primarily by hunting and gathering. Anthropologists have also commented that the transition from foraging to farming may have increased the workload and burden placed upon women because enhanced food security increases fertility and reduces the spacing between births. Conversely, it is speculated that women in foraging bands bear fewer children during the course of their lifetimes because high mobility would lead to reduced body fat content, and the intensity and duration of breastfeeding, combined, would contribute to amenorrhea. In this scenario women breastfeed on demand and wean infants only when they become toddlers. Likewise, the nomadic nature of many foraging societies would increase mobility and reduce body fat among women.

This Neolithic model, in part, can apply to the Guajá as modern hunter–gatherers transition to farming. The dynamics of modern foragers compress evolutionary time but, indeed, may mimic some of the pathways experienced by Neolithic hunter–gatherers; however, we must also consider the fact that the Guajá and other hunter–gatherers across the globe are embedded within developing nation states hooked up to the rapid pace and networks of globalization (Lee, 1992). After being contacted and settled by the National Indian Foundation (FUNAI) they currently live in four seminucleated communities and practice a host of mixed subsistence strategies and are now considered wards of the state. Current farming practices were passed on to them by FUNAI and, as previously noted, calories derived from crops now comprise the bulk of their diet, accounting for nearly 60% of their intake. The biggest staple crop is manioc (*Manihot esculenta*), grown in consortium with corn, rice, sweet potatoes, yams, melons, beans, and other cultivars. These new subsistence practices have, indeed, increased their resource options, but regional development has cordoned the Guajá within their current reserves and rendered them charges of the Brazilian state, under the tutelage of FUNAI. As such, they have had to subordinate many of their beliefs and practices to state development agendas and ideologies. While they are ensconced on reserves, relatively out of harm's way, marriage practices are being altered and work regimes are often tailored to the needs of FUNAI.

According to Keegan (1986), the transition from foraging to farming does increase the number of available resources yet eventually leads to a reduction in food options. As agricultural practices expand, there is a funneling of the resource base toward carbohydrate-dense crops. In the case of the Guajá, their transition to farming has followed this course. Although foraging provides most groups with a broad-spectrum diet (Binford, 1968; Flannery, 1969), the transition to farming initially expands the gamut of resources, but, with increased sedentarization, the dependence on crops increases, resource options dwindle, and health can become compromised. Coupled with this, the archaeological record also shows a deterioration in dental health as carbohydrates convert to sugars, increasing the rate of caries (Cohen & Armelagos, 1984). Sedentarization also increases the risk of bone deterioration and other pathologies.

In addition to the polyandrous marriages observed among the Guajá, the men in this community are absorbing a heavier burden during this transition. Time allocation and nutritional studies reveal that both women and children enjoy more leisure time than men, and they also enjoy a better nutritional status. As the Guajá recover from the initial impacts impinged by interethnic contact with mainstream Brazilian society, they are investing in their future through these series of mechanisms. Thus, men are engaged in most of the subsistence tasks and also lend their services to the Indian agency charged with administering their affairs, FUNAI.

On the whole, relations between men and women among foraging societies are egalitarian, but in the shift from foraging to farming both the resource base and management of natural resources change, invariably altering power relations. Among the Guajá, we are witness to relatively equal footing in gender relations. Both polygynous and polyandrous marriages occur, and women have a choice in marriage partners, even if they are betrothed. Similarly, men and women will defer to one another in the decision-making process. Thus, decisions on subsistence practices are discussed and women can often dictate if their men should hunt, gather, fish, or farm on a given day. This scenario, however, is changing as FUNAI engages more frequently with Guajá men. Contact between Western and indigenous societies offers many historical and ethnographic examples of the shift in power relations as state agents interact more with men than women. Over the course of time, indigenous men learn the mainstream language, deal with outsiders more frequently than women, and gain better access to resources and power in these exchanges (Posey, 1994). Eventually, women are relegated to a lower status and are left without the former networks and engagements that previously benefitted them. The extended family networks often encountered among traditional societies frequently give way to an atomization of families. This change transforms traditional kinship ties into nuclear families, modeled after European and North American ideals of family social structure and organization, with men at the head of households.

When the balance sheet is drawn, we are witness to a series of push and pull factors that both contribute to and conspire against the well-being of women and children. On the one hand, the flexibility of Guajá social organization and their reproductive ideology would conceivably permit them to regroup and rebuild their society during this critical transition period in their history. On the other hand, the advancing frontier and unbridled development in the Amazon have enveloped the Guajá and are contributing to their forced assimilation into mainstream society. The results of this interaction await further analysis as longitudinal studies are currently underway among the Guajá to assess future directions in maternal and infant well-being.

As noted earlier, Guajá women will breastfeed their infants until the toddler stage. The weaning process now involves introduced foods from a new resource base, occasionally including sugar, salt, coffee, canned goods, and other foodstuffs. Thus, introduced food items have not only deteriorated the dental health and reduced dietary fiber among mothers, but children, too, can contract caries in their first set of teeth. At best, FUNAI has provided only scant preventive health measures among the Guajá, and dental practitioners serve more as tooth pullers for this community. Ambulatory health crews from Brazil's National Health Foundation (FUNASA) periodically make brief visits to indigenous communities to administer vaccines; take routine blood, urine, and fecal samples; and maintain a basic dispensary. However, budgetary problems, fraud, and inconsistency have fraught this agency with a number of problems in delivering adequate health care for mothers and children, and the Guajá in general.

Generally speaking, the traditional practices and pharmacopeia of the Guajá have helped them prevent, heal, and anticipate illnesses and diseases within their repertory. Yet some traditional practices have also had unintended and undesirable consequences. For example, it is customary for Guajá women to care for pets and breastfeed them. Guajá women breastfeed monkeys, baby peccaries, agoutis, pacas, and other animals. Even if they are not breastfeeding directly, lactating women will squeeze out milk from their breasts to feed other pets. The Guajá obtain these pets mostly in the course of hunting. When hunters fan out to the forest and kill their prey, they take these slain animals back to their villages, along with the orphaned young, who are then raised as pets. Some authors have even pointed out that there are religious and mythological reasons to explain why women would raise and breastfeed young pets, especially howler monkeys (Cormier, 2003). In the act of breastfeeding, both the pets and the mother's children will share her breast and, as a result, microbes will be exchanged. One of the ailments that may beset infants during this exchange may be moniliasis (*sapinho* in vernacular Portuguese), a fungal infection. FUNAI nurses are aware of this possibility and administer medicines to help the infant along. Wet nursing is also practiced among the Guajá and, again, the exchange of microbes can create some unintended illnesses for infants.

CHAPTER 12 Maternal–Infant Care in the Brazilian Amazon

Granted, some of these practices have unforeseen consequences, yet they should not detract from the fact that the advantages of multiple caretakers, by far, outweigh their disadvantages. Sharing tasks of child care translates into extra leisure time and better nutritional status that Guajá women and children enjoy, as we previously pointed out. The sharing of caretaking responsibilities relieves mothers of burdens and helps to engage children earlier in socializing. Yet, as observed earlier, in the wake of contact with mainstream society, many of these beliefs and practices are eroding, and mothers cannot rely on this traditional network to assist in caretaking.

PAHO Health Study

As noted in our introduction, this particular study was conducted in six municípios of Pará state. It was commissioned by PAHO to revise and develop dietary guidelines based on the study results of mother–infant feeding practices. The study team was composed of an anthropologist, a nutritionist, and two students from the Universidade Federal do Pará. The study communities were visited over a period of 3 months in 1998, and households with mothers and infants up to 24 months of age were selected for interviews. At first, project coordinators requested that only two communities be selected to carry out this study, the state capital of Belém and one of the rural municípios of Pará state. Later, this sample was expanded to include other communities in an attempt to more accurately portray the variegated profile of Pará state to embrace different ecological zones, integration to markets, and indigenous communities. In this manner, the fine-tuning of our sample would more accurately reflect the diversity of Amazonian communities. Mothers were interviewed on dietary recall, infant health history, household infrastructure, food stores, income, and education. Heights and weights were taken for both mothers and infants. In the case of infants, a stadiometer was used to measure the length of the child while lying down.

We report on the more general findings of this particular study in order to draw a broader picture of factors contributing to the variability in mother–infant well-being and health. Results of this particular case study showed that, during the weaning process, the median age infants began eating introduced foods was 2.7 months. Most of the introduced foods were gruel mixed with water. There was a marked decline in the health and nutritional status when weaning began. Because our sample was analyzed in cohorts of 6 months, our analysis showed a marked decline in growth velocity and heights and weights after the first cohort of 0–6 months. And as infants grow, the disease load and illnesses increase. The direct factor leading to this scenario, of course, is diminished breastfeeding, compromised living conditions and infrastructure, and accessibility to health care. Yet expanded to the larger picture, the intervening variables are altered lifestyles brought on by the dynamics of Amazonian development.

As with the Guajá, these communities are experiencing a rapid course of change brought on by the intense development and transformations of the Amazon region. Some of these communities have experienced out migration because of large land-consolidation ventures, often being siphoned off to the larger cities of this region, such as Belém and Manaus. This regional mobility has undermined some mothers' ability to adequately care for their children because they often have to absent themselves from their homes and begin the weaning process early. Still, many mothers are the moral heads of households because the men of the family have to take leave for a variety of reasons, most of which are working as migrant laborers and seasonal jobs.

Public health campaigns have promoted the benefits of breastfeeding throughout Brazil, but their effectiveness can be compromised by a weak dissemination and an abstract language. Although public health campaigns have their benefits, we also have to be mindful that the reception of the medicalized discourse does not always sit well with indigenous and peasant communities. Medicalized discourses and practices may often disorient and bemuse people undergoing treatment and orientation on health issues. Similar to the Guajá, many of the non-Indian Amazonians have their own concepts of ethnomedicine. As such, they have their own constructs for health, curing, illness, dying, and disease.

Thus, when health professionals attempt to convey their standards for breastfeeding, weaning, treating diarrhea, and so on, their discourse is often not contextualized or sensitized to the nuances of native and peasant communities. Many of the health practices are relatively new and are introduced to each community with a top-down approach and, often, these directives may encounter resistance. In one instance, we witnessed a health worker in the town of Itupiranga berate a mother on the way she was breastfeeding her child. In truth, the health worker was unfamiliar with how the mother breastfed her child yet still assumed an authoritative posture to scold and lecture the mother on correct breastfeeding practices. As she put it, "don't use your breast like a pacifier; let the baby nurse until he's satisfied!" Afterwards, the health worker turned to us and remarked that one has to be callous with mothers and caretakers lest they not learn the proper orientation and techniques of child care. Although this person may have had a point, her authoritarian approach was equally as alienating.

CHAPTER 12 Maternal–Infant Care in the Brazilian Amazon

Similar situations were encountered among the Guajá who were undergoing treatment with FUNAI and FUNASA. In the early days of contact, a number of Guajá contracted malaria. As FUNAI began administering antimalarial medicines, their methods and administration of medications were abrasive. Language barriers also created a problem, and it was difficult to inform the Guajá how prescriptions should be taken. During illness, it was difficult to keep the Guajá close by, under observation, because they frequently fan out to the forest to forage for their livelihoods.

For instance, if the Guajá would contract the vivax strain of malaria, they would stop taking their medications when they felt better. The vivax strain, while less deadly than the falciparum strain of malaria, is more treacherous because patients exhibit cycles of fever and pain, followed by brief periods of improvement. The Guajá will interpret these periods as full recovery from the illness and stop taking their medications. In turn, they will trek out to the forest to their hunting camps, leaving FUNAI agents anguishing for them to return and terminate treatment. When they are out in the forest, the bouts of fever and pain return and they no longer have access to their medications. In some instances this suspension of treatment can be fatal, and what ensues is a tense situation between FUNAI personnel and the Guajá. Mystified by the death of friends and family members, the Guajá will resist further treatment and, for their part, FUNAI agents will act more authoritarian and demand that the Guajá obey their orientation.

In this scenario, both peasant and Indian communities may languish in a state of malaise. Although most communities actively seek out treatment and are willing to try new medications and methods of treatment, they may still find reason for resistance in light of the heavy-handed discourse and procedures administered in treatment by state agents and policies. Berry (2008, p. 167) comments on a similar situation in Guatemala where women are distrustful of some health professionals and prefer staying at home than visiting obstetricians at local health clinics to deliver their babies, claiming that hospital staff "do not attend to you."

Echoing Scott (1985), Wolf (1990, p. 590) noted that subordinated peoples often resist through various forms of behavior; these may include foot dragging, lying, gossip, sabotage, forgetfulness, intrigues, and other mechanisms to not conform to mainstream efforts to forcibly assimilate them. For sure, these "weapons of the weak" can undermine attempts to improve health care for mothers and infants, but they also have the potential to serve as a diagnostic feature in assessing their health and create new venues of concern in public health policies.

The work of Sheper-Hughes (1992) in the Brazilian northeast helps portray some of these points more vividly. The Brazilian northeast is an area often stricken by drought and misery. In fact, this region as a whole exhibits Brazil's worst human development index (HDI), an indicator of the region's low status and well-being. Women in this region often find themselves subjected to conditions of squalid poverty, yet they bear a large number of children. Survival is a key issue, and when infants show little response and undergo many bouts of illness, mothers are prone to gradually withdraw support for the child. Thus, women will not invest wholeheartedly in the child and not respond attentively to the child's needs. Ultimately, this response translates into a form of triage where a child will not get fed on time, and subtle neglect will drag on to the point of a child passing on. As Sheper-Hughes points out, a "death without weeping" (1992, p. 394) follows, and women justify the passing of the child as the will of God.

Forline's previous work in a coastal fishing village of Maranhão showed a similar trend. During 8 months of fieldwork, 12 children died from dehydration occasioned by intestinal maladies. In one instance, the parents of the deceased child asked to have photographs taken of the ritual wake. In one of the photographs the child's mother was visibly smiling. On the surface, her reaction seems insensitive and a confession of being relieved of a burden. Perhaps this is an unfair characterization, yet on another level, we can interpret her behavior as a coping mechanism against very adverse odds. Much of the passive aggression we are addressing here speaks to a structural violence that mothers encounter in their daily lives, and they adopt these behaviors and attitudes as a coping mechanism against a dynamic that literally cannibalizes them and their children.

REFLECTIONS AND RECOMMENDATIONS

The studies presented in this chapter provide a continuum of responses and health conditions experienced by communities in Brazil's eastern Amazon region. These communities included indigenous groups that were recently contacted by the Brazilian state and those that have been assimilated into Brazilian mainstream society. For their part, peasant communities of the region represent a group of people undergoing rapid change as well. Already integrated into Brazilian mainstream society at the lower rungs of the socioeconomic ladder, these groups have adopted a mixed set of livelihoods as a class of unskilled laborers. In their case, reduced infrastructure, poor purchasing power, education, and socioeconomic status contributed to the quality of health care and well-being

CHAPTER 12 Maternal–Infant Care in the Brazilian Amazon

of mothers and infants. While the foci of development are more targeted to the goals of nation building and income generation, public policy has sporadic trends of improvement in terms of infrastructure development and health care.

Each of the communities examined in this chapter must be treated individually, within the parameters of its own history, ecology, and influences of local development. Yet in our attempt to show a broader perspective of the Amazonian experience, we provided some insight into the general and specific dynamics influencing most communities of this region for comparative purposes. All told, these communities are experiencing a similar series of external pressures that are altering their lifestyles and contribute to inconsistent and sporadic health care for mothers and infants. As mothers are forced to wean at earlier intervals, children lose the benefits of breastfeeding and begin to experience a number of ailments. Food security is also compromised and is frequently accompanied by a reduction in nutritional quality.

In an effort to propose food pyramid guidelines, a number of criteria were made to formulate suggestions that would contribute to food alternatives. In order to recommend foods that could be embraced in a revised food guide pyramid, the criteria of compatibility, accessibility, and feasibility were taken into consideration. Other considerations also assessed the bias of current food guide pyramids that are in vogue because they can tilt toward a diet more compatible with other regions of Brazil, in addition to being based on a North American and European model for dietary practices. Additionally, a number of health professionals now acknowledge the influence of political lobbying in the elaboration of dietary guidelines (Nestle, 2002; Harris & Ross, 1987). These factors not only influence the types of food people eat, they also undermine and marginalize healthy alternatives to eating.

Another factor must also be considered in evaluating alternative recommendations. The recent publicity given to tropical forest products is on the rise, often accompanied by an aggressive advertising campaign to market products that would improve the livelihoods of local residents, increase economic opportunities, and save the rainforests. One such product is the açaí palm (*Euterpe oleracea*). This tree provides local residents with building materials, fodder, and food. The most common of these food items is the açaí berry juice and palm hearts. The former is now encountered in a number of products sold in retail supermarkets in North America and Europe. Berry juice, yogurts, beverages, ice cream, and jam are but a few of the açaí products sold and, in southern Brazil, the açaí drink is touted as a healthy energizer for athletes. In North America it is also marketed for its antioxidants and medicinal uses.

For their part, indigenous and peasant communities of the Amazon rely on açaí berry wine as a main staple in their diets. Riverine dwellers often prepare the wine without sweeteners to accompany a meal of fish and manioc flour. This berry wine is rich in calories, vitamin A, iron, oil, and protein. As this forms part of the local Amazonian diet, where mothers often introduce it to infants in the weaning process, our team recommended including açaí as an alternative in the food pyramid guideline. Not only would this recommendation lift açaí from its relegated status, its inclusion in the food pyramid would legitimize it as a viable and affordable alternative, an alternative with relatively easy access for peoples of the Amazon. Unfortunately, the recent hype given this product has promoted a big run on açaí stands, compromising the sustainability of this resource as a natural product.

In view of this scenario, we see that a food once relegated, or unnoticed, in terms of dietary recommendations is now thrust onto the market in what would seemingly benefit all parties, including local resident stakeholders and the tropical forest. Yet after it was transformed into a global commodity, we saw this item begin to dwindle and become beyond the reach of peasant and indigenous groups. Thus, such a lobbying and publicity effort eventually expropriates a valuable subsistence resource that can lead to a monopoly on açaí landscapes and their fruits, restricting its access for traditional stakeholders (Brondizio, Carolina, & Siqueira, 2002).

CONCLUDING REMARKS

In this paper we showed a continuum of Amazonian communities ranging from little contact with Brazilian mainstream society to those that are squarely enmeshed in the machinations of development policy and, by extension, the mechanisms of globalization. In each case, the well-being of mothers and infants is challenged as the rapid and unfettered pace of Amazonian development takes to the wing. While the administration of president Luiz Inácio Lula da Silva (Lula) was lauded for its efforts to transform Brazil into a more just and equal society, it mimicked and embraced the heavy development posture set in motion by previous administrations that adhered to neoliberal policies and agendas. As Brazil enters the 21st century, it aspires to place itself squarely in the league of developed nations and situate itself in the global economy. Thus, even if praised as a promoter of community development, enhancing the quality of life for disenfranchised people, the benefits that would accrue to Amazonian peoples are subordinated to Brazil's aspirations to be a leader in the global community.

And as globalization proceeds at full speed, the stakes increase as foreign players also pitch in to invest in Amazonian development. In light of these developments, we have provided some insights to the realities of indigenous and peasant communities vis-à-vis mother and infant health, reflecting on their prospects and diagnosing some features that could be examined for future reference. While the internal mechanisms of these societies have helped them cope accordingly, these still have to be assessed in face of the speed, velocity, and intensity of Amazonian development and globalization.

Discussion Questions

1. Explore the influence of the ecological landscape of the Amazon region on the belief systems and health practices of the Guajá.
2. a. Compare the implications of the concept of multiple paternity for female sexuality to that of women in your own country.
   b. Do the same for paternal responsibility.
   c. How has contact with the outside world changed gender relations among the Guajá?
3. Modernization has changed the lifestyle and nutritional patterns of the Guajá. Explain how this may influence fertility and child rearing patterns.
4. Compare and contrast the health status and practices of the Guajá with the mostly peasant communities in the PAHO study. Speculate about the reasons for these differences and similarities.
5. Consider that FUNAI nurses treat moniliasis with medication. Do you think this encourages the nursing of pets? If so, what do you think they should do instead, and why?
6. What are some of the challenges presented to public health professionals who use medical anthropology as a source of information about the health practices of societies that are so vastly different from their own?

REFERENCES

Beckerman, S., & Valentine, P. (2002). The concept of partible paternity among native South Americans. In S. Beckerman & P. Valentine (Eds.), *Cultures of multiple fathers: The theory and practice of partible paternity in lowland South America* (pp. 1–13). Gainesville, FL: University of Florida Press.

Berry, N. (2008). Who's judging the quality of care? Indigenous Maya and the problem of "not being attended." *Medical Anthropology, 27*(2), 164–189.

Binford, L. (1968). Post-Pleistocene Adaptations. In S. Binford & L. Binford (Eds.), *New perspectives in archaeology* (pp. 313–341). Chicago, IL: Aldine.

Brondizio, E., Carolina, S., & Siqueira, A. (2002). The urban market of açaí fruit (*Euterpe oleracea Mart.*) and rural land use change: Ethnographic insights into the role of price and land tenure constraining agricultural choices in the Amazon estuary. *Urban Ecosystems, 6*, 67–97.

Cohen, M., & Armelagos, G. (Eds.). (1984). *Paleopathology at the origins of agriculture.* New York, NY: Academic Press.

Cormier, L. (2003). *Kinship with Monkeys: The Guajá Foragers of Eastern Amazonia.* New York, NY: Columbia University Press.

Davis, S. (1978). *Victims of the miracle.* Cambridge, MA: Cambridge University Press.

Flannery, K. (1969). Origins and ecological effects of early domestication in Iran and the Near East. In P. Ucko & G. Dimbleby (Eds.), *The domestication and exploitation of plants and animals* (pp. 73–100). Chicago, IL: Aldine.

Harris, M., & Ross, E. (Eds.). (1987). *Food and evolution: Toward a theory of human food habits.* Philadelphia, PA: Temple University Press.

Keegan, W. (1986). The optimal foraging analysis of horticultural production. *American Anthropologist, 88*(1), 92–107.

Laraia, R. (1974). "Polyandrous adjustments" in Suruí Society. In P. Lyon (Ed.), *Native South Americans: Ethnology of the least known continent* (pp. 370–372). Boston, MA: Little, Brown.

Lee, R. (1992). Art, science, or politics? The crisis in hunter–gatherer studies. *American Anthropologist, 94*(1), 31–54.

McDonald, D. (1977). Food taboos: A primitive Environmental Protection Agency (South America). *Anthropos, 72,* 734–748.

Nestle, M. (2002). *Food politics: How the food industry influences nutrition and health.* Los Angeles, CA: University of California Press.

Posey, D. (1994). Environmental and social implications of pre- and postcontact situations on Brazilian Indians: The Kayapó and a new Amazonian synthesis. In A. Roosevelt (Ed.), *Amazonian Indians from prehistory to the present* (pp. 271–286). Tucson, AZ: University of Arizona Press.

Ramos, A. (1984). Frontier expansion and Indian peoples in the Brazilian Amazon. In M. Schmink & C. Wood (Eds.), *Frontier expansion in Amazonia* (pp. 83–104). Gainesville, FL: University of Florida Press.

Scott, J. (1985). *Weapons of the weak: Everyday forms of peasant resistance.* New Haven, CT: Yale University Press.

Sheper-Hughes, N. (1992). *Death without weeping: The violence of everyday life in Brazil.* Berkeley, CA: University of California Press.

CHAPTER 12 Maternal–Infant Care in the Brazilian Amazon

Sponsel, L. (1989). Farming and foraging: A necessary complementarity in Amazonia? In S. Kent (Ed.), *Farmers as hunters* (pp. 37–45). Cambridge, MA: Cambridge University Press.

Treece, D. (1987). *Bound in misery and iron: The impact of the Grande Carajás Programme on the Indians of Brazil.* London, England: Survival International.

Velho, O. (1995). *Capitalismo autoritário e campesinato.* Rio de Janeiro, Brazil: Zahar.

Wagley, C. (1974). The effects of depopulation upon social organization as illustrated by the Tapirape Indians. In P. Lyon (Ed.), *Native South Americans: Ethnology of the least known continent* (pp. 373–376). Boston, MA: Little, Brown.

Wolf, E. (1990). Distinguished lecture: Facing power. *American Anthropologist, 92*(3), 586–596.

CHAPTER 13

Mbyá Grandmothers, Mothers, and Granddaughters

Motherhood and Upbringing throughout Generations

Carolina Remorini, PhD

Location: National University of La Plata (UNLP), Argentina, South America

Name of Project: Culture, environment, and health. Ethnographic and cross-cultural study about child rearing and healthcare practices in rural and aboriginal populations.

Sponsoring Organization: National Council for Scientific and Technical Research (CONICET)

Target Population: Children aged 3 years and younger and their caregivers in Mbyá Guaraní communities (Misiones Province, Argentina) and Molinos population (Salta Province, Argentina)

Project Goal: The ethnographic research explores representations and daily child rearing practices in two rural populations of two contrasting ecological contexts in Argentina—Mbyá Guaraní indigenous communities located in the northeast rainforest (Misiones Province) and creole communities from Molinos (Salta Province)—in the highlands and semiarid areas of the Argentinean northwest

CHAPTER 13 Mbyá Grandmothers, Mothers, and Granddaughters

> **Project Objectives:**
> 1. Identify and characterize ecocultural factors that influence child development and health–illnesses processes in various populations in Argentinian territory
> 2. Make a comparative analysis of the impact of ecocultural factors on child development and health–illnesses processes
> 3. Develop and contrast hypotheses about the differential value of these factors with regard to their impact on the populations studied

INTRODUCTION

The information in this chapter is the result of research[1] carried out between 2001 and 2005 in Mbyá Guaraní communities in the province of Misiones, Argentina, that focused on the study of health–illness processes in the first stages of the life cycle (Remorini, 2008). Based on that, the aim of this chapter is to analyze both the discourse and practices of women of different ages about experiences such as pregnancy, delivery, the postpartum period, and child rearing. In order to do so, our study is based on the results of combined and complemented applications of different qualitative techniques, including daily observation (Lewis, 1985), genealogies, and semistructured interviews. The use of observation and discourse allowed information triangulation and enabled us to contrast the hypotheses that emerged throughout the research.

Working with women belonging to different generations allowed us to gain access to the way they speak about changes in their knowledge and practices related to pregnancy and delivery, as well as health–illness processes during these stages of their life cycle, within the context of transformations in the Mbyá way of life.

In this chapter, we consider three cases, based on the information obtained from interviewing three women of different ages and the observation of their everyday activities. By means of this selection we attempted to show the diversity of life courses inside the Mbyá society, where the different perspectives, customs, projects, and decision-making criteria can be seen. This allows us to transcend the homogeneous and static way of seeing Mbyá women that appeared in classical literature about this ethnic group so we could perform analyses focused on these women's everyday life, taking into account their numerous present contexts. We will particularly focus on their health conditions, their opportunities to access health services, and their views of those services.

This chapter aims to contribute a different outlook on everyday life and expectations of these indigenous women about both their children's and their own health care within a context of deep ecological, economic, political, and cultural changes.

MBYÁ CHILDREN AND WOMEN: HEALTH CONDITIONS AND THEIR ACCESS TO SANITARY SERVICES AND PROGRAMS

At present, there are some communities, scattered throughout Argentina, Brazil, and Paraguay, that belong to the Mbyá people. The total population is about 19,200 individuals (Assis & Garlet, 2004). In our country, according to the Complementary Survey of Indigenous Peoples (ECPI) in 2005, there are about 3,975 people who recognize themselves as belonging to the Mbyá Guaraní people in Misiones Province. The Mbyá language is spoken within these communities, and most adults and schoolchildren also speak Spanish and, less frequently, Yopara (Paraguayan Guaraní) and Portuguese. The Mbyá communities where we developed our research settled on land that is considered a private reservation, Valle del Arroyo Kuña-Pirú, which belongs to UNLP, in Misiones Province between Cainguas and Libertador General San Martín departments. Provincial Route Number 7, which connects these settlements with neighboring localities and other Mbyá communities on the basin of Cuña Piru I and II streams, goes through the northern part of the reservation. According to a census we made in May 2003, both communities constitute a total of 280 people. These figures may have changed due to the constant movement of individuals and families among the different settlements as part of their life strategies. From a demographic point of view, it is a young population, with most individuals between 0 and 14 years of age (54%).

The present subsistence strategies combine traditional activities—horticulture, hunting, fishing, and gathering in the *monte* (forest)—with new ones that have emerged from their relationship with several sectors of national society. At present, craft selling and temporary paid jobs in *colonias* (rural settlements devoted to the production of yerba mate, tea, tobacco, and tung) contribute to

CHAPTER 13 Mbyá Grandmothers, Mothers, and Granddaughters

the subsistence of most households. Some individuals receive allowances, and others get a salary for being teaching assistants or sanitary agents. The money obtained from either activity allows them to obtain supplies (flour, sugar, pasta, rice, beans, cold cuts, soda, and candy, etc.), which has resulted in a lesser degree of commitment to traditional food-gathering activities and important dietary changes (Remorini, 2008). Consequently, according to our research, the most frequent illnesses in indigenous populations are respiratory, gastrointestinal, and nutritional (Navone, Gamboa, Oyhenart, & Orden, 2006; Remorini, 2008; Sy, 2008). The relationship among infection by geohelminths, malnutrition, and anemia has been shown in numerous research papers (Navone et al., 2006; Sy, 2008; Sy & Remorini, 2009).

In Ka'aguy Poty community there was a sanitary station until 2000. It had two permanent staff members: a nurse and a sanitary agent (aborigine). A doctor who provided primary health attention (PHA) paid a weekly visit. At present, a doctor from the Dirección de Asuntos Guaraníes visits the communities to deliver PHA, but not on a permanent basis. This is done with the help of the local sanitary agent. The doctor generally has medicine (antibiotics, antifever, antiparasite, pain killers) to solve the most common problems. The sanitary agent is a member of the community and is appointed by the Health Ministry of Misiones Province, within the framework of the Program for the National Support of Humanitarian Actions for Indigenous Populations (ANAHI). His job involves distributing medicine (under a doctor's supervision) and recording and distributing powdered milk granted by the provincial government to pregnant women and children younger than age 2 years, whose weight and health state are checked. Work in the Sanitary Unit was extended to nearby communities, such as Yvy Pytã and Ka'a-Kupe.

The Mbyá population in this area goes to urban centers to solve health problems that cannot be solved within the community by local specialists.[2] One of the most frequently attended health centers is Unidad Sanitaria Aristóbulo del Valle, which has doctors, odontologists, and biochemists on its staff. This unit is about 14 kilometers from both communities. Less frequently, the population also goes to the Hospital de Jardín América (30 kilometers), which has more advanced services. Other alternatives are the hospitals in Oberá and Posadas, which are situated farther away from the communities (58 and 147 kilometers, respectively). The latter, although it is farther away, has the advantage of being near the government organization (Dirección de Asuntos Guaraníes) that offers accommodation to members of aborigine communities (Sy & Remorini, 2008).

Sanitary programs in indigenous communities were recently established (within the past 10 years), and their development and results have been influenced by the discontinuities that are characteristic of public policies in Argentina. In spite of the state's interest to reach the indigenous population with programs (e.g., ANAHI of the National Health Ministry 2000–2005; the Community Team for Originary Peoples; Plan Nacer; and Techaî Mbyá—Indigenous Health—Province Health Ministry), there are serious barriers to accessing health assistance.

Experts on the subject agree that the main obstacle to improving the health situation in indigenous communities is the lack of specific information about epidemiology within the Guaraní population in the province. This makes it difficult for us to accurately analyze the distribution of health indicators among the Mbyá Guaraní. Even though a higher appeal to biomedical health services has been recorded, aborigines face a lot of difficulties related to their interaction with the staff. Among these barriers is the homogenization of the target population, the lack of culturally acceptable strategies, the poor training of sanitary staff to work with indigenous populations, the difficulties to mutual communication and understanding, the aboriginal expectations about medical diagnosis and treatment, and the distant locations of health services (Foro de Investigación en Salud de Argentina, 2008; Sy & Remorini, 2008).

BACKGROUND OF MOTHERS AND WIVES: MBYÁ WOMEN IN THE ETHNOGRAPHIC LITERATURE

The Guaraní are one of the ethnic groups in South America that have been most written about; descriptions of their beliefs and customs can be found in the early records of naturalists and missionaries in the 17th and 18th centuries. Beginning in the 20th century, anthropologists have also shown interest in Guaraní linguistic differences and lifestyles, due not only to their wide mobility and geographic dispersion, but also because of their contact with other societies throughout time (Clastres, 1993; Metraux, 1927, 1948a, 1948b; Müller, 1989; Schaden, 1991; Susnik, 1983). Moreover, some ethnographers have accounted for the common aspects, beliefs, and practices that make the Guaraní a cultural unit beyond regional variations (Schaden, 1991).

With regard to the Mbyá in particular, Cadogan's extensive work is the most obvious starting point to approach any subject related to the Mbyá from Paraguay. Cadogan examines in various papers, through their myths and accounts, the Mbyá's beliefs and practices related to health care in different stages of the life cycle, mainly during gestation and childhood (1948, 1949, 1950, 1971, 1997). His main text (1997) contains some very significant passages about the human being's constitutional process and the events that may cause illnesses and death in different stages of the life cycle. Cadogan stresses the importance ascribed to pre- and postbirth care (mainly in terms of respecting taboos and performing traditional rituals) for the newborn's health and the individual and collective consequences of that care.

We also found in other papers some references to child rearing and health care associated to life cycle characterization, where beliefs about conception, the soul, birth, and puberty rituals are described and compared in Guaraní ethnic groups (Metraux, 1948b; Susnik, 1983). Many of these authors devote only a few paragraphs to childhood. The way they treat childhood is limited to describing games and puberty initiation ceremonies (Metraux, 1948b; Müller, 1989).

Not much is mentioned about motherhood. There is very little reference to the mother's health, which is sometimes limited to describing delivery and listing a few taboos during gestation and the postpartum period (Cadogan, 1950, 1997; Susnik, 1983). Occasionally these appear as only superstitions or magical beliefs without an in-depth study of their meaning and their relationship to other aspects of the culture. Conversely, a lot has been written about the Guaraní women and their traditional roles of wife and mother. Susnik states that since historical times, "a Guaraní woman's ideal has always been her role as hai, mother-breeder, the guarantee of community continuity (teyy)" (1983, p. 16). In every ethnographic paper, the importance the Mbyá ascribe to maternity is reinforced, as is a child's birth because it enables the society's continuity. The Mbyá's desire to have a lot of children is attributed to this, as is the social undervaluation of an infertile woman (Cadogan, 1950, 1997) and the fact that an individual achieves Karai or Kuña Karai status, as an adult, only after his or her first child is born (Cadogan, 1997). Therefore, parenthood is an event that marks an important transition in any individual's life cycle.

Likewise, the literature reinforces women's relationship with the domestic realm, which is linked to child care, food preparation, and looking after the fire. Therefore, according to Cadogan, "The Guaraní woman's duty within her culture may be defined as 'being next to the fire'" (1971, p. 113). It is in this sense that women are considered to be oriented to the inside (home, the community), and men are oriented to the outside, that is, they go into different spaces that are, supposedly, exclusively male (the monte, or rainforest), and they go out to other communities and cities to work or participate in political meetings.

This characterization of traditional roles and activities seems to hide other roles that women perform, but at the same time they offer a static and stereotyped image of themselves. In fact, the long-time, exclusive use of male informants (in part due to linguistic issues) and the predominance of spoken sources over observational records of everyday activities has led to Mbyá women becoming invisible. It is only in the past years that an interest has arisen to describe the women's actions in different contexts than the domestic one, as shown in the documentary and bibliographic revision work by Dos Santos Landa (1995). Ciccarone, in turn, published a thesis (2001) focused on the character of a Kuña Karai (shaman woman) in a Brazilian village and analyzed her performance in different spheres of the village everyday life and her leadership while moving to different places in search for better life conditions. This work turns out to be particularly interesting because there are scant references to women's performance within the domain of religion and therapeutics. In that respect, Martínez, Crivos, and the author of the present chapter have extensively dealt with the old roles of women, their everyday activities, and their contribution to the domestic group's subsistence, as well as child rearing and health care and welfare of all community members due to their therapeutic and religious knowledge (Martinez, Crivos, & Remoini, 2002; Remorini, 2005, 2006).

We have recently found a paper by Enriz and García Palacios (2008) that focuses on describing the process by which a girl becomes a woman, that is, Kuña, Karai and points out the changes that take place in roles and social relationships among women, and among women and men, from the moment of a woman's first menstruation.

In short, we do not have any systematic ethnographic studies on Mbyá women in Argentina, except for the ones quoted. The studies on child rearing and health care are also scarce, and it is difficult to find official data on Mbyá children and women's health in our country. The research developed by the author (as described in the Introduction) contributes by making these subjects visible, along with the problems affecting their development possibilities.

DIFFERENT STORIES, THE SAME CULTURE: INTRACULTURAL VARIABILITY AND GENERATIONAL CHANGES

As we said at the beginning, using three cases (Kerechu, Jachuka, and Para) will allow us to develop different aspects of women's everyday life, as well as their

CHAPTER 13 Mbyá Grandmothers, Mothers, and Granddaughters

knowledge, expectations, and practices related to their own and their children's health care. It is necessary to clarify that these cases were not chosen for being representative of statistics, but because they offer the possibility of exploring convergences and differences about the aspects we pointed out. Through them, we can account for generational perceptions of beliefs and practices in health care during pregnancy, delivery, and the postpartum period.

Kerechu: "I Am Guaymi, That's It, We Are from the Past"

Kerechu is the Mbyá name of AC (50). She was born in Garuhape Mini village (El Alcazar locality), and she lived in Leoni, Yvy Pytã and then in Ka'aguy Poty, where we interviewed her. She is married (*acompañada*) to Adolfo, 51, and they have two children: Francisco and Santa. Kerechu had her first child at the age of 18 years. Three of her daughters died very young.

> (How many children do you have?) three alive and . . . let's see . . . three dead ones . . . one died of, of measles, one of diarrhea . . . the other died of . . . I don't know what it was . . . (How old was she?) one died when she was one year old, the one with diarrhea, the one with measles died when she was 7 months old . . . the other also died when she was 7 months old . . . (Where did they die?) They died . . . the first one, in El Dorado . . . and the other one, the one with diarrhea, died near . . . Intercontinental, that is near Brazil (Did they die at the hospital or at home?) No, at home because I was never at the hospital, you see, I never had my children at the hospital, they were all born at home, all of them. My mum help me and some other woman, a midwife.

Francisco is married (acompañado) and has a 3-month-old daughter. Another daughter had previously died 15 days after birth from respiratory infection. Francisco and his wife live with his grandmother in 1º de Mayo, a faraway village. Santa, who is also married, has two children (a 2-year-old daughter and an 11-month-old son). She lives with her family in Concepción, close to the southern border with Corrientes Province. Both Santa's and Francisco's children were born in state hospitals. Their children's and their granddaughter's deaths were caused by the health problems we previously described, that is, infectious-contagious and gastrointestinal diseases that have a greater impact on children's morbidity and mortality.

Kerechu defines herself as *guaymi*, an elderly lady from the past—that is, she leads the same kind of life her ancestors led. Her speech focuses on traditional patterns and practices in relation to women's health care from their first menstruation, during pregnancy and delivery, and caring for the newborn child. She emphasizes that she never gave birth at the hospital, and she usually assists other women in her community, as other woman assisted her in her own youth. This is how she explains the midwife's task during delivery and the mother's care afterwards:

> You have to rub the belly and movements for the baby to go down; she must be sitting . . . and the woman who helps her has to know where the baby's head is, and if you have found the head, then you must make it go down . . . then we give her a herb tea so that it doesn't hurt. She must go on taking the tea for three days, for the belly not to hurt.

The massage they perform to place the child in the right position for birth; the administration of "remedies" favoring delivery and relieving postdelivery pain; the provision of smoking tobacco (*sahumados*) to scare away evil spirits (*mbogua*) who may harm both the mother and the child; and the advice these women usually give to the laboring woman (rest, proper food, etc.) cause them to be highly valued specialists within the community.

According to the information obtained from two sets of fieldwork, in both communities 90% of babies were born in hospitals, and most of their mothers were born within the community environment, which accounts for a generational difference in terms of their use of healthcare services. Although most of them choose hospital delivery, some women still choose to have their babies within the community because they feel safer and calmer in the company of the midwife and other women in their family. That is, they prioritize emotional support over arguments about the higher risk they will be exposed to in the community (see the following discussions of Jachuka and Para).

Although most elderly women, like Kerechu, favor delivery in the community, some of them find it beneficial to have assistance at the hospital. No adult or elderly men expressed being in favor of that practice. Younger men (between ages 20 and 30 years), on the other hand, believe it is up to the woman to decide where she would like to get help. In general, those who choose the hospital have been trained as sanitary agents or nurses. Those who prefer delivery in the community give preference to two factors: (1) more emotional support and more attentive care to the woman when she is surrounded by her relatives, and (2) the ability to have women of different ages watch during the delivery, which favors intergenerational transmission of traditional practices.

Going back to Kerechu's account, she highly values the fact that she almost never went to the hospital. This is quite ordinary among elderly people. They

CHAPTER 13   Mbyá Grandmothers, Mothers, and Granddaughters

usually say, "I never got ill and I never went to hospital." That is, the absence of illness is associated with the fact that they never go to the hospital. This does not imply that they never got ill, but this argument is used to enhance a generational difference in relation to health conditions ("there was less illness in the past") and to young people's decisions ("now they all go to hospital"). In speaking about her own health, Kerechu says that she was ill a few times. Nevertheless, she remembers suffering from great depression when her first son died and had to be admitted to the hospital:

> When I was 18 I was admitted I don't know what about, and I had a relapse, you see, after that . . . never again, because when I had the first one who died, I got bad, I got sad, I went in hospital, I was admitted. . . . for a long time, yes . . . a month, I got saline solution, injections, pills, but I don't remember the name (And after that you never had any illness?) no, never, a few times . . . I had a headache or flu, or a fever, but not bad, I cured very soon, with *yuyo* (medicinal herbs) . . . well, there are illnesses, you see, but when you take care you don't get ill very often, if you believe in God you don't get ill and nothing happens to you. God looks after you.

From her perspective, though she has suffered from some illnesses, she does not believe them to have been serious. She was able to solve them within the community, using medicinal plants.

Finally, and in relation to little children's health care, Kerechu advocates the need to respect food prohibitions, consume food that is "light" (not heavy) or "ours" (of Mbyá culture), and avoid sexual intercourse for some time.

> *Mbaipy* or some *locro*[3] we prepare, with a mortar take all the kernel corns, take the kernels off the cob and we put them in the mortar . . . sometimes some kind of bean is put, and when some tatú meat can be found, that is put, too, because that is our own food, also some coatí or some deer from the forest. [Otherwise] you can catch some illness, some relapse or headache, dizziness, then you look after her, she doesn't get up for some days, you look after her, give her something to eat, but she mustn't get up.

Apart from food restrictions, the prohibition of sexual intercourse between spouses is indicated to avoid another pregnancy. Among the reasons for the prohibition are the woman's need to devote herself exclusively to feed and nourish the child. It would be difficult for her to look after more than one breastfeeding baby at a time. The baby's vulnerable condition during this time justifies the need to guarantee a long breastfeeding period as a way to avoid illnesses. It is worth mentioning than some of the elderly women's main criticisms about young mothers is that they do not breastfeed their children for as long as "the ones from before" did, and they sometimes choose to give bottled milk, which, from their point of view, does not feed or protect the infants in the same way. Kerechu says that she breastfed her children until they were 1 year old and supplemented their diet with a milk bottle and bee honey. Changes in child rearing patterns and their consequences on health are considered, by the women in Kerechu's generation, the result of a break in intergenerational transmission of Mbyá knowledge and practices:

> The old ones are the ones who know the most, how the Mbyá live before, and now everybody, almost nobody knew nothing else, history, children know almost nothing, Mbyá history . . . before, the mother gave them advice, to the girls, how they had to live, when they had the menstruation, they talked to the mothers, the aunts "you are my daughter, you're going to be a woman, you are no child any more, go around like a lady, do your lady things . . . work as a lady does and then, when you find someone you are interest in . . . marry."

Jachuka: Keeping Tradition and Participating in Changes

Jachuka (29) has seven children and lives with them, her husband, and her mother-in-law in Ka'aguy Poty, where her parents live, as well as her uncles, aunts, grandmothers, and eight siblings. Jachuka's husband was trained in educational and sanitary institutions and was a sanitary agent for a few years. Her two grandmothers are prestigious old ladies because of their knowledge as traditional therapists and midwives. Jachuka's house is somewhat apart from her family's, but there is permanent traffic of mainly women and children. Her everyday activities basically consist of performing domestic chores—with her mother-in-law and children's help—and making crafts for sale.

In several ways, Jachuka's everyday life and accounts reflect the continuity of traditional patterns for rearing children and for mother and child health care. When it comes to little children's nourishment, for example, she tells us about the food that is allowed and forbidden at a certain age:

> I always breastfeed them until one year and five months, so, because if they have teeth it hurts already, well, to some I gave until two years (And if they have teeth they may start with something solid?) yes, when they were six months old they already had a little soup, rice, corn meal, beans too, but in soup, AnD already eats, now she likes eating everything, meat too, chicken, always chicken, boiled, beef is also eaten (and pork?) no, not pig because it is bad for children, they say, I don't

CHAPTER 13   Mbyá Grandmothers, Mothers, and Granddaughters

> know why, that's why we, Mbyá, don't give pig for one year and five months (Why is it bad for babies?) well, because it gives diarrhea, some babies have diarrhea because some are fed at 5, 6 months things they can't eat and they get ill, they catch parasites, the older people say (And before they are one year old, what do you give them?) only milk (And who gives you advice on these things?) my granmother, old ladies are the ones who always advise moms.

The pregnancy period (*mitã yrui*) and the 2 months after birth (*mitã*[4] *pyta*) are considered extremely vulnerable for both the mother and the baby, and there are a lot of restrictions in terms of diet, everyday activities, and the spaces they should stay in and go about, which also affect other members of the domestic group. It becomes obvious from Jachuka's accounts that breaking the rules may cause illnesses in the child that will require traditional specialists' intervention or consulting health services, depending on the kind of illness:

> (How should mitã yrui be looked after?) well, you don't have to do any heavy job . . . you may go to the stream but not bring soaked clothes . . . that is heavy, I always go with somebody else, you can clean, but slowly, go and fetch water, you can, cook too . . . some of them go, it depends on the person, I went to the stream and I almost fell and I was hit, the baby was somewhat bad, that's why I had to be admitted and stay at the hospital in Obera for two days . . . it hurt and I could barely walk . . . I had an ultrasound (at the hospital) everything to see if it was all right (And is there any other thing that is forbidden?) well, you shouldn't take any yuyo (herbs) medicine when you're pregnant, there are some that are very strong (And who advises on which remedies can be taken?) well, sometimes my mum, but sometimes my husband says, because my husband knows everything, too, because he attends courses on all that (And does he explain to you why they can't be taken?) yes, well, that it is for the baby to be born healthy and for me too.

It is interesting to note that when they are asked about what should or should not be done during that period, informants (between 20 and 30 years old) refer to a set of restrictions that have been respected since "the old people's times" (*el tiempo de los antiguos*) to avoid damaging the child's health or to avoid complications during delivery (the most frequent restrictions are to avoid contact with "twin" elements, do not link or tie things, and do not weave baskets, along with the ones already mentioned). Nevertheless, when we intend to go deeper into the consequences of these restrictions, only a few people can account for the connection between the rule and its effects on the child's health. Most of them, including Jachuka, have admitted they do not know the reasons behind such prohibitions, resorting to explanations like "it's our custom," "according to the elders it is like this," or "it is our system."

In her speech, Jachuka overvalues the possibility of having access to the knowledge and resources of scientific medicine and, at the same time, she recognizes the pertinence and efficiency of traditional knowledge and practices, passed on by her grandparents and parents. Moreover, she takes into account the knowledge provided by her husband, Alberto ("because my husband knows about health things, he trained for that"), and accepts what he says as a valid explanatory alternative or solution to a health problem. Alberto, though he prioritizes biomedical knowledge over that of grandparents, does not discard the possibility of the grandparents' knowledge being pertinent, and he seeks a way to integrate that knowledge into an explanation of the causes of his children's illnesses by taking into account various factors. As an example, we quote a passage of an interview he participated in:

> Because I think that is true, because there you have my daughter, who has parasites, and my wife said that was because we ate coatí's meat too soon, and pig's, and that is true, it has been proved, you see. But to me, and I know, in some way it has to do with cleanliness too. (AD, 32, Ka'aguy Poty, Aboriginal Sanitary Agent, 2001)

In other words, when he retrospectively looked for the causes that led to his daughter's illness, he recognizes the need for still respecting dietary taboos concerning the parents while the child is "new" (mitã pyta), thus reasserting its validity ("it has been proved") and at the same time incorporating another factor (lack of hygiene), which is prioritized by biomedical experts as a main cause for enteroparasitoses.

Let us continue examining Jachuka's speech about mother and newborn child care:

> Mothers must always be cared for because they shouldn't go around the cold, the water, the stream, because if they went around the water before two months, their belly hurts, and the head too ... and babies must be cared for a lot too, they must be cleaned and they mustn't be outside all the time, in el yard, because of the wind ... well, sometimes until thirty days if age they can't be taken a long way ... because of the wind, it's bad for them, they say (And the mum, where must she stay?) just in the house, she can't go out or a long way, she must stay at home and slowly clean around the house, one must be still, the brothers and sisters too (the newborn's) they have to be still because otherwise illness comes through the little head, it gets on its head (the baby's), in Mbyá it is called ojeo

CHAPTER 13   Mbyá Grandmothers, Mothers, and Granddaughters

ke´a, like he can't look well and he cries too, he cries and he can't be peaceful and he can't sleep, he cries a lot . . . just born, must be looked after until ten months, until the head is open, here (she points to the suture of the frontal bone with the parietal ones) . . . I don't know what they call it because it takes time to close the head bone, and the navel is dangerous too, it doesn't close (And if that happens, can it be cured?) yes, it is cured, with remedies, chamomile, tuna (And did that ever happen to any of your children?) yes, it happened to AD and to OD (And did you know how it had to be cured?) no, well, OD is the first one, that's why I didn't know and my mum taught me and now I know (And when that happens you don't take him to hospital?) I did take to hospital but doctors don't know about that (And do you take them to the opyguã when that happens?) no, I sometimes asked for that but she (her mother) never took to the opyguã, now they almost don't take, but before they always took to the opyguã, and then sometimes the children died, older ones too . . . because they didn't go to the doctor before, but now . . . if it is something serious I always take to hospital . . . but if you have kamby ryru jere not any more (Is that an illness?) yes, it is an illness the babies catch, they have diarrhea with vomiting and it doesn't stop, it doesn't stop and it can't eat, it becomes skinny, small, it can die, it's not like any diarrhea . . . it happened twice to AD, my grandmother cured him here . . . in hospital they gave him medicine but didn't cure.

The most worrying illnesses are those affecting the gastrointestinal system (diarrheas, parasites) and those considered specific to infancy: ojeo ke´a and kamby ryru jere, which can be treated only by local healers. Regarding gastrointestinal ailments, parasitoses are the higher-risk ones for little children's health, due to their consequences on growth and development. In this sense, recurring parasitoses and diarrhea during the first months of life lead to the child being "skinny," "undernourished" (*ipirui*), "without any strength," and vulnerable to other illnesses. Another important symptom is the delay to walk, which produces great concern because it is the start of free vertical walk that indicates a change in children's status (Remorini, 2008).

Ojeo ke´a consists of a subsidence of the frontal fontanel, or its late closing.[5] To describe this ailment, it is often said that the child has "his little head split open." Typical symptoms are irritability and crying. Although this illness is not very frequent, unlike respiratory and gastrointestinal conditions, its occurrence causes great concern, and most of the time experts are consulted for treatment. It may have different origins and is not generally attributed to only one cause. It may have originated in "stress" prior to birth or because taboos may have been ignored in the family environment (Remorini, 2008).

Different Stories, the Same Culture

Kamby ryru jere (literally, "rotating stomach") is an illness affecting only unweaned babies. Our informants often said that babies are exclusively breastfed until they are 5 or 6 months old, and then some solid food and bottled milk are incorporated. In this sense, kamby ryru (milk stomach) is the name for the unweaned babies' digestive organ. This ailment occurs when babies receive a strong blow or when they fall on the floor. The risk of being affected by this is the main reason why Jachuka does not want to leave the baby in the care of her younger children: "that's why one can't leave the children looking after the little ones, at least until they are 7 or 8, because they may drop them and they may get kamby ryru jere."

The diagnosis is made by observing the length of the child's legs, that is, if one leg is shorter than the other, it means the stomach has rotated toward that side. The symptoms also include vomiting and diarrhea. In that case, the diarrhea is "like water," that is, it is watery, without any consistence, which leads to recognizing "it is not *any* diarrhea." The treatment differs according to each expert. Some of them use medicinal plants, and others cure it with tobacco smoke in addition to massaging the child's legs until they are a normal length. When the child is made to lie down on the dorsal decubitus and the feet are at the same level, the child is considered cured (Remorini, 2008; Sy, 2008). Because of the uniqueness of this treatment, parents do not consult a doctor for this pathology.

On the other hand, Jachuka expresses her preference for hospital attention in cases when, in her view, traditional experts' participation does not prove effective—in particular, when it comes to facing "serious" illnesses or those requiring a fast solution. As other interviewees state, scientific medicine is preferred in those cases because, even though local therapeutic resources (medicinal plants and ritual procedures) are considered effective, a longer time is required for them to be effective. It is clear that their access to medical intervention can prevent some deaths that could not be avoided in the past. Another situation where the hospital appears to be a more efficient alternative is delivery. The arguments in favor of choosing the hospital include that it is "safer" for the woman in case she has severe hemorrhaging, her recovery is faster, the child's height and weight is controlled, and the child receives obligatory vaccinations. Likewise, many Mbyá women and men justify their choice on the grounds that there are a few old women in their community who may serve as midwives.

It should be taken into account that there are no private vehicles in these communities. Therefore, if a woman starts to feel labor pains in the early hours of the morning, she will probably give birth right there because there is no access to any kind of public transport at that time. It is interesting to notice, then, that the decision to go to the hospital does not necessarily include the possibility of having a traditional midwife. Jachuka and two of her sisters decided to go to the hospital to have all their children, in spite of the fact that their grandmothers are experienced midwives. When asked about the reason for this, Jachuka said the following:

> I'm afraid to have, now there are a few midwives and it may be dangerous because sometimes it comes in the wrong way, or sometimes it is not born normal, a lot died at birth, sometimes, if the baby comes in the wrong way, nothing can be done in the community... Guaymi i (old women) think that women go to hospital and they don't want to give birth in the community (And your mum, for example, what does she think?) my mum agrees because... she had a baby at home before and I don't know what happened, my mum almost died because of that, then they always went to hospital... I saw one baby died, my mum almost died.

Para: Articulating the Inside and the Outside

Para (22) lives with her husband, Carlos (29), and her three children in a dwelling near her mother-in-law and her sisters-in-law. Every nuclear family has a different house (four altogether) that are separated by a few meters. The women, youth, and children in this extended family, whose referent is Silvia (60), Para's mother-in-law, spend most of the day together, preparing food, looking after the children, playing, talking, doing crafts, and watching television. Carlos and his brother spend most of the week away from the community, working in Posadas (a city). Silvia and one of Para's sisters-in-law are in charge of looking after the children when she goes out to study at Jardín América (a city).

Before her second child's birth, Para decided to "change" during the last months of her pregnancy and give birth in the *Chapa i* community. Her decision was based on her need to be near the women in her family she has a closer bond with, which is very valuable in these situations. Her other children were born in the hospital.

Para's life story is marked by her constant circulation between Mbyá communities and cities. Para considers this "coming and going" a way to gain access to new knowledge and opportunities. She has studied to become a health agent, and in 2003 she was training to become a professional nurse at a private institution. Her interest in community health has led her to take charge of negotiations to get appointments for people at hospitals and to get medicine for them, though she has not been officially appointed as a sanitary agent. Her training at biomedical institutions allows her to have a somewhat critical position in relation to some beliefs "from the grandmothers," though she finds much of their advice effective. In her speech, an integration of biomedical terms is noticed, as well as the elaboration of traditional beliefs in light of scientific knowledge. This is the way Para recounts some illness episodes she went through during and after pregnancy:

> This happened to me in 2000, I felt weak, when I walked I didn't feel my feet, I was anemic . . . Chichote (her son) was very little, it was after delivery. They told me it was because I didn't look after myself (where did they tell you that?) here, in the community . . . Silvia (her mother-in-law), SB (opyguā). Because after delivery one has to beware of the cold, not to go out if it is windy, not to wash oneself with cold water. For example now, at the hospital, when I was in Posadas they told me, don't be afraid of cold water, the grandmothers of the past tell all lies, said the doctor, then I washed myself, and that time, I don't know, nothing happened, and then, with my second (son), I again wanted to do that, wash myself in the stream and the water was cold, I washed the clothes too . . . (grandmothers say that) after 15 days you can, but not after five, six or seven days, because the cold catches you, and all your blood deviates, they say, and a clot of blood is formed, it is called *tuguy roicha*, that means the blood gets cold, then when you begin to have problems there, because every time I washed myself with cold water, there I began to feel that, cold . . . and it was like this that I began with the bladder problem . . . because after your blood gets cold you suffer the consequences, that's why we are always forbidden to have cold food, cold drinks, watermelon, fruit you can't eat, sodas is cold, too. Because we are forbidden to eat like that mixing salty and sweet. One has to be careful for one month, if not you get internal hemorrhage (And with the next child, were you careful?) yes, I don't feel bad, because I was in bed for a week, resting.

Studying allows Para to get new knowledge, which widens her criteria for decision making. This marks a contrast with other women in her own generation. Her perception of the factors influencing her health and that of her children is strictly related to her contact with medical professionals. In the previously quoted passage, she establishes analogies between Mbyá and biomedical diagnostic categories.

Nevertheless, when a bladder problem arises, she consults both traditional specialists and doctors. The doctors diagnose "stones in the bladder" and advise her to get an operation to remove them. Surgery was not an option for Para at the time, and she decided to find a treatment within her community. Therefore, she visited the Opyguā, who diagnoses *ita* (stones), an ailment caused by intentional

CHAPTER 13   Mbyá Grandmothers, Mothers, and Granddaughters

damage from another living person or by the action of some supernatural agent (*mbogua*, spirits of the dead). These entities cause evil by means of material elements; this time they are stones introduced in the affected person's body. This new diagnosis, which is consistent with the Mbyá belief system, is reflected in what she says about the allopathic medicine diagnosis. This illness episode allows her to recall previous experiences that she finds meaningful. Therefore, based on elderly people's ways, she found that her illness was due to her neglect of certain requirements after delivery. However, at the same time, and based on what the doctors said, she had some doubts about the truth of these assertions. The value she places on traditional and biomedical knowledge and practices depends on the whole circumstance; one approach is preferred and more acceptable than the others, apart from their accessibility and truth.

With regard to children's health, Para, like Jachuka, emphasizes the events during pregnancy and the first months of life as explanatory factors of the health trajectory later in life. Likewise, she stresses the family's group responsibility in the fulfillment of the elders' recommendations:

> There are some mothers who pay no attention and children get sick, perhaps they eat pig meat 15 days after birth and that's the way they say the illness comes to them, that's why it is banned after delivery to all of them, the dad too, the little brothers and sisters already know what they don't have to do, after the brother is born, what they can't eat (And who teaches that to children?) we, the parents or the grandparents and there they grow up already knowing that.

When thinking about her children, the one who worries Para the most is the eldest, because of her low height and weight in the past 2 years. This is how she recounts the facts that, from her own perspective, led to the girl's health deterioration:

> This girl was born big, but now it looks as though she doesn't want to grow up, ndokakuaa, she fell off a bed and had a fever and the fever infected all her blood and I had to take her to Oberá for 15 days and left her alone, and there it was when she lost weight, because I couldn't breastfeed her, I was bad because she was skinny, and then she didn't recognise me, and she started to cry, she didn't feel well with me (no se hallaba), she was 8 months old, we took her to Posadas to the hospital too, but she didn't recover, she stayed like this, skinny, small, because she was born well and fat . . . but afterwards, every little thing she had made her ill, she got diarrhea and then she didn't recover. doctors forbade me to breastfeed her, because they say that if you stop one day you can no longer feed them because your milk is no use,

she can get a fever, diarrhea . . . She was bad for a long time and now, she started to eat well, to put on some weight, and she has got better.

Ndokakuaachy, that is, "he/she doesn't want to grow," is an expression that is often used by parents when describing their children's health problems. Saying that a child "doesn't want to grow" means that he or she doesn't show any evidence of normal growth and development, and that the child is weak, skinny, and is permanently getting ill. They also speak of some symptoms having to do with the child's emotional state, such as weepy, sad, or doesn't find him- or herself (*no se halla*). In the previous paragraph, Para describes the reason for her daughter's successive illnesses and the doctor's advice to not breastfeed her. Breastfeeding is considered by Mbyá women—according to biomedical advice—a practice that favors the child's health and avoids exposure to illnesses. As we saw in the previous account, stopping breastfeeding or the early addition of other kinds of food cause complications in children's health and have short-term and long-term consequences. Moreover, the girl's admission to the hospital without her mother's company is considered to affect both the child's and the mother's emotional state, as well as the bond between them that is believed to be so important for the child's health.

Although biomedicine seems to be an accessible and efficient alternative of treatment for Para's family on some occasions, traditional knowledge remains the reference framework to find the causes for the illness and a healing resource when she is faced with illnesses that biomedicine cannot diagnose:

> There are things that only the opyguā know what they are, also the older ones, people like my mother-in-law, she once had a dream, and nobody paid attention, and they didn't look after the children and they got ill . . . I listen to her dreams, because I don't go to pray at the Opy (Mbyá traditional church), because the younger ones don't understand what the elders say . . . they speak with words we don't understand, with old words.

LESSONS LEARNED

We would like to finish this paper by drawing a few conclusions. What do these life stories teach us? Which relevant aspects can we identify in terms of mother–child health care? What have we learned after all these years of working among the Mbyá Guaraní?

First, and according to other contributions about the Guaraní and research developed in other Latin American societies, the woman's relevance is enhanced—both

CHAPTER 13 Mbyá Grandmothers, Mothers, and Granddaughters

in the past and in the present—with regard to taking care of their children and other members of the family group. As we noted early in the chapter, Guaraní women have always been described as mothers and wives. Although we have recorded a set of transformations in their activities, roles, and status, the motherly function is still the core of her everyday life.

From an ethnographic observation of a day of life, it turns out that women are the ones in charge of looking after their babies during most of the first months of life. They never delegate this task to other people, except in very special situations. As the child grows up, his or her care is shared with other members of the domestic group, including other children, and the child may even be raised by other relatives on a regular basis for some time (Remorini, 2005). During the first months of life, the relevance of the mother's breastfeeding requires mothers to carry their babies with them wherever they go, for example, when they go to other cities to sell their crafts.

Moreover, it is the mothers themselves who perceive and explain in detail a wide range of symptoms and even explain the probable causes leading to a diagnosis of their children's illnesses. That does not mean that parents or other adults have no participation—quite the contrary. The whole domestic group is usually involved in the healing and care of a sick child. Men are usually in charge of the search and collection of medicinal plants because they are usually found in the monte (rainforest), a space that usually belongs to men (Remorini, 2008). Nevertheless, it is the domestic group of women who have the greater responsibility in the care of family members' health. Our results agree with those of Price (1997), Módena (1990), Daltabuit Godás (1992), Ryan and Martínez (1996), Bronfman (2001), Osorio Carranza (2001), Loyola (1984), Queiroz (1993), Pícoli and Adorno (2006), Scheper-Hughes (1990), and Crivos (2004), to give a few examples. That is, ethnographic observation confirms this behavior as a general pattern.

Second, these cases demonstrate many strategies when facing illness. Different ways of explaining the causes and methods of healing are combined and articulated in these accounts. The availability and preference of some therapeutic resources over others depends on the person's health trajectory (Sy, 2008) and the particular situation. In their speech and practices, these women appeal to tradition, call on the advice of the elders, and rely on their previous experiences. They also consider the availability of a particular resource to justify their decisions. The Mbyá women's decision-making criteria when dealing with illness and possible remedies is simplified when there is a dichotomy between traditional versus biomedical knowledge or indigenous versus nonindigenous people (Remorini,

2008). This dichotomy, which is usually present in the women's speech—mainly that of the community elders and political and religious leaders—must be considered an element that tends to reinforce their ethnic identity in situations like an ethnographic interview.

Third, and closely related to what was previously noted, these cases reflect some points of intragenerational and intergenerational agreement and disagreement. A respect for taboos that affect people's behavior during gestation and delivery, and after delivery through the child's first living months, is emphasized both in young women's and old women's speech. The intimate connection of grandmothers, mothers, and granddaughters, as well as the continuity of their knowledge, values, and practices related to motherhood and child rearing, is favored by traditional family organization and residence patterns that are still in force (extended families and uxorial locality). As Traphagan points out, it is common in indigenous and rural societies (unlike industrial societies) to find old women providing care, more than receiving it: "particularly, as they enter into middle and old age, women often become caretakers of the collective well-being of the family" (2003, p. 127). That is, they have the responsibility for the welfare of the next generations, due to their handling of knowledge that the others cannot access.

Although we have recorded the sharing of some positions in generational terms, the elders of Mbyá communities do not represent a homogeneous sector. As Bataille and Sands (1986) point out, the women's role in indigenous societies is mostly seen as being responsible for preserving and reproducing tribal tradition. From our interviews with women of different ages, it emerges that their perspective about certain subjects does not come solely from their position in their life course or from the models they encountered in their early socialization. More than tribal tradition, what ultimately guides and justifies their actions and points of view can be found in their past experience. Tradition involves more than what is established in myths and their ancestors' legacy. It does not relate to a set of beliefs detached from everyday actions, but to a common past of shared experiences. As Malinowski (1964) pointed out, the agreement about what proved to be effective in the past specifies the possible alternatives in the present.

In spite of recognizing the symbolic, moral, and practical value of tradition, which is noticeable in the statements we gathered, the young people's actions in certain situations have moved away from the ideal prescribed by "the old ones." Their choice for alternatives that are nearer to those of the *jurua* ("the white ones") is evident (Remorini, 2006). Therefore, tradition, which is associated with their

CHAPTER 13 Mbyá Grandmothers, Mothers, and Granddaughters

grandparents' lifestyle, is starting to be questioned, and the efficiency of some practices becomes doubtful when they are compared to new knowledge and biomedical technology. Likewise, some young girls express their ignorance of the basics of traditional rules. There is a breakdown in intergenerational transmission, accompanied by access to formal education and new knowledge and values, where the media is a key factor. Para's statement about the relevance of listening and paying attention to what is revealed in old women's dreams and the nearly exclusive attendance of old people at *Opy* meetings shows the old people's role of translating the incomprehensible code of the ancient ones for young people. This is evident in a commonly used expression, "they say," to explain the causes of an illness. This emphasizes their intention to reproduce other people's sayings, though they do not necessarily make them their own. There is a certain tendency of young informants to restate what others say or is known in the community, thus they do not commit themselves when it comes to deciding the truth of what is stated (Crivos, 2004).

Nevertheless, young people admit that when they face uncertainty about the risk of an illness, they turn to the knowledge and experience of the old ones, and this is a key factor in their decision making. This represents for them a necessary anchor point. Likewise, they admit that certain illnesses affecting children are neither identified nor treated by biomedicine, which means that the old people's knowledge is the only valid resource.

Fourth, the old women's speech, like that of Kerechu, emphasizes transformations in health conditions and the worsening of some illnesses that have increased the child morbidity–mortality rate. Continuous reference to the fact that there was less illness before and there are new illnesses now justifies their utilization of biomedicine. It is interesting to note that this perception of the past and the elders is consistent, in part, with the present social–sanitary and ecological situation, though a certain idealization of the past times is noticeable. Transformations in the forest, sedentarism in intensively exploited spaces, the decrease in horticulture activities, the scarcity of wild animal resources, and the higher consumption of industrialized food increase the Mbyá people's vulnerability to infectious and nutritional diseases and has a high impact on children (Sy & Remorini, 2009).

Beliefs are not unchangeable explanatory systems; they are susceptible to being transformed and given a new meaning (Sy, 2008). The Mbyá women's beliefs account for the plasticity of these communities to incorporate, and they ascribe a new meaning to and complement knowledge and resources from different origins. Role transformations and new opportunities to access to formal training, together with a change in the recognition of indigenous women's opportunities and rights—favored by international movements—encourage Mbyá women to look for new alternatives for rearing and caring for their children and grandchildren, articulating the inside and the outside, and going through and communicating different contexts.

We hope our work will contribute to a greater ethnographic visibility of indigenous women and awareness of the present mother–child health conditions to foster initiatives aiming at improving this people's quality of life.

ACKNOWLEDGMENTS

This research was supported by CONICET. I wish to express my acknowledgment to Dr. Marta Crivos, Dr. María Rosa Martínez, and Dr. Anahi Sy. I am indebted and especially grateful to all members of Ka'aguy Poty and Yvy Pytã communities for their cooperation and warm hospitality. I wish to dedicate this work to all Mbyá women who shared their knowledge with me.

Discussion Questions

1. How do the Mbyá integrate modern and traditional models of medicine? (Consider Para in particular.)
2. If you were to work in this community, how would you decide what traditional methods of taking care of mothers and infants should be kept and which should be replaced with modern methods? Would you see this as your role? Why or why not?
3. What do you think accounts for 90% of babies being born in a hospital, given the low rates of hospital births in many traditional communities around the world?
4. How can the hospitals that serve the Mbyá provide the emotional and psychological care for the other 10% who want to and choose to stay at home?
5. Is there a low-cost way to provide the safety of a hospital birth with the comfort of a home birth in this community?

CHAPTER 13 Mbyá Grandmothers, Mothers, and Granddaughters

NOTES

1. I did this research within the frame of my thesis to obtain my doctorate in natural sciences at UNLP, funded by CONICET.
2. In every community, some individuals—generally elderly men and women—are recognized as therapeutic experts, known in the Mbyá language as *Karai* or *Kuña Karai poro poāno va'e*, an expression that generically refers to people (men and women, respectively) who have the ability to cure. Moreover, some of these Karai are also recognized as religious leaders within the community, in which case they are called *Pai* or *Opyguā* (Remorini, 2008).
3. Traditional Argentinian food. Stew with different vegetables and some meat.
4. *Mitā* means, generically, "child." Within this category, *avai* is used to refer to male children and *kuña i* is used to refer to female children. For information about the categories used to refer to different stages of the Mbyá Los indios Jeguaká Tenondé (Mbyá) del Guairá, Paraguay life cycle, see Remorini (2008).
5. These illness can be consider analogous to those in other Latin American societies that are called *caída de mollera* (fallen fontanel).

REFERENCES

Assis, V., & Garlet, I. J. (2004). Análise sobre as populações Guaraní contemporâneas: Demografía, espacialidade e questōs fundiárias. *Revista de indias, LXIV*(230), 35–54.
Bataille, G. M., & Sands, K. M. (1986). *La Mujer India Americana: Historia, vida, costumbres.* Barcelona, Spain: Mitre.
Bronfman, M. (2001). *Como se vive se muere. Familia, redes sociales, y muerte infantil.* Buenos Aires, Argentina: Lugar Editorial.
Cadogan, L. (1948). Los indios Jeguaká Tenondé (Mbyá) del Guairá, Paraguay. *América Indígena, VIII*(2), 131–139.
Cadogan, L. (1949). Síntesis de la Medicina Racional y Mística Mbyá-Guaraní. *América Indígena, IX*(1), 21–36.
Cadogan, L. (1950). La Encarnación y la Concepción; la Muerte y la Resurrección en la Poesía Sagrada esotérica de los Jeguaka Tenonde Pora-güe (Mbyá-Guaraní) del Guaira, Paraguay. *Revista do Museu Paulista Nova Serie, IV*, 233–246.
Cadogan, L. (1971). *Ywyra ñe'ery: Fluye del árbol la palabra.* Asunción, Paraguay: CEADUC-CEPAG.
Cadogan, L. (1997). *Ayvu Rapyta. Textos Míticos de los Mbyá-Guaraní del Guaira.* Asunción, Paraguay: Biblioteca Paraguaya de Antropología. CEADUC.

References

Ciccarone, C. (2001). *Dama e Sensibilidade. Migracao, Xamanismo e Mulheres Mbyá-Guaraní.* (Tesis Doctoral). Sao Paulo, Brazil: PUC/SP. MS.

Clastres, H. (1993). *La Tierra Sin Mal. El profetismo tupi-guaraní.* Buenos Aires, Argentina: Ediciones del Sol.

Crivos, M. (2004). *Contribución al estudio antropológico de la medicina tradicional de los Valles calchaquíes (Provincia de Salta).* (Tesis Doctoral). Facultad de Ciencias Naturales y Museo. Universidad Nacional de La Plata, Buenos Aires, Argentina. Retrieved from http://sedici.unlp.edu.ar?id=arg-unlp-tpg-0000000083

Daltabuit Godás, M. (1992). *Mujeres Mayas. Trabajo, nutrición y fecundidad.* Mexico City, México: Instituto de Investigaciones Antropológicas UNAM.

Dos Santos Landa, B. (1995). *A mulher Guaraní: Atividades e cultura material.* (Disertación de Maestría). PUC. Rio Grande do Sul. Porto Alegre. MS.

Enriz, N., & García Palacios, M. (2008). Deviniendo Kuña va'era. En S. Hirsch (Coord.), *Mujeres indígenas de la Aregtina* (pp. 205–230). Buenos Aires, Argentina: Editorial Biblos.

Foro de Investigación en Salud de Argentina. (2008). Resumen Ejecutivo. Situación de Salud, intervenciones y líneas de investigación para la toma de decisiones en salud con pueblos indígenas. Silvia Kochen (Coord.). Buenos Aires, Argentina: Cámara Argentina del Libro.

Lewis, O. (1985). *Antropología de la pobreza. Cinco familias.* México DF: Fondo de Cultura Económica.

Loyola, M. A. (1984). *Médicos e Curandeiros—conflito Social e Saúde.* São Paulo, Brazil: Difel.

Malinowski, B. (1964). El problema del significado en las lenguas primitivas. En C. K. Ogden y L. A. Richards (Coord.), *El significado del Significado. Una investigación acerca de la influencia del lenguaje sobre el pensamiento y de la ciencia simbólica* (pp. 312–360). Buenos Aires, Argentina: Paidos básica.

Martínez, M. R., Crivos, M., & Remorini, C. (2002). Etnografía de la vejez en comunidades Mbyá-Guaraní, provincia de Misiones, Argentina. En Guerci y Consigliere (Eds.), *Il Vecchio allo Specchio. Vivere e curare la vecchiaia nel mondo* (Vol. 4) (pp. 206–222). Geneve: Erga Edizione.

Metraux, A. (1927). Migrations historiques des Tupi-Guaraní. *Journal de la Societé des Americanistes, 19*, 1–45.

Metraux, A. (1948a). The Couvade. In J. Steward (Ed.), *Handbook of South American Indians* (pp. 369–374). Washington, DC: Smithsonian.

Metraux, A. (1948b). The Guaraní. In J. Steward (Ed.), *Handbook of South American Indians* (Vol. 3) (pp. 60–94). Washington, DC: Smithsonian.

Módena, M. E. (1990). *Madres, Médicos y Curanderos: Diferencia cultural e identidad ideológica.* Tlalpan, México DF: Ed. Casa Chata.

Müller, F. (1989). *Etnografía de los Guaraní del Alto Paraná.* Buenos Aires, Argentina: CAEA.

Navone, G. T., Gamboa, M. I., Oyhenart, E., & Orden, A. (2006). Parasitosis intestinales en poblaciones Mbyá-Guaraní de la Provincia de Misiones, Argentina: aspectos epidemiológicos y nutricionales. *Cadernos de Saúde Pública, 22*(5), 1089–1100.

Osorio Carranza, R. M. (2001). *Entender y atender la enfermedad. Los saberes maternos frente a los padecimientos infantiles.* México DF: CONACULTA-INI-CIESAS.

Picoli, R., & Adorno, R. C. F. (2006). A Saúde de crianças Kaiowá e Guaraní: reflexões. En *Anais do 2º Seminário Internacional: fronteiras da exclusão.* Campo Grande.

Price, L. (1997). Ecuadorian illness stories. In D. Holland & N. Quinn (Eds.), *Cultural models in language and thought* (pp. 313–342). Cambridge, MA: Cambridge University Press.

CHAPTER 13 Mbyá Grandmothers, Mothers, and Granddaughters

Queiroz, M. S. (1993). Strategies for consumption of health care by working-class families. *Cadernos de Saúde Pública, 9*(3), 272–282.
Remorini, C. (2005). Mujeres Mbyá: vida cotidiana y cuidado infantil. Estudio etnográfico en comunidades Mbyá del Valle del Cuña Pirú (Misiones). *Cuadernos del Instituto Nacional de Antropología y Pensamiento Latinoamericano, 20*, 301–316.
Remorini, C. (2006). Las relaciones intergeneracionales en la vida cotidiana. Sobre el rol de los abuelos en las actividades de cuidado infantil en comunidades Mbyá (Misiones, Argentina). *Actas del VIII Congreso de Antropología Social, Simposio 14: Cultura y envejecimiento. Abordajes multi e interdisciplinarios.* Universidad Nacional de Salta, CD-ROM. Salta: EDUNSa.
Remorini, C. (2008). *Aporte a la caracterización etnográfica de los procesos de salud-enfermedad en las primeras etapas del ciclo vital, en comunidades Mbyá-guaraní de Misiones, República Argentina* (Tesis de Doctorado). La Plata: Universidad Nacional de La Plata, Edulp, 1st ed. ISBN 978-950-34-0602-1.
Ryan, G. W., & Martínez, H. (1996). Can we predict what mothers do? Modeling childhood diarrhea in rural Mexico. *Human Organization, 55*(1), 47–57.
Schaden, E. (1991). *Aspectos Fundamentales de la Cultura Guaraní.* Asunción, Paraguay: CEADUC. Biblioteca Paraguaya de Antropología.
Scheper-Hughes, N. (1990). *Death without weeping: The violence of everyday life in Brazil.* Berkeley, CA: University of California Press.
Susnik, B. (1983). *Los Aborígenes del Paraguay. Tomo V: Ciclo vital y estructura social.* Asunción, Paraguay: Museo Etnográfico "Andrés Barbero."
Sy, A. (2008). *Estrategias frente a la enfermedad en dos comunidades Mbyá Guaraní (Ka'aguy Poty e Yvy Pytã, Provincia de Misiones). Aporte del estudio de casos a la investigación Etnográfica de los procesos de Salud-enfermedad* (Tesis de Doctorado). Facultad de Ciencias Naturales y Museo. Universidad Nacional de La Plata.
Sy, A. & Remorini, C. (2009). Hacia un abordaje integral e intercultural de la salud de los niños Mbyá. Contribuciones de la investigación etnográfica y desafíos para la gestión pública. En M. B. Noceti (Comp.), *Oportunidades. Caminos hacia la protección integral de los Derechos del niño* (pp. 83–104). Bahía Blanca, Argentina: Libros en Colectivo.
Traphagan, J. (2003). Older women as caregivers and ancestral protection in rural Japan. *Ethnology, 42*(2), 127–139.

CHAPTER 14

Introducing Nursing Students to Childbearing Practices in Rural Guatemala

Catherine Carr, CNM, DrPH, FACNM
Amy Levi, CNM, WHNP-BC, PhD, FACNM

Location: San Lucas Toliman, Solola, Guatemala, Central America

Name of Project: Student experiences in rural Guatemala

Sponsoring Organization (and Funders): San Lucas Mission, Solola, Guatemala (the participation of our students and us was primarily self-funded). Partial scholarships were provided by the University of Washington School of Nursing from the Citizens of the World program.

Target Population: Rural Guatemalan women with no access to regular prenatal care

Project Goal: Provision of prenatal care to women in rural Guatemalan communities

Project Objectives: Network with local health promoters and *comadronas* to set up antenatal clinics in health offices and private homes to provide prenatal care

CHAPTER 14 Introducing Students to Childbearing Practices in Rural Guatemala

BACKGROUND

Students of the health professions increasingly identify an interest in global maternal child health because there continues to be no improvement in international maternal morbidity and mortality rates (Miller, 2009). In addition, the increasing number of immigrants to the United States has required the education of health professionals to meet the needs of a population of patients from a variety of cultural and ethnic backgrounds, which further underscores the need for curriculum content that includes an international perspective. In 2004, the U.S. Census Bureau estimated that 12% of the population in the United States was comprised of foreign-born immigrants; 53.5% of this population comes from Latin American countries (U.S. Census Bureau, 2004). As healthcare providers are encountering increasing numbers of immigrants in their patient populations, the educational programs that prepare them are developing curricular responses to support the needs of this growing demographic (Foster, 2009). These additions to the curriculum vary from short-term immersion experiences in existing healthcare programs abroad to *clinical tourism*, in which students have a short exposure to care in another country with no preparation or follow-up (Levi, 2009). Student experiences designed to increase the culturally appropriate awareness of future healthcare providers must properly prepare students to make a contribution to the community they serve and integrate them into an existing structure of services that is both sustainable and valued by the population being served.

CULTURAL COMPETENCY VERSUS CULTURAL HUMILITY

The identification of a need to embrace the sociocultural aspects of a patient to ensure the best care gave rise to the concept of *cultural competence* on the part of the provider and healthcare system (Betancourt, Green, Carillo, & Aneneh-Firompong, 2003). Betancourt and colleagues define cultural competence as follows:

> Understanding the importance of social and cultural influences on patients' health beliefs and behaviors; considering how these factors interact at multiple levels of the healthcare delivery system (e.g., at the level of structural processes of care or clinical

decision-making); and, finally, devising interventions that take these issues into account to assure quality healthcare delivery to diverse patient populations. (p. 297)

For a provider to best be able to meet the needs of a patient from a different cultural and ethnic background requires familiarity with the concept of cultural competence and the ability to implement it in practice. Tervalon and Murray-Garcia (1998) underscore the importance of the provider's self-reflection and acknowledgment of the power imbalance inherent in the patient–provider relationship as imperative to the delivery of culturally appropriate care; she uses the term *cultural humility* to describe this self-assessment as the basis for patient–provider relationships. Both cultural competence and cultural humility should be embraced to ensure the interaction that transpires to support a patient's well-being meets that person's level of need and includes a holistic view of the patient that includes sociocultural preferences for care.

SERVICE LEARNING TO REDUCE HEALTH DISPARITIES

One of the approaches to incorporating cultural awareness into the education of healthcare professionals is service learning. Service learning is a concept that provides students an opportunity to offer needed services to underserved populations while they learn about cultural humility and explore concepts of culturally competent care. Service learning incorporates community service into an educational program for the purpose of enhancing both the richness of the student's educational experience and the quality of life of the community in which the student lives and learns. The roots of service learning lie in initiatives in undergraduate education that encouraged students to use their communities as sources of learning (Seifert, 1998). In 1993, President Clinton signed legislation creating the Corporation for National and Community Service, which spawned the development of a large network of educators and community agencies that participate in partnerships to promote service learning; this was supported in 1995 by the Pew Health Professions Commission's creation of the Health Professions Schools in Service to the Nation program (Seifert, 1998). This stimulated the growth of a large number of national and international community and campus collaborations that support the value of bringing students into closer contact with communities.

CHAPTER 14 Introducing Students to Childbearing Practices in Rural Guatemala

The application of service learning to international programming in the health professions has been widely utilized to increase cultural awareness and understanding (Bentley & Ellison, 2007). Because service learning encourages contribution to the community as well as enhancement of the students' educational experience, it is important that such programs also provide a tangible benefit to the communities that are being served. Ideally, programs that sponsor students from the United States should provide services in countries at the invitation of a care system that can best utilize the services and incorporate them into the system so they can continue to be provided after the program participants have gone (Foster, 2009).

PRACTICAL STRATEGIES FOR SERVICE LEARNING AND TEACHING

This section examines how students are prepared to participate in an ongoing service learning experience in the western highlands of Guatemala. This small project involves three returning faculty from different universities and rotating groups of students that visit a small city and its surrounding villages for short-term (2-week) service learning experiences. Over the years our group has found that careful preparation for students and faculty prior to departure makes the trip successful, which keeps the welcome mat out for return visits. During the 2-week stay, students participate in prenatal care clinics organized by the health promoter of the Catholic parish in the town where the service learning occurs, and they attend births at the parish clinic with the faculty. Approximately 90 to 100 women attend the prenatal clinics; they receive simple screening procedures and referrals to local resources as appropriate. Students from the three institutions visit the community four times a year to provide services to support the health promoter's efforts to ensure that pregnant women get the level of care they need for a healthy pregnancy.

Pretrip Work
Promotion
When the trip is promoted, it is critical to be transparent and realistic about what will happen. The first informational e-mails sent to the student body set the stage for the experience. It is particularly important to be clear that the trip is to provide work and service rather than a vacation to an exotic location. A

brief description of what the work will likely be and a description of the cultural, political, and environmental setting are included. Upfront knowledge helps students self-select for this type of trip. An excerpt follows:

> This is an immersion experience in a developing country, so flexibility and a willingness to "see how it unfolds" are paramount. The area is also very conservative and students will be expected to act and dress in a way that does not offend the culture (e.g., no shorts, tight clothes, or sleeveless tops even when "off duty"). Students who are fluent in Spanish will be given priority. It will be possible to take some non-Spanish speakers, but it is more difficult for them to participate since there is virtually no English spoken outside the staff.
>
> Conditions: Poverty, rural environment, different standards of health care, exposure to enteric parasites, etc. This is not a malaria or cholera zone. Rural Guatemala is subject to sporadic violence, mostly related to drug traffic. Students will be expected to adhere to local advice regarding personal safety.

Selection of Students: What Is Needed and What Is Desirable

The trip director, who has an understanding of the site realities, sets basic criteria for applicants. Review of applications by a committee is valuable for reducing bias and bringing issues to the surface. English is not spoken outside the group and we must provide our own interpreting; as a baseline, we try to have at least one Spanish speaker for every three non-Spanish speakers. Limiting selection solely by language skill prevents participation by students who may be strong assets and who could find the opportunity transformative. International living and working experience, like language skills, may be preferred, but international learning can open up lives. Student flexibility, willingness to be open to new experiences, and curiosity are far more important characteristics.

It is crucial that the applicants understand the authority of the program director. If decisions have to be made on the ground, they will be made by the program director. There are clear written expectations about alcohol and drug use, behavior—including sexual behavior—and any other specific issues that would warrant expulsion from the trip and self-paid return to the Unites States.

Course Work

Required pretrip coursework is important for a successful experience. Readings and discussions prepare the participants for what to expect and provide background knowledge that will deepen their ability to understand the experience.

CHAPTER 14 Introducing Students to Childbearing Practices in Rural Guatemala

The schedule includes three seminars prior to leaving and one on return. The seminars include a variety of readings, with some selected to raise questions that may be uncomfortable, such as articles about clinical tourism. Even students who have traveled extensively may be fairly naïve about the effect of globalization and the impact of do-gooders on small environments.

One of the first topics of discussion answers the question, why are we going? Frequently students have the idea that they can help make a difference by providing education in such areas as healthcare practices, nutrition, and hygiene. It is important for the discussion to facilitate examination of the role of Western volunteers, both helpful and harmful. Both faculty and students reflect on what a service learning experience brings to the setting and the importance of cultural humility on the part of the visiting group. Institutions and students obviously benefit from international service learning trips, but there is far less clarity of the benefit accrued to the host setting. It occasionally surprises participants that there was health care in the Guatemalan highlands before visiting providers began to arrive. An awareness that any visiting group is highly unlikely to be either the first or last tempers expectations of making large or lasting changes over a short time.

Readings about culture and history are critical, particularly in this strongly traditional area. Some cultural mores tend to be more difficult for U.S. visitors and are discussed openly before the trip. Students often find it difficult to work within a culture where the role of women is extremely different, particularly if women are seen as not having decision-making authority. Arriving with some preparation and knowledge of cultural and political realities adds credibility and helps minimize blunders. We repeatedly stress the importance of trying to understand the context of culture as it exists rather than trying to fit it into our Eurocentric model.

It is important for visitors to understand the history of the United State's relations with Guatemala, a history that is not always pleasant to discover and is usually surprising to students. Although the great majority of Guatemalans are very clear about the difference between government policy and individual volunteers, criticism of the United States is not uncommon. Particular weight is given to discussing the history of the recent civil violence and ongoing tensions. This may bring a new consciousness to students who have never been exposed to sectarian conflict or war. In Guatemala, the 36-year civil conflict ended in 1996, but the scars remain, as does residual violence. Special attention is given to a discussion of the role of indigenous Mayans in the domestic conflicts that continued through the 20th century.

Faculty Preparation

Typically there are two instructors per group: the program director and one other instructor. The faculty is responsible for all care provided by students, and therefore the clinical expertise of the faculty has to fit both the setting and the student level. In Guatemala, the program directors are certified nurse midwives (CNMs), and the second instructor is usually a CNM but is sometimes an advanced practice clinician with strong expertise in women's health. Instructors must be flexible, good humored, and willing to work in challenging circumstances. Instructors who have prior experience working internationally and in low-resource settings find it much easier to cope with daily discomforts and challenges. Spanish speaking ability is a high priority.

Scope of Work

It is tremendously tempting for students to exceed their appropriate scope of work in a resource-poor setting. They may be politely invited to participate in patient care activities that are beyond their legitimate practice and understanding—whether it is delivering a baby without supervision, administering unfamiliar medications, or diagnosing common ailments. We specifically state that students may participate in care to the limits of their scope *as students* and that one of the instructors must be present for anything other than observation. It is quite common to see other volunteer healthcare groups that do not operate under these limits, and the repercussions can be significant. Over time our groups, collectively known as "the midwives," have developed a community reputation for being different because we work within the local systems and make a practice of consulting with the health promoter who acts as our liaison and informally as a valued cultural broker.

Avoiding Unintentional Harm and Stupid Mistakes

We devote considerable time to discussing avoidance of unintentional harm—what it is and how to avoid common pitfalls. Participants quickly begin to see examples of how harm can come from good intentions. Some of the main examples are listed in the following paragraphs.

Assuming that No One Understands English

Time and again we have heard disparaging remarks made in public settings by English speakers who do not know their audience. Although many Guatemalans do not feel comfortable speaking English, most have some understanding and many are reception fluent and quite able to figure out content.

Beware of Giving Gifts

Giving gifts is a high-risk behavior because gifts have particular potential for harm. Gifts of labor, however meaningful, may take someone's job in a very poor area with high baseline unemployment. Gifts to individuals may cause unintentional harm by upsetting a fragile balance of community hierarchy. One of the authors provided simple scales for the midwives to weigh newborns. Having missed some of the local midwives, the remaining scales were left with the health promoter to distribute. Rumors quickly flew that he was hiding large amounts of donated equipment in his house and offering it only to certain midwives. We have seen candy thrown from the back of an open pickup (by a dental group!) to children scrambling in the streets to get their share. The unavoidable image is that of tossing birdseed—how does this promote dignity and self-respect? The only allowed gifts for children are ones that can be used in groups: pads of paper and markers for drawing (the child gets to keep the picture, not the tablet or set of markers), soap bubbles, soccer balls that are donated to schools, books for the community library. It is always important to consider the counterfactual question "Would I do this in my community at home?"

Not All Donations Are Good

A commonly seen problem is inappropriate donations from the Northern Hemisphere, usually because the donors want to give specific items that have not been requested, are not needed, or are simply useless in the setting. We have seen full-sized wheelchairs destined for rural communities that have no paved roads (sometimes no roads at all) and where houses are far too small to accommodate a wheelchair. A local community-initiated library project that needed middle-school science and history books in Spanish received Protestant religious tracts in English. Health teams have brought antipsychotic drugs to a community that lacks a psychiatric provider and frilly baby bibs and diaper covers (made for disposable diapers) to a setting where bibs are unknown and diapers are made from old rags. Inappropriate donations can be very expensive to a host community that may have to pay for customs fees and shipping and then ultimately for storage or disposal of unusable items.

Using Scarce Resources

This is a behavior that unknowingly can cause harm. In an arid environment it may be seen as wasteful to use water for frequent hand washing, showers, or laundry. A practice often seen as wasteful is the use of gloves to give injections, start IVs, and clean contaminated areas. Rather than ignore universal precautions we bring a large supply of gloves; this avoids using scarce resources and provides a contribution to the host site. Some items are easily bought locally, and purchasing on-site directly benefits the community. Creating excessive waste by overuse of disposable items can create problems of waste disposal, particularly of contaminated items.

Give Me a Little Respect! Recognizing (Lack) of Respect

Respectful behavior is nonnegotiable on service learning trips. What constitutes respect varies from place to place, even within the same general region. In the area of Guatemala we visit, courtesy requires shaking the hand of every person in the room on entering—though in other parts of Guatemala, as well as other Central American countries, acquaintances meet and part with a kiss on the cheek. The same "respect" would be appalling across genders in a conservative Muslim setting.

Less obvious but no less important respectful behavior can be thought of as visual respect. Clothing should blend in, loosely cover the appropriate body areas, and neither be worn out nor obviously luxurious. In Guatemala, it is very common to see children heading to school dressed in spotless uniforms, even if they are from extremely poor families without indoor plumbing. When it is so apparent that looking clean and neat is a high priority, it would be insulting to do otherwise. We warn students that T-shirts with stains or holes and torn pants are not appropriate. In countries that have experienced civil conflict, camouflage clothing may be a painful reminder of violence.

Respect also includes working within the culture. The local decision-making hierarchy may seem inexplicably complex and cumbersome. The Eurocentric value of autonomy is of little consequence if decision makers are the family elders. Decisions may have to wait until husbands return from the fields, parents and in-laws are consulted, or permission is obtained from the village leader.

The direct approach in communication is valued by North Americans, and is quite literally part of our language. Spanish is more indirect, and in fact has

CHAPTER 14   Introducing Students to Childbearing Practices in Rural Guatemala

a number of tenses devoted to the indirect use of language. In Guatemala, both the language and the culture value courtesy and indirect communication. For example, a "yes" answer may mean any of the following:

- I hear what you are saying.
- I don't understand you.
- I will go home and think about it.
- I agree.
- I disagree but will say yes to make you go away.

Cultural humility requires participants to look for what is beyond and around the surface, and in doing so they find a world of nuanced meaning that adds richness and context. This not only deepens and enhances their immediate journey but also prepares them to work in a world that is made up of cultures other than their own.

Awareness of Bigger Issues

Self-Reflection

On-site structured seminars are important to help participants critically self-reflect and integrate their experiences. Each evening we have reflections on a specific topic or issue. Pairs of participants take turns leading some of the sessions; other sessions feature local guests speaking on such topics as the education system, local politics and history, or are led by faculty with a focus on an emergent topic or issue. Subjects have ranged from a review of interpreting auscultated fetal heart tones to the ethics of international adoption. The informal evening setting and adherence to the adult learning axiom of "all are teachers, all are learners" supports airing of ideas and concerns that might otherwise remain unspoken.

The Hardest Things to Do Are Nothing and Waiting

Slowly watching and waiting as events unfold is not something that Unites States clinicians are accustomed to, and it can provoke both anxiety and anger in students who feel that they are helpless to fix something that to them may seem obvious. Conditions that we would consider emergent may not be thought of in the same way; actions have to work within a fragile, low-resource microsystem. Participants find it difficult to support a person within that system who, by all their education, seems wrong. Care decisions may require consultation with several family members, and the final answer may be not to act. Children with reparable heart defects may not be allowed to go to the city; a woman with severe preeclampsia may opt to go to the market instead of the hospital; the traditional healer may be called for cancer treatment. Decisions are made for many and complex reasons, but refusal to act is very unlikely to be because the family does not care. Cultural humility demands a willingness to be present even when we cannot understand and may not agree.

We frequently discuss the "baby in the well" situation of rescuing an individual and ignoring the setting and community. We ask students to consider what happens when a family decides something completely different from what we think of as sound, evidence-based advice—does this affect our relationships with the individual, family, and community? Do they become "those people who . . . ?" A local nurse who has lived in the area for many years tells students that it is not possible to truly understand someone else's life, but by walking with that person you share something greater that enables support and communication on a far higher level. We remind students of the old question, "What is the hardest thing to do with your hands at a birth?" The answer is "Nothing."

Sustainability and Change

It is easy to feel trapped in a rut of returning to the same place to do the same thing with the same expectations. But needs change over time. Over the past 10 years we have seen many changes, including the advent of cell phone towers, Internet cafes, and *tuk tuks* (motorcycle taxis). The colorful hand-woven *huipile* blouses are less common now, and polyester is clearly ascending in popularity. Cell phones are ubiquitous, and even the most traditional-looking woman is likely to have one tucked inside her shirt. Romanticizing the good old days of any culture is uncomfortably similar to visitors from Europe or Asia expecting to see cowboys riding the range in Texas and prospectors panning for gold in California. But it's important to remember that the beautiful huipiles take a month to weave, are costly to buy, and are heavy and hot to wear. *Ropa americana*, Western-style clothing, is very cheap and easily available. Visible changes in clothing and the adoption of technology lead to conversations about romancing the culture and what it says about respect if outsiders try to insist that a culture not change.

Measuring success needs to be realistic. The local midwives may be able to recognize a problem, but if there is no access to the next level of care, it is not likely to help. Balancing the need for a longitudinal view with the desire to solve immediate problems is not easy, particularly with time pressures from funding, institutions, or students. Accountability is critical in even the smallest things, and rarely has much accountability been demanded from outside sources. U.S.

nongovernmental organizations (NGOs) need to partner with local or country NGOs. Sustainability is improved with long-term commitments from the sending institutions that continue to build on existing relationships.

We emphasize that building relationships begin with preparation and continue with observing, asking questions, and responding with respect. We ask students to notice behaviors that connote respect or, conversely, a lack of respect. For example, if a woman closes the shutters before an exam, the next time the healthcare provider should ask if they should be closed. If no one ever points with a finger, then others should use their hand. People who have lived in an environment for a long time have developed complex behaviors and skills that are locally adapted, usually for very good reason. Avoiding disruption of them is an important place to start.

LEARNING ABOUT GLOBAL MATERNAL HEALTH CARE THROUGH SERVICE LEARNING

There are many reasons to support international student experiences in health care. It promotes cultural understanding, exposure to a variety of socioeconomic lifestyles, and an introduction to a diversity of health beliefs and behaviors. It also provides an opportunity for students' self-reflection on the meaning of culture to health status. Students may also begin to understand the role of the healthcare culture in their own clinical practice—how the beliefs of the dominant healthcare culture affect the well-being of individuals who have their own paradigm of health, based on their community, family, economic status, or belief systems. All of these reflections can improve the quality of care that students will ultimately provide to the immigrant populations that are an increasingly large proportion of the U.S. population.

Designing programs that promote student experiences in international health require an understanding both of the students' needs and expectations, and the community in which the students will be getting experience. Faculty need to be prepared to act as culture brokers for the students to understand the community where they will be, as well as the health care and illness care experiences of community members. It is vital to engage students in preparation prior to experiences abroad in order to explore their beliefs, expectations, and biases, and to help them anticipate the kind of situations they may encounter. Additionally, students need to understand their responsibility as ambassadors of the mores of the Northern Hemisphere.

> ### Discussion Questions
>
> 1. Outline the challenges and opportunities of an international service component in the learning experience of professionals in maternal and child health.
> 2. List some of the essential elements of the preservice component of an international service learning course, and explain why you think they are essential.
> 3. The authors have students examine "the role of Western volunteers, both helpful and harmful." Do the same within the context of ethical practice.
> 4. Develop strategies to prevent or minimize each of the ways students can cause unintentional harm.
> 5. Explain the role of reflections in the service learning experience.
> 6. Explore the concept of sustainability in the context of a short-term learning experience.

REFERENCES

Bentley, R., & Ellison, K. J. (2007). Increasing cultural competence in nursing through international service-learning experiences. *Nurse Educator, 32*(5), 207–211.

Betancourt, J. R., Green, A. R., Carillo, J. E., & Aneneh-Firompong, O. (2003). Defining cultural competence: A practical framework for addressing racial/ethnic disparities in health and health care. *Public Health Reports, 118*, 293–302.

Foster, J. (2009). Cultural humility and the importance of long-term relationships in international partnerships. *Journal of Obstetrical, Gynecological, and Neonatal Nursing, 38*(1), 100–107.

Levi, A. (2009). The ethics of nursing student international clinical experiences. *Journal of Obstetrical, Gynecological, and Neonatal Nursing, 38*(1), 94–99.

Miller, S. (2009). Cultural humility is the first step to becoming global care providers. *Journal of Obstetrical, Gynecological, and Neonatal Nursing, 38*(1), 92–93.

Seifert, S. D. (1998). Service-learning: Community-campus partnerships for health professions education in medicine. *Academic Medicine, 73*, 273–277.

Tervalon, M., & Murray-Garcia, J. (1998). Cultural humility versus cultural competence: A critical distinction in defining physician training outcomes in multicultural education. *Journal of Health Care for the Poor and Underserved, 9*(2), 117–125.

U.S. Census Bureau. (2004). Population profile of the United States: Dynamic version 1. Retrieved from http://www.census.gov/population/www/pop-profile/profiledynamic.html

PART VII

Medical Interventions in Birth

Although birth is one of the most primal events in human life, there are times when nature needs help. Across the world the standards for medical intervention in labor and delivery varies for a wide range of reasons which are primarily related to social and cultural values, payment systems, professional roles and training, and the availability of technology. In countries with few technological or human resources, there is less likely to be intervention simply because it is not available. In other countries with lots of access to medical technology, the tendency is to use technology to intervene with birth. Cost systems that make hospital stays expensive also predispose toward intervention because the speed of labor and delivery impacts the bottom line.

It is ironic that women in prosperous countries are pushing for more home births while public health professionals push for more clinic and hospital births in poorer countries. However, this is based on the availability of a skilled attendant at a home birth in prosperous countries and the very low likelihood of such an occurrence in poorer countries. In poorer countries, medical interventions are less likely to be technologically advanced, and therefore can be delivered by less skilled personnel in low-resource settings, and yet they can have a significant impact on the outcomes of pregnancy and birth in places where skilled birth professionals are few.

In places where the number of nurses, doctors, and midwives are insufficient, the role of volunteers becomes critical to the delivery of any medical intervention on a large scale, especially in rural areas where distances are a barrier to efficient service delivery. Thus the roles of literacy, training, and supervision become the key strategies to effective intervention at the community level—whether in the actual delivery of service or to educate the populace about risks and warning signs that are precursors to intervention.

Of course, the major barrier to medical intervention in low-resource countries is cost. Many countries are highly dependent on donors for the provision of technology and the training related to medical intervention. Except for emerging economies such as Brazil, India, or China, most countries do not produce the medical technologies they need, so the variable costs of importing and the unreliability of supply chains, combined with the reliance on donors, make medical intervention in birth a luxury in many settings.

CHAPTER 15

Saving Newborns at the Community Level

Delivering an Innovative Treatment Model through the Government System in Nepal

Christina Lagos Triantaphyllis, MSc

Location: Morang District, Nepal, Asia

Name of Project: Morang Innovative Neonatal Intervention (MINI)

Sponsoring Organization (and Funders): Saving Newborn Lives, a program of Save the Children-USA, funded by the Bill and Melinda Gates Foundation and implemented by JSI Research and Training Institute Inc. and the District Public Health Office in Morang. Additional funding from USAID-Nepal Family Health Program for expansion and ongoing technical assistance and cost sharing.

Target Population: Neonates and young infants (less than 2 months of age)

Project Goal: Implement and assess the effectiveness of community-based management of neonatal infections within existing government health infrastructure

CHAPTER 15 Saving Newborns at the Community Level

> **Project Objectives:** MINI was designed to examine whether existing community-based female community health volunteers (FCHVs) and the most peripheral community health workers under the Ministry of Health and Population could perform a set of activities that would result in the improvement of early identification and management of neonatal infections.

When they are called, they respond at all hours of the day and night. They often walk for hours, traversing unforgiving terrain and steep hills. They counsel mothers, examine neonates, and treat sick children in the flatlands, hills, and mountains. They are volunteers, mothers, wives, heroines. Many are illiterate and most have not completed secondary school. Nepal's Female Community Health Volunteers (FCHVs) have once again proved that lives can be saved within a government's existing health infrastructure and without expensive technologies (**Figures 15-1** and **15-2**). "I serve my community because of the satisfaction I bring to mothers now that I can save newborn lives," said one FCHV in Nepal who delivers newborn care services through the Morang Innovative Neonatal Intervention (MINI), a program model addressing Nepal's persistently high neonatal mortality rate.

BACKGROUND

Nepal is a landlocked country in South Asia and is the world's youngest republic. It is bordered to the north by the People's Republic of China, and to the south, east, and west by India. It has a population of approximately 30 million. Nepal ranks 144th on the Human Development Index of 182 countries ranked. The mountainous north contains 8 of the world's 10 highest mountains, including the highest, Mount Everest. The fertile and humid south is more heavily urbanized than the mountainous region or the hill region, although the belt of hills in between includes the Kathmandu Valley, the country's most urbanized area. Nepal is predominantly rural, with only 10% of the population living in urban areas. The majority of the population resides in the flatlands (Terai) (49%) and the hills (45%) (Save the Children, 2002). For development, Nepal has been divided into 75 districts. The districts are further divided into mostly rural village development committees (VDCs) and urban municipalities.

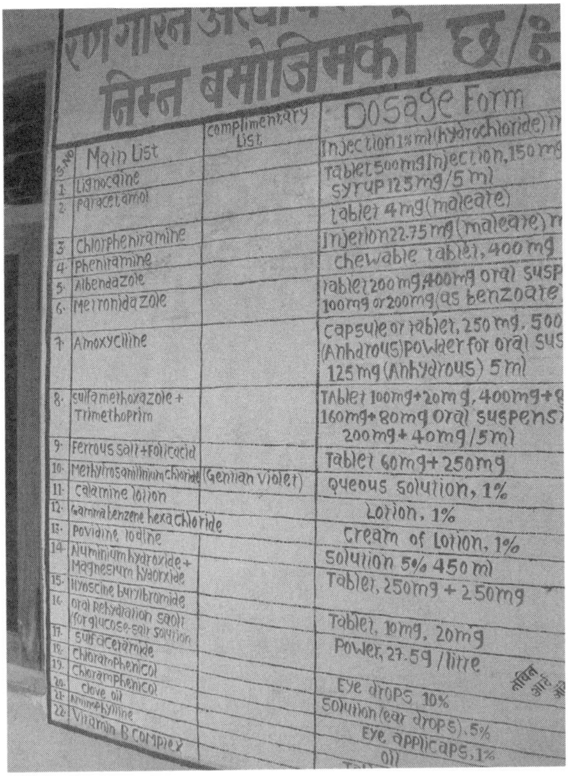

Figure 15-1 Pharmacy inventory and appropriate dosages on display at village development committee health posts for health personnel.

Political History

After having a monarchy throughout most of its history, reforms in 1990 established a multiparty democracy in Nepal, but economic progress continued to stagnate. Beginning in 1996, the constant conflict between the Maoists and the elected government resulted in the displacement of the population across Nepal, leading the king to dissolve the government in 2005 and declare a state of emergency. However, a decade-long People's Revolution by the Maoist Communist Party of Nepal in 2006 culminated in a peace accord. Yet the leadership continues to change frequently, and such political struggles and instability continue to pose challenges for health and development efforts.

CHAPTER 15 Saving Newborns at the Community Level

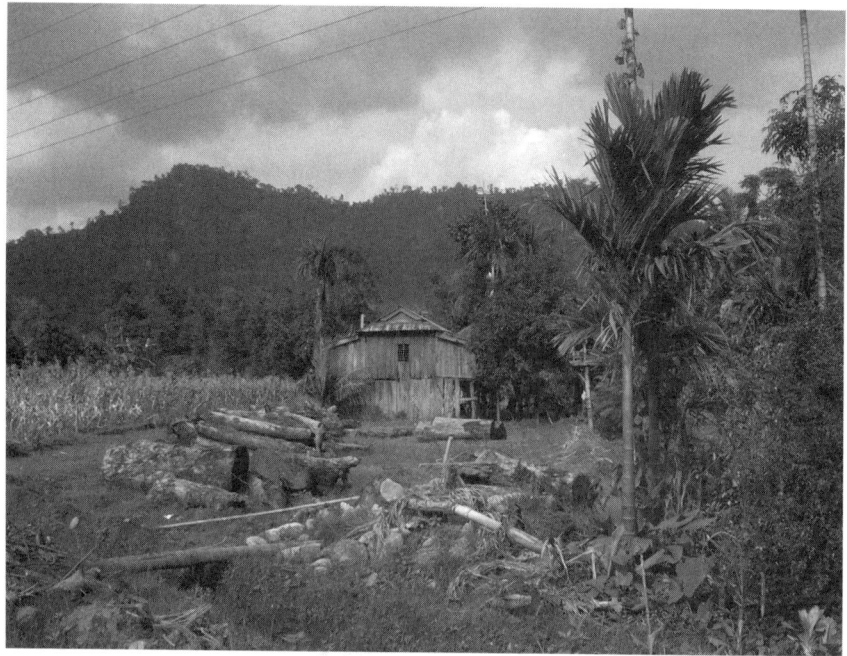

Figure 15-2 Often in remote corners of village development committees, FCHVs travel to traditionally-built homes such as these to visit and care for newborns.

Religion and Culture

By some measures, Hinduism is practiced by a greater majority of people in Nepal than in any other nation. Buddhism, though a minority faith in the country, is linked historically with Nepal as the birthplace of the Buddhist tradition. Nepal is also home to small Muslim and Christian minorities, with some ethnic groups also following animistic religions. Despite Nepal's tumultuous political history, this diversity has been preserved, and multiple ethnic and religious groups continue to coexist.

Development

Nepal is a low-income country in which 78% of the population lives on less than US$2 a day; 86% live in rural and often remote areas. Its diverse ecological regions, multiethnic population, and unstable political situation create challenges for systematizing healthcare delivery. Nepal remains deeply dependent on foreign aid, which makes up 25% of the state budget and more than two-thirds of Nepal's total development budget. The female literacy rate is 55%, and about one-quarter of men and half of women have never attended school, although the percentage of men and women with no education has declined since 2001 from 32% to 23%. Poverty, the lack of education, and poorly developed transportation and communication systems create tremendous challenges for public health interventions.

Neonatal Health in Nepal

Although data from the 2006 Nepal Demographic and Health Survey show that infant mortality has declined by 41% over the 15-year period preceding the survey (from 82 to 48 deaths per 1,000 live births), and under-five mortality has declined by 48% (from 118 to 61 deaths per 1,000 live births), the corresponding decline in neonatal mortality (33% over the 15-year period) has not been as dramatic (**Figure 15-3**). Consequently, neonatal mortality has risen from 40 to 60% as a proportion of infant mortality. Neonatal mortality in the most recent period, 2001–2005, is 33 deaths per 1,000 live births; 69% of infant deaths in Nepal occur during the first month of life. Any efforts to further reduce infant and child mortality in Nepal will have to focus on addressing factors contributing to neonatal mortality (Ministry of Health and Population, New ERA, Macro International Inc., 2007).

Because neonates do not represent a large proportion of patients presenting to health facilities, it is rare that districts record or maintain data on neonates (Save the Children, 2002). Based on evidence available globally and in Nepal's hospital-based studies, the direct causes of these neonatal deaths are birth asphyxia, infections, prematurity, low birth weight, hypothermia, and congenital anomalies (Save the Children, 2002). Contributing factors include inadequate antenatal care, lack of skilled attendance at delivery, staff shortages, and inappropriate newborn care practices in the family and in the community, in addition to the nutritional status of mothers and the educational and general status of women in the family (Weber et al., 2003).

Political Mobilization

Political attention for newborn survival has developed steadily in the past 10 years. Global health policy and advocacy organizations, foreign assistance programs, and child survival activists built on the momentum of the Millennium Development Goals (MDGs) established in 2000, and especially goal 4 to reduce child mortality. The Ministry of Health stated priority for achieving

CHAPTER 15 Saving Newborns at the Community Level

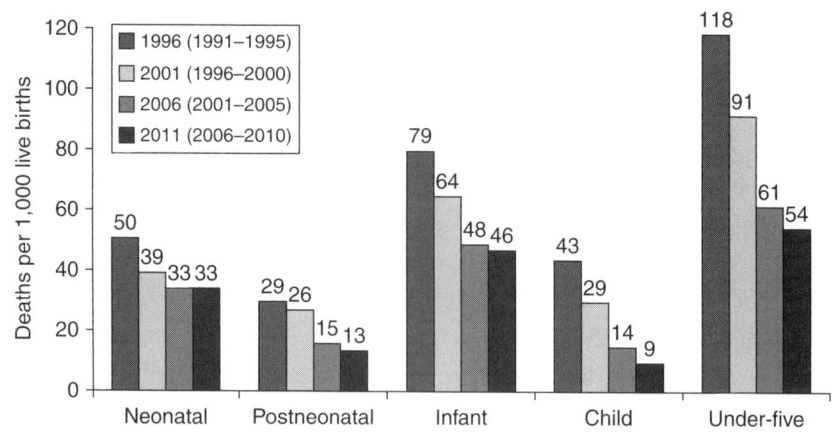

Figure 15-3 Trends in childhood mortality, Nepal (1991–2010).
Source: Reproduced from Ministry of Health and Population (MoHP) [Nepal], New ERA, and ICF International, Inc. (2012). Nepal Demographic and Health Survey 2011. Kathmandu, Nepal: Ministry of Health and Population, New ERA, and ICF International, Calverton, Maryland. Retrieved from http://measuredhs.com/pubs/pdf/FR257/FR257%5B13April2012%5D.pdf. Page 114.

the health MDGs in the Nepal Health Sector Implementation Plan (Ministry of Health, 2004), and in 2004 the Ministry of Health and Population (MoHP) endorsed a National Neonatal Health Strategy. Given that more than 80% of births take place in the home in the absence of a skilled attendant (MoHP et al., New ERA, Macro International Inc., 2007), proven interventions addressing causes of maternal and neonatal complications at family and community levels were the strategy's primary focus.

PUBLIC HEALTH SYSTEM

In VDCs, health posts, subhealth posts, and primary healthcare centers comprise the most important segments of Nepal's health system and were the central health facilities for MINI's activities. The nearest paid health worker to most newborns is a traditional birth attendant, a maternal and child health worker, a village health worker, or an auxiliary health worker. The nearest health facility is the subhealth post or health post. In some cases, a hospital with neonatal services may be available, but the majority of newborns do not receive care at health facilities with necessary or quality services. Although pregnant mothers are encouraged to deliver in health facilities, the realities at the community level are complex and unpredictable. The latest interventions have focused on encouraging institutional deliveries while providing support and care in communities for mothers and newborns.

Health Posts

Currently there are 611 health posts in the country. The role of the health post is to provide integrated preventive and curative primary healthcare services. Health post staff provides supervision and training to subhealth post staff and community-level workers (including FCHVs) and attends normal deliveries at home. Subhealth posts are established at the level of VDC; each one is staffed by an assistant health worker (AHW), a maternal and child health worker (MCHW), and a village health worker (VHW). The subhealth post (from an institutional perspective) is the first contact point for basic services.

Primary Healthcare Outreach Services

Primary healthcare outreach clinics are an extension of health post and subhealth post services operating at the community level. These institutions send their staff—mainly MCHWs, VHWs, and at times, even AHWs—to conduct clinics at predetermined places in a VDC once a month. Outreach clinics provide a basic minimum service package that includes health education, family planning, basic maternity services, child health services, referral, and follow-up.

District Public Health Office

As the coordinating and governing body for health activities at the district level, the District Public Health Office (DPHO) is responsible for managing public health activities related to vaccination, nutrition, acute respiratory infection (ARI) control, control of diarrheal diseases, safe motherhood, family planning, tuberculosis control, malaria, and the FCHV program.

Payment for Health Services

In general, health care provided at peripheral government health facilities is free of charge. Patients pay only at the district government hospitals for consultation and for medicines. Any medicines on the government's essential drug list are provided free to all, and families under MINI's care are not charged for any type of service provided.

CHAPTER 15   Saving Newborns at the Community Level

THE MINI STORY: LEADING THE WAY IN COMMUNITY-BASED CARE FOR NEONATES IN NEPAL

MINI has taught us that simple measures implemented by dedicated individuals can save newborn lives at community level.

—DISTRICT PUBLIC HEALTH OFFICER, MORANG

Evidence Base

In Nepal and throughout the developing world, sepsis—a severe illness in which the bloodstream is overwhelmed by bacteria—is a leading cause of death among neonates (Weber et al., 2003). More than one-third of the estimated 4 million neonatal deaths around the world each year are caused by severe infections, and a quarter are due to neonatal sepsis or pneumonia alone (World Health Organization [WHO], 2009). Many factors contribute to the high number of neonatal deaths from infection. These include underrecognition of illness, delay in care seeking by the family, and lack of access to high-quality services to manage the illness (WHO, 2006).

In Gadchiroli, India, in 2005, a field trail performed by SEARCH, included community-based identification and treatment of possible severe bacterial infection (PSBI)[1] within a larger package of neonatal and perinatal interventions, conducted by trained VHWs who were hired by the project. The study demonstrated a 62% reduction in neonatal mortality (Bang et al., 2005). A similar home care approach was used for infection management in Sylhet, Bangladesh, and showed a mortality reduction of 34% (Baqui et al., 2008). Although both of these studies contributed significantly to the body of knowledge on community-based management of newborns, health workers trained outside the government system were instrumental in the implementation of these research programs. MINI was the first of its kind to partner with a district government to train existing government staff and volunteers for its model.

Funding

The Saving Newborn Lives (SNL) initiative, led by Save the Children–USA, is funded through a generous grant from the Bill and Melinda Gates Foundation. SNL promotes affordable and sustainable solutions to maternal and neonatal health issues in countries where neonatal death rates are highest (Save Children, 2002). The initial funding for JSI Research and Training Institute to implement MINI began in 2004 under Save the Children's SNL Initiative I. After MINI's initial successes from 2004–2006, the United States Agency for International Development (USAID) funded an expansion of the program in late 2006 and provided ongoing technical assistance and logistical support. Save the Children resumed funding from 2007 under SNL Initiative II. The external funding ended on December 31, 2009.

Morang District

Morang District, located in the southeastern part of Nepal adjacent to the Indian border, was selected as the site for MINI (**Figure 15-4**). Morang is primarily low-lying, flat agricultural land with some adjoining hills and has an area of 1,855 square kilometers. It has a population of 914,799, 80% of which is rural (Sharma, Joshi, & Bhandari, 2007). The per capita income for Morang is US$297, and the overall literacy rate is 56% (female 47%, male 67%) (International Centre for Integrated Mountain Development, Central Bureau

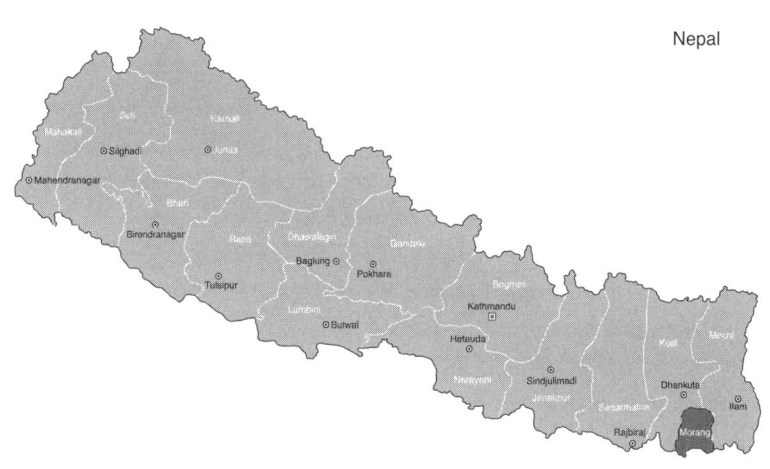

Figure 15-4 Map of Nepal with the zones, capital cities, and the Morang district highlighted.

Source: © Volina/ShutterStock, Inc.

CHAPTER 15   Saving Newborns at the Community Level

of Statistics, & Netherland Development Organization, 2005; United Nations Development Programme, 2005). One of the most diverse districts in Nepal, Morang, is home to more than 14 major ethnic groups. Morang was selected as the first district to implement community-based management of neonatal sepsis because of its accessibility and its success as an early ARI program district experienced in training FCHVs to treat children.

Initially, 21 of Morang's 65 VDCs were selected for the MINI program model, but after demand from local government and governing bodies, the program was implemented in all 65 VDCs (including eight hill VDCs) by the end of 2006. There is only one hospital in the area providing referral care for young infants. Each VDC has one government health facility staffed with some combination of VHWs, AHWs, MCHWs, and ANMs serving an average population of 14,219 people, and nine FCHVs (one per ward) are working in their immediate community and serving an average population of approximately 1,200 people. In Morang, only 18% of deliveries are conducted at health facilities. Among those deliveries conducted at home, only 6% are attended by health workers. Prior to the initiation of MINI, only 6% of expected neonatal sepsis cases were recorded as seen at health facilities, and little is known about their care.

Partners

The MINI partners include the following:

- DPHO, Morang: Leaders at the DPHO were partners in earlier community-based programs. It was acknowledged that this was an unmet need because no program was addressing infants younger than 2 months of age. The DPHO had partial ownership of the effort from the onset.
- MoHP, Kathmandu: The Child Health Division supported MINI as an extension of what FCHVs were already active in doing through the ARI program in diagnosing and treating pneumonia with sulfamethoxazole and trimethoprim (Cotrim). The MoHP, Nepal, approved MINI's work, and ethical approval to conduct this program model was obtained from the Western Institutional Review Board (WIRB) in the United States.
- JSI Research and Training Institute, Nepal: JSI has been working on child and family health programs in Nepal continuously since 1981, providing support to the Ministry of Health for strengthening various health programs primarily through USAID-funded bilateral projects.

- Nepal Family Health Program: Under the Nepal Family Health Program (NFHP) cooperative agreement, JSI continues to work with multiple partners to assist the MoHP in an expanded role to strengthen the delivery and use of high-impact family planning and maternal and child health services delivered at the household and community level.
- Save the Children–USA, SNL, Nepal: In June 2000, SNL identified Nepal as one of six target countries. Early on, SNL staff familiar with JSI's previous success with integrated management of childhood illnesses and community-based pneumonia programs gathered a team of potential partners to propose an initiative to attempt community-based management of neonatal sepsis in Nepal. A proposal was subsequently developed by JSI and funded by SNL to begin in Morang.

The MINI Model

The fact that MINI was implemented in complete partnership with the local government and through the existing channels and functions of the health system makes the model unique and successful.

—MINI Field Coordinator, July 2009

The idea and motivation behind MINI was that it is possible to manage neonatal infection within a government's existing health infrastructure in communities where access to district hospitals or primary healthcare facilities may be difficult. In rural areas, Nepal's health system is sustained by the most peripheral community health workers based in health posts and subhealth posts and a strong cadre of FCHVs.

Implementation

MINI's philosophy from the program's onset was to partner with the local government at each stage to ensure support and ownership for the eventual sustainability of the model. MINI partnered with the government to provide funding and technical support in logistics and supply management, data management, training, supervision, and monitoring. The MINI program model was envisioned to test a sustainable and replicable approach for the MoHP to implement at a smaller scale. Hence, it was conducted through the existing government infrastructure (**Figure 15-5**).

CHAPTER 15 Saving Newborns at the Community Level

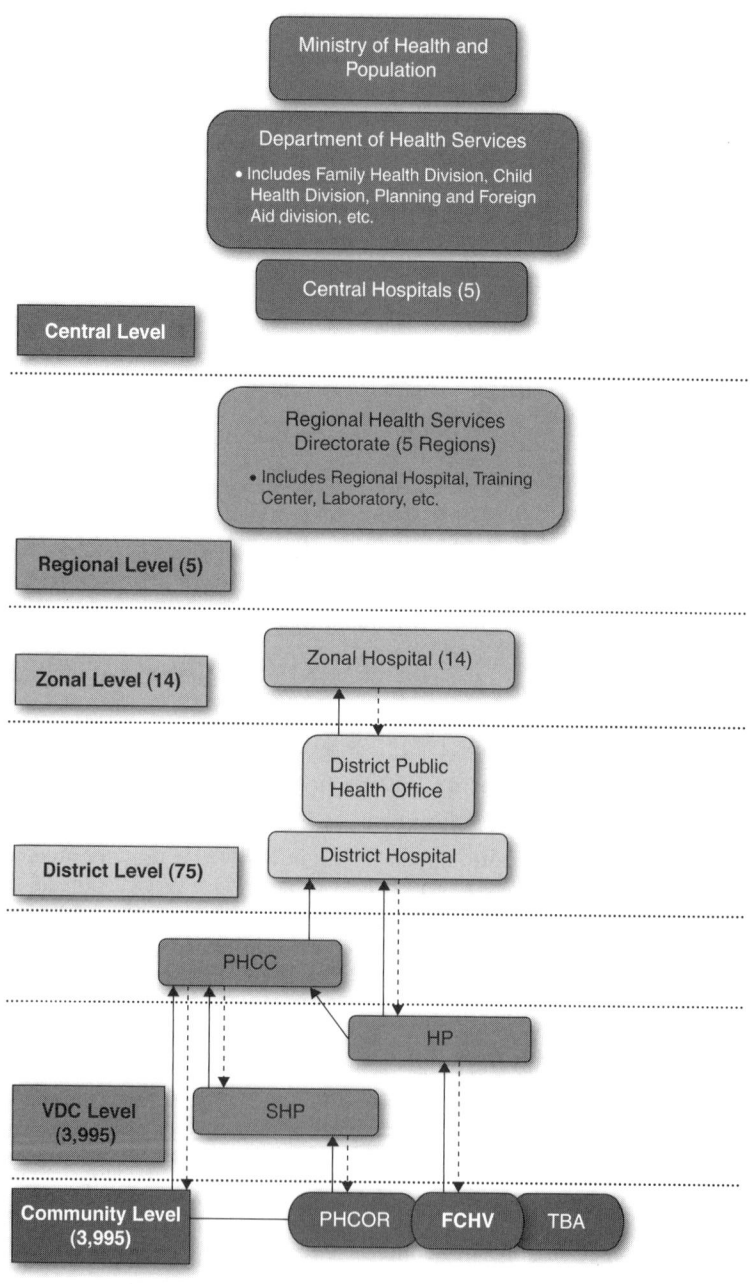

Figure 15-5 Central and local health system.

Human Resources

FCHVs: MINI Champions

It's about serving and contributing to the nation. Now that I can treat newborns, I feel that I have earned the respect and faith of my community more than ever before.

—FCHV in Morang, July 2009

FCHVs are local women who serve in all wards (the lowest administrative unit) of Nepal. They are the frontline health workers in communities and are, in most cases, the first point of contact with the health system for mothers and newborns. They receive basic training (18 days) and periodic refresher and program-specific trainings. Since the FCHV program was established in 1988, FCHVs have been given responsibility by the MoHP for health promotion and some limited service provision. Because they reside in the communities they serve, they are likely to know about pregnancies and deliveries and are thus able to record births.

Though many are illiterate, more than 50,000 FCHVs have been trained to detect and treat a range of childhood illnesses, and they often provide life-saving advice and treatment where no other health services exist (UNICEF, 2007). FCHVs have led awareness efforts for national immunization campaigns and administered polio vaccinations and vitamin A supplements, and they have provided advice and iron–folate supplements to pregnant women. In cases of severe childhood diarrhea, they provide oral rehydration therapy and zinc tablets. They support family planning activities and have also been trained to identify and manage pneumonia with oral sulfamethoxazole/trimethoprim pediatric tablets (Cotrim Pediatric) in children older than 2 months of age in most of Nepal.

Since FCHVs are not paid government employees, they often make sacrifices in their homes and family life to serve their communities. Despite these challenges, many FCHVs have stated they gain personal satisfaction from serving their communities, saving newborn lives, and promoting safe motherhood programs among new and expecting mothers. FCHVs must have the support of their husbands and other family members because their work often compromises responsibilities in the home. It seems that some FCHVs and their husbands agree that the work is a worthwhile undertaking because it is related to dharma, the Hindu and Buddhist spiritual and religious term that means one's righteous duty or any virtuous path. FCHVs do not face cultural and social barriers that

CHAPTER 15 Saving Newborns at the Community Level

prevent males from entering a home to provide maternal and child health services. FCHVs in Nepal are not usually compensated in any way for their work, although small incentives such as tote bags, umbrellas, flashlights, ID cards, and certificates were provided by MINI for motivation.

Facility-based Community Health Workers (FB-CHWs), a purely descriptive term for MCHWs, VHWs, and AHWs, are the most peripheral paid government health workers. Their basic education varies from grade 8 to grade 10, and they receive in-service training, which includes injection skills. They were involved in facility-based parts of MINI's program but had no specific skills to manage neonatal infections prior to the program.

Leadership

Dr. Penny Dawson, a physician and public health champion with more than 25 years of experience in child survival in Nepal, assumed JSI's senior leadership position on the MINI team. She served as the principal investigator and technical advisor for MINI. Having achieved tremendous success with earlier community-based ARI programs in Morang and throughout Nepal, her experience in implementing community-based programs in collaboration with government health officials facilitated MINI's integration in existing child health programs in Morang and provided the expertise necessary to design an effective training program for newborn infection management.

In Morang, the program was supported by numerous District Public Health Officers due to quick turnover in leadership. They were instrumental in introducing the program to political parties and in building support for MINI and coordinating government efforts at the district level. MINI funded the trainings, and the DPHO provided the personnel and support to conduct the trainings.

Field Staff

At its peak, MINI had eight field supervisors (with full district coverage) who served as the direct supervisory link between FCHVs, FB-CHWs, and MINI's program staff. These field supervisors were at the level of auxiliary health workers with 1 year of paramedical training and experience at the community level.

The importance of supportive and trusting relationships between the field supervisors and the FCHVs and health workers in each VDC cannot be overstated. MINI's most recent project director made the following comment:

> When it comes to working with volunteers and community-based programs, the motivation and dedication of each health professional and health volunteer stems

from the commitment of the trainers and field supervisors who mentor, support and spend time on a consistent basis listening to the concerns and issues in each community, whether directly involved with MINI's activities or not.

Training and Supervision

Training, communication, and data recording materials were developed by the MINI team with support and input from NFHP staff and the DPHO, Morang. Taking into consideration the semiliterate status of many FCHVs, pictorial materials were drafted, pretested, and revised before finalization. A total of 189 FCHVs and 83 FB-CHWs were initially trained on the assessment and management of neonatal infections and essential newborn care (ENC) messages. The FB-CHWs were trained for 4 days, and the FCHVs were trained for 5 days. Allowances for training were paid according to government rules and regulations, but no cash incentives were provided for service delivery. Because of the program's initial success and proven training model, in late 2006 the remaining 396 FCHVs in Morang and the health facility staff were trained to expand the program throughout the district. Regular supervision for program implementation was provided through the existing government system. In addition, MINI field supervisors provided support to reinforce clinical skills of FCHVs and FB-CHWs and to collect specific data as part of the model's expanded monitoring system.

Treatment and Management of Sick Young Infants

Before MINI, we were only treating children between the ages of two months and five years. Now we can fill that gap and we have the tools and knowledge to help an infant less than two months old and that is a very good thing for mothers, for families, and for our communities.

—FCHV, Morang, July 2009

The main objective of MINI was to test a replicable model for community-based management of infections in neonates and young infants within the existing government health system. The specific objectives were to demonstrate the following:

- FCHVs can identify births, correctly assess sick neonates and young infants, initiate oral antibiotic treatment, and facilitate referral for injectable antibiotics for PSBI.

- FB-CHWs can respond to referrals in a timely fashion and administer an injectable antibiotic for PSBI.

A technical working group (TWG) was established to guide all technical aspects of MINI implementation. The TWG and national neonatal experts approved the clinical algorithm[2] for PSBI, which was based on those used in SEARCH/India and the World Health Organization Young Infant Studies (Bang et al., 2005; Weber et al., 2003). Oral sulfamethoxazole and trimethoprim (Cotrim Pediatric) tablets, dissolved in breast milk, were given twice daily for 5 days. In addition, intramuscular gentamicin injection was given once daily for 7 days using insulin syringe (WHO, 2003). The treatment classification card that was used by the FCHVs is shown in **Figure 15-6**.

FCHVs had antenatal contact with pregnant women to provide iron–folic acid tablets, advise them on antenatal care, and counsel them on ENC messages and danger signs for the newborn. The ENC messages included the following: immediate breastfeeding after birth; immediate drying and wrapping of the newborn; applying nothing to the cord; and delaying bathing for at least 24 hours after birth. MINI trained FCHVs to conduct a postnatal visit for all births in her ward, ideally within 24 hours of delivery. She weighed the newborn, recorded the birth, encouraged the mother to register the birth with the VDC, counseled the mother on ENC, and assessed the baby for signs of infection. If any signs of PSBI were present, she initiated treatment and gave the mother a referral. The program model is illustrated in **Figure 15-7**.

Low birth weight infants were also identified and managed by FCHVs. Given the varying levels of literacy among FCHVs, MINI modified the Salter scale by coding weight ranges with colors to simplify measurement. After an infant was classified as low birth weight or very low birth weight (less than 2000 grams), families were counseled further on ENC, and the FCHV then conducted four follow-up visits.

If the infant became sick at any time within the first 2 months, the FCHV was called to examine the baby for danger signs. If any single danger sign was present, she classified the illness as PSBI. After obtaining informed consent, the FCHV assisted the caretaker in giving the first dose of oral sulfamethoxazole and trimethoprim (Cotrim Pediatric) tablets and provided the family with tablets to be given twice daily for 5 days. After giving the first dose of antibiotic, she completed a call form and directed a family member of the sick baby to call the

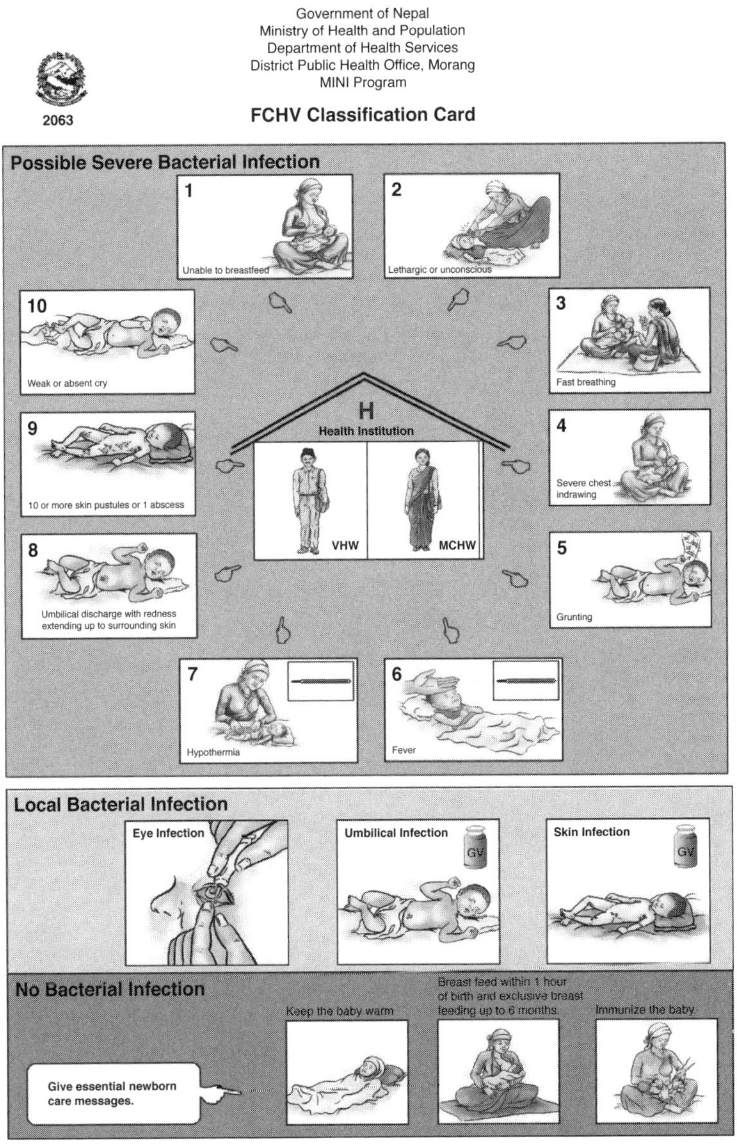

Figure 15-6 FCHV classification card.
Source: Courtesy of Morang Innovative Neonatal Intervention Program, JSI Research and Training Institute, Inc.

CHAPTER 15 Saving Newborns at the Community Level

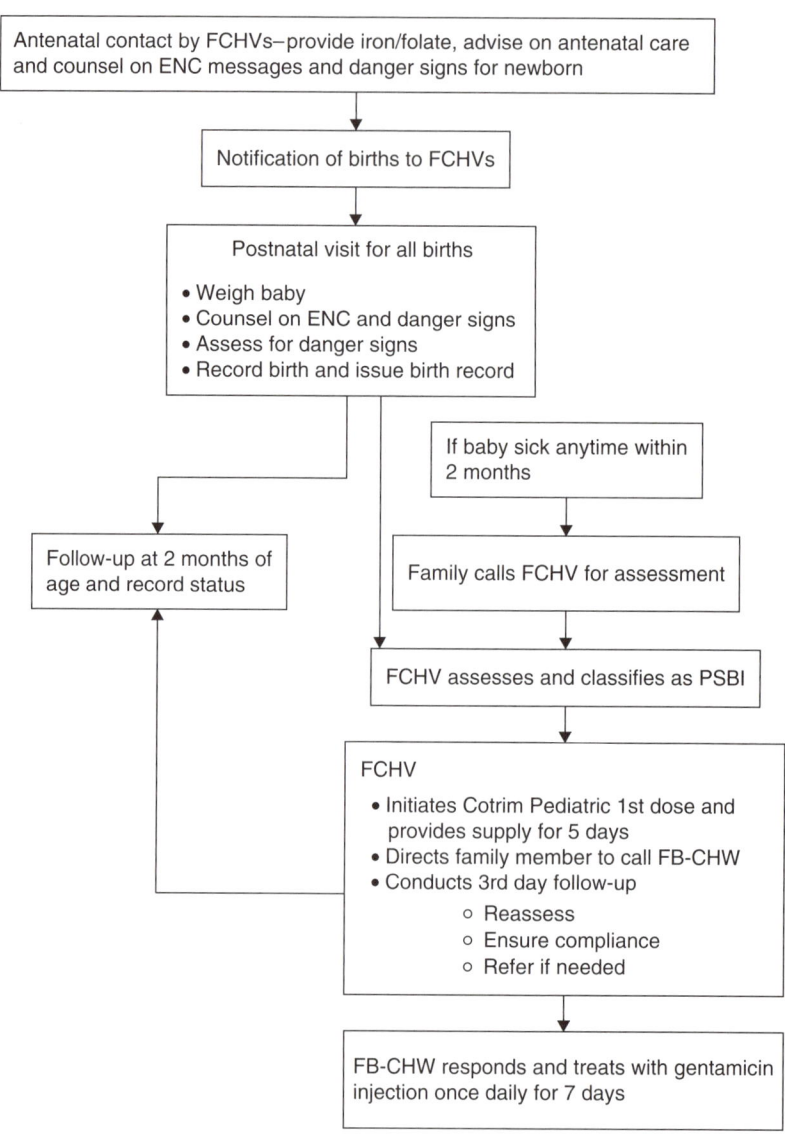

Figure 15-7 MINI program model.

Source: Courtesy of Morang Innovative Neonatal Intervention Program, JSI Research and Training Institute, Inc.

FB-CHW, who was trained and qualified to give intramuscular gentamicin injections. The FCHV subsequently made a third-day follow-up visit, reassessed the baby for danger signs, and ensured that gentamicin had been initiated and that sulfamethoxazole and trimethoprim (Cotrim Pediatric) was being given correctly. If she identified any new danger signs or perceived deterioration in the baby's condition, she immediately referred the baby to the nearest health facility.

All babies whose births were recorded during the study period were enrolled as participants in MINI. The FCHV conducted a 2-month follow-up visit to all identified newborns to determine the child's vital status and the outcome of any treatment. All FCHV and FB-CHW services were recorded in registers designed specifically for MINI, thus creating a longitudinal database for all recorded births.

Information Management

There is very little information available on neonatal health and the management of neonatal infection for most communities in Nepal. Most deliveries occur at home, few have a birth record, and many neonatal infections and deaths are not reported. Thus, an extensive system was developed to monitor a variety of indicators that would ultimately help provide the Ministry of Health with a set of recommendations for scaling-up MINI's activities. FCHVs and FB-CHWs used registers specifically developed to record all data related to the MINI program model, and they reported through the existing government reporting system.

Supply Chain Management

MINI relied on existing supplies provided through the government. FCHVs were already equipped with timers for counting respiratory rate and were already distributing sulfamethoxazole and trimethoprim (Cotrim Pediatric) for pneumonia management. MINI provided color-coded scales, registers, thermometers, pricking needles, and gentamicin. Insulin syringes were provided to health facilities, and ARI timers, and sulfamethoxazole and trimethoprim (Cotrim Pediatric) tablets were resupplied as needed to FCHVs and health facilities. After initial support through MINI, supplies were gradually distributed and financed through the DPHO to stimulate the existing government system and promote sustainability. Because of political disturbances, there was a potential for supply disruptions, but on the whole, health facilities were well stocked and field supervisors carried backup supplies in case stock shortages were encountered. To the extent possible, these supplies were provided through existing DPHO channels for distribution to FCHVs. Gentamicin is now on the approved essential drug list for subhealth posts, which allows immediate implementation of community-based treatment of neonatal sepsis in future districts.

Decreased Supervision Model

The extensive supervision and monitoring that was done by MINI field supervisors in the first phase of implementation was followed by a decreasing supervision model to learn the effects of supervision as the program matured and to provide a model for future implementation of a similar program to other districts. Under MINI's second phase, a streamlined supervisory support model was tested to assess program performance when external supports are decreased.

Achievements

I sincerely believe that MINI is an effective, necessary program that is appropriate for Nepal's context. I have faith that while the MINI field staff will be no longer with us, MINI activities will become a regular program and will continue.

—VHW, Morang District, July 2009

MINI proved that through strong partnerships, community relationships, and effective program implementation, FCHVs and FB-CHWs in rural villages can successfully identify and treat infections in newborns and provide care to those who previously had no other option at the community level.

Impact Indicators

The impact of MINI is summarized as follows:

- Before the intervention in Morang, only 6% ($n = 98/1663$) of expected episodes of PSBI in young infants were recorded and addressed at government health facilities, and after 2 years of MINI activities, the percentage of expected episodes that were treated at health facilities increased to 29%.
- Among 48,753 live births recorded between May 2005 and April 2009, 3,446 episodes of PSBI were identified in young infants.
- A total of 10,013 young infants were treated through MINI's program from May 1, 2005, to April 30, 2009, including both local bacterial infections and PSBI.

- Additionally, 56% (of the 48,753 live births) were treated by FCHVs. When taking into account the number that were seen by FCHVs, the total expected cases treated within Ministry of Health infrastructure was 78% of all cases.
- The FCHVs' overall diagnosis of PSBI matched that of the more highly trained FB-CHWs in 100% of cases, when assessed on the same day.
- The timing of treatment for PSBI is important, and MINI attempted to ensure early treatment. During the intervention period, 85% of PSBI episodes identified by FCHVs or FB-CHWs had gentamicin injections initiated within 2 days of identification.
- For the same time period, there were 3,448 total PSBI cases identified. Of these, 2,988 (94%) received all 7 doses of gentamicin.
- Treatment was initiated in 90% of PSBI episodes.
- The case fatality in fully treated episodes was 0.3%, compared to 18.2% in untreated episodes and 11.3% in partially treated episodes.
- Less-privileged groups, as classified by the government, accounted for 61% of the total population served by MINI.

The results show that one of the major causes of neonatal mortality can be effectively managed, within an existing government system, by utilizing an existing cadre of community health workers and volunteers with limited or no education. Through the use of a simple algorithm for identifying PSBI, focused training, regular supervisory and logistics support, and improved coordination between community and facility-based workers, an increased number of young infants can receive treatment for a potentially life-threatening infection, and the most disadvantaged groups can comprise the majority of the population served.

Demonstrating a Model for Scale-Up

By demonstrating that it is not necessary to create a parallel body of health workers or a new cadre of staff solely for the purpose of neonatal PSBI management, MINI serves as a replicable and scalable model for other districts in Nepal and similar settings throughout the world. In addition to the impact FCHVs have had on their communities through MINI and other programs, there have been important shifts in practices that previously prevented newborns from receiving appropriate treatment. Typically, family members do not take the newborn child to a doctor for at least 11 days (Save the Children, 2002). Now, throughout Morang it is more acceptable for neonates to leave the home before a name is given, and it seems that more mothers are leaving the home shortly after delivery to seek care if their newborn is sick, and it is increasingly more common for infants to be brought forward earlier and to more readily receive essential vaccines.

The knowledge and hope transmitted through MINI has also resulted in an increase in awareness for mothers on ENC. There has been a significant increase in knowledge of the importance of breastfeeding, wrapping, drying, delaying bathing, and appropriate cord care among mothers under MINI's care. This has likely contributed to a documented improvement in behaviors that may also be preventing infections and deaths previously caused by inappropriate newborn care practices.

Harnessing the Strength of Existing Programs

Community-Based Integrated Management of Childhood Illnesses (CB-IMCI)—MINI was able to assure community buy-in of the program by building on the strength of the FCHV program and the community networks through which they work. MINI was designed from the onset in close collaboration with the longstanding CB-IMCI program, making it a logical fit for future expansion neonatal infection management at the community level. In this way, moving forward in other districts may be more streamlined by incorporating the MINI model within the existing CB-IMCI program.

As one health post VHW expressed, "Of course mothers' groups are successful in promoting programs like MINI. Anything heard in a gathering of women is sure to spread throughout the village. No such thing happens if men are to gather and discuss things." Meetings were held monthly, and health facility staff supported the FCHVs in informing mothers about their new knowledge and the fact that they could now assess and initiate treatment for sick neonates. This became a powerful way for FCHVs to disseminate their new knowledge, spark behavior change, and connect with the pregnant and expecting mothers who they would serve in the future.

Indirect Benefits: Social and Economic Impact

Apart from saving newborn lives and preventing deaths attributed to sepsis, families involved in MINI's interventions have benefited in ways not directly related to MINI's intended outcomes. Families have reported cost savings through MINI because they would have otherwise spent money on expensive visits to distant clinics for newborn illnesses. This is in addition to time away from jobs and the cost of traveling to distant health facilities.

Additionally, there seems to be a more reliable system for birth recording in place, an essential part of identifying and treating sick young infants. This facilitates the formal birth registration through the government or local VDC. Through MINI, FCHVs weigh newborns, and this seems to be an important entry point, not only for recording a birth, but also for other postnatal care elements.

FCHVs have assumed a more curative role through MINI. They take pride in their contributions to saving newborn lives and are motivated by this important responsibility. Empowering and raising the status of these dedicated volunteers has been an indirect benefit of MINI's activities that is difficult to quantify, but it impacts all FCHV activities. Similarly, giving VHWs the tools and knowledge to treat PSBIs with injectable antibiotics has raised their status and their confidence in treating very young infants.

Challenges and Opportunities

One of the main challenges that this community-based neonatal infection intervention will face as it transitions to become a DPHO program without an external supporting organization is the decreased level of supervision at the VDC level. Although the government has already demonstrated the will and ability to assume full responsibility for MINI's activities and reproduce them in other districts, there is limited capacity to provide close supervision for every program. To achieve impact at a national level, Nepal's government has announced its support of a Community-Based Newborn Care Package (CB-NCP), of which the MINI model is a core component. CB-NCP will consist of seven components to be implemented across all districts to decrease neonatal mortality: (1) antenatal care, (2) promotion of institutional deliveries, (3) postnatal care, (4) asphyxia management, (5) low birth weight management, (6) infection management, and (7) hypothermia management.

MINI, as a proven model for infection management, is therefore being transformed into a core part of a national initiative to reduce neonatal mortality and will have a future home in a broader national initiative for maternal and newborn health. Because funding for gentamicin syringes, weighing scales, and treatment registers has come from MINI throughout the program's implementation, the government will need to assume responsibility for funding to ensure sustainability and replication in other districts. The District Public Health Officer in Morang remains confident that the central government will provide support for the continuation of community-based newborn care, but the officer claims that if support falters, the program can continue in Morang with support from other nongovernmental

CHAPTER 15 Saving Newborns at the Community Level

Exhibit 15-1 MINI Snapshot: UNIJECT

Technology and Innovation for Neonatal Health — maximizing outcomes in remote areas

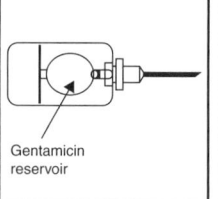

Gentamicin reservoir

The device pictured to the left is called Uniject, an injection device developed by PATH in Seattle, which is little more than a small bubble of plastic attached to a needle. It cannot be reused, which eliminates one route of disease transmission and it is precisely prefilled by the manufacturer with a single dose, which ensures that the correct amount of medicine is delivered. This device has been used for vaccine and contraceptive medicine delivery in many countries, and for the first time, it has been filled with gentamicin and used in field trials in Morang. Since many peripheral health workers in Nepal such as FCHVs are illiterate, this device can be used in areas where no other health workers exist.

UNIJECT was piloted in some of Morang's villages with support from USAID through the Nepal Family Health Program II (Cooperative Agreement No: 367-A-00-08-00001-00) in order to assess FCHVs' ability to administer gentamicin on their own when referral//travel to the health post is not possible and also to study the acceptability of FCHVs as an injector by the community. Approved by the government of Nepal before initiation, this is the first time FCHVs have administered an injectable treatment for children in Nepal. Preliminary results and conversations with FCHVs reveal that nearly all young infants completed the full 7 doses of injections of gentamicin administered by FCHVs using the UNIJECT device in the pilot area. When assessing other modalities for community-based management of sepsis across Nepal, perhaps UNIJECT can be incorporated into neonatal interventions as a strategy in the hill and mountain regions where more localized approaches may be necessary.

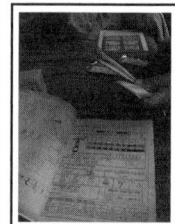

organizations, plus government funding for supplies and VDC and local community commitment through local resource mobilization. Currently, the DPHO in Morang regularly supplies gentamicin to health posts, and funding for syringes (**Exhibit 15-1**) will continue to come from MINI until CB-NCP is active. Regular data collection, although decreased from the volume that MINI collected, is flowing in via the regular government Health Monitoring Information System.

LESSONS LEARNED

The lessons learned from the MINI project are summarized as follows:

- Synergies: From the outset, MINI was not introduced as a separate project or undertaking, but rather a natural addition to other DPHO activities related to CB-IMCI and maternal and newborn health. Thus, the commitment of DPHO and health post staff was a natural extension of existing activities, and the strengths of both implementing partners were harnessed in the process.

- Commitment: Local level VDC commitment was crucial. Supporting incentives for FCHVs—such as monthly stipends, bicycles, and a revolving fund for FCHVs in each VDC to allocate as they wished—provided them with choice and flexibility in their own lives to devote more energy and time to the families they were monitoring.
- Dedicated personnel: FCHV and community health worker training and supportive supervision was a key link to the community. Although FCHVs in Nepal were unpaid volunteers, it seems feasible that in another country a paid cadre of health workers could also carry out these functions. However, if other countries create a new, paid cadre of health workers to carry out these and other tasks, they should be trained and operate within an existing government health system program to take the intervention to scale. Although task shifting was not a motivation in MINI's implementation, the existing function of FCHVs provided an opportunity to address the gap in access to care for neonates in a critical time when no other options for postnatal care may be feasible. The tremendous results seen in young infants treated by FCHVs may provide evidence for settings in which the policy environment for task shifting is less readily acceptable than in Nepal.
- Effective partnerships: Flexibility and effective communication with supporting partners was important at the community, district, and central level.
- Planning for sustainability: Working alongside existing government efforts, involving DPHO in all parts of the process, and preparing for decreased support from JSI as an implementing partner through a decreased supervision model were critical in preparing for the complete transition of MINI management to government. The program's success facilitated DPHO commitment to future needs, such as supplying gentamicin regularly after the model was proven.
- Relationships: Relationships were built between local communities and FCHVs. MINI became more than a job at each level of implementation. These relationships motivated FCHVs, field supervisors, and health facility staff to commit to saving newborn lives. The important bond among field supervisors, FCHVs, and FB-CHWs cannot be quantified, but the qualitative impact was tremendous for morale and momentum.
- Patience and persistence: When asked what they would tell other women who have just begun treating neonates, FCHVs in Morang explained that, "It is important to realize that you may not remember everything at once and that you may have difficulty or nervousness to start, but there is constant

CHAPTER 15 Saving Newborns at the Community Level

support and advice from health workers and field personnel." The persistence displayed by FCHVs was prevalent throughout MINI's system and allowed trust to build among those involved at every level of implementation.

The lessons learned from MINI's experience are further evidence that the political, geographic, and human resource challenges facing developing countries such as Nepal can be countered by the resilient spirit and dedication of female community volunteers, many of whom are illiterate or semiliterate. FCHVs, when supported by communicative field staff and when equipped with the knowledge and resources to carry out simple interventions in rural villages, have proven that saving newborn lives where no physician exists is possible.

NOTES

1. PSBI is a term MINI uses to define infections identified at the community level through a diagnostic algorithm based on the presence of any of the following 10 symptoms: more than 10 skin pustules, hypothermia ($\leq 35.5°C$), fever ($\geq 37.5°C$), unable to feed, redness around umbilicus, grunting, fast breathing, severe chest indrawing, weak cry, and lethargic or unconscious.
2. The final algorithm defines PSBI as the presence of any one of the following signs: unable to feed; lethargic or unconscious; fast breathing (60 or more breaths per minute); severe chest indrawing; grunting; fever (auxiliary temperature $\geq 37.5°C$); hypothermia (axillary temperature $\leq 35.5°C$); redness around the umbilicus; more than 10 skin pustules or 1 large abscess; and weak or absent cry. The TWG also approved the antibiotic regimen for PSBI, based on modified World Health Organization guidelines.

Discussion Questions

1. How does working within the Ministry of Health influence sustainability? What are some of the challenges presented by this approach?
2. What are some of the implications of dependency on female volunteers for the delivery of health services in general, and to maternal and child health services specifically?
3. Suppose female literacy was an outcome of this program. How would it have changed the training of volunteers?
4. Describe some of the issues related to scaling up a model that is volunteer driven.

REFERENCES

Bang, A. T., Bang, R. A., Stoll, B. J., Baitule, S. B., Reddy, H. M., & Deshmukh, M. D. (2005). Is home-based diagnosis and treatment of neonatal sepsis feasible and effective? Seven years of intervention in the Gadchiroli field trial (1996 to 2003). *Journal of Perinatology, 25,* Suppl. 1, S62–S71.

Baqui, A. H., El-Arifeen, S., Darmstadt, G. L., Ahmed, S., Williams, E. K., Seraji, H. R., . . . Projahnmo Study Group. (2008). Effect of community-based newborn-care intervention package implemented through two service-delivery strategies in Sylhet district, Bangladesh: A cluster-randomized controlled trial. *Lancet, 371*(9628), 1936–1944.

International Centre for Integrated Mountain Development, Central Bureau of Statistics, & Netherland Development Organization. (2005). *Districts of Nepal: Indicators of development 2003.* Kathmandu, Nepal: Authors.

Ministry of Health and Population, New ERA, & Macro International Inc. (2007). *Nepal demographic and health survey 2006.* Kathmandu, Nepal: Author.

Ministry of Health, His Majesty's Government of Nepal. (2004). *Nepal health sector program—implementation plan 2004–2009.* Kathmandu, Nepal: Author.

Save the Children. (2002). State of the world's newborns: Nepal. Retrieved from http://www.healthynewbornnetwork.org/sites/default/files/resources/State%20of%20the%20World%27s%20Newborns%2C%20Nepal%202002.pdf

Sharma, N. K., Joshi, S. R., & Bhandari, H. (2007). *District profile of Nepal.* Putalisadak, Kathmandu, Nepal: Intensive Study and Research Centre.

UNICEF. (2007). 'Miracle women' help combat under-five mortality in Nepal. Retrieved from http://www.unicef.org/infobycountry/nepal_42078.html

United Nations Development Programme. (2005). Nepal human development report 2005: Empowerment and poverty reduction. Retrieved from http://www.undp.org.np/publication/html/hdr2005/hdr2005.php

Weber, M. W., Carlin, J. B., Gatchalian, S., Lehmann, D., Muhe, L., Mulholland, E. K., & WHO Young Infants Study Group. (2003). Predictors of neonatal sepsis in developing countries. *Pediatric Infectious Disease Journal, 22*(8), 711–717.

World Health Organization. (2003). Explore simplified antimicrobial regimens for the treatment of neonatal sepsis. Retrieved from http://whqlibdoc.who.int/hq/2003/WHO_FCH_CAH_04.1.pdf

World Health Organization. (2006). Neonatal and perinatal mortality: Country, regional and global estimates. Geneva, Switzerland: Author.

World Health Organization. (2009). Neonatal sepsis—a major killer to be tackled in communities. Retrieved from http://www.who.int/child_adolescent_health/news/archive/2009/19_01/en/index.html

CHAPTER 16

The Nonpneumatic Anti-Shock Garment in Nigeria: The Tension Between Research and Implementation

Oladosu Ojengbede, MBBS
Elizabeth Butrick, MSW, MPH
Hadiza Galadanci, MBBS, MSc
Imran Oludare Morhason-Bello, MBBS
Carinne Brody, DrPH
Titi Duro-Aina, MBBS, MHSc
Adetokunbo Fabamwo, MBCLB
Suellen Miller, PhD, CNM

Location: Nigeria, Africa

Name of Project: The Nonpneumatic Anti-Shock Garment (NASG) for Obstetric Hemorrhage

Sponsoring Organization (and Funders): Safe Motherhood Program, Bixby Center for Global Reproductive Health at the University of California, San Francisco in collaboration with the Centre for Population and Reproductive Health, College of Medicine/University

CHAPTER 16 The Nonpneumatic Anti-Shock Garment in Nigeria

College Hospital, University of Ibadan, Nigeria. Funding provided by the John D. and Catherine T. MacArthur Foundation.

Target Population: Nigerian women suffering from obstetric hemorrhage

Project Goal: Reduction of maternal mortality in Nigeria through research and dissemination on the use of the NASG for obstetric hemorrhage

Project Objectives: Test the effectiveness of the NASG for obstetric hemorrhage in Nigeria using a pre-post design. Scale up from the initial pilot study by expanding to several facilities in northern Nigeria.

BACKGROUND

With the inception of the Safe Motherhood movement, ignited by an international meeting in Nairobi in 1987, global leaders have been working toward the elimination of maternal mortality. These efforts were reaffirmed by the establishment of the Millennium Development Goals (MDGs), wherein goal 5 calls for a reduction of maternal mortality by 75% by the year 2015 (United Nations, 2000).

Nigeria, with 2% of the global population, accounts for 10% of maternal deaths (World Health Organization, 2007). This most populous African country has one of the highest maternal mortality ratios (MMR) in the world, with national figures officially at 1,100 maternal deaths per 100,000 live births (World Health Organization, 2007). The leading causes of maternal death in Nigeria, as in many other developing countries, include hemorrhage, eclampsia, sepsis, and incomplete abortion (Ujah et al., 2005). Hemorrhage alone accounts for at least 34% of deaths (Khan, Wojdyla, Say, Gülmezoglu, & Van Look, 2006; Ujah et al., 2005).

In 2004, researchers from the University of California, San Francisco (UCSF) teamed up with researchers from the University of Ibadan, University College Hospital (UCH) in Ibadan, Nigeria, to investigate a new technology to decrease deaths from hemorrhage. The approach involved using an old device in a new way. The Nonpneumatic Anti-Shock Garment (NASG) is a simple neoprene and Velcro lower body compression device that is used to stabilize patients experiencing obstetric hemorrhage, consequently affording more time for patients to

Background

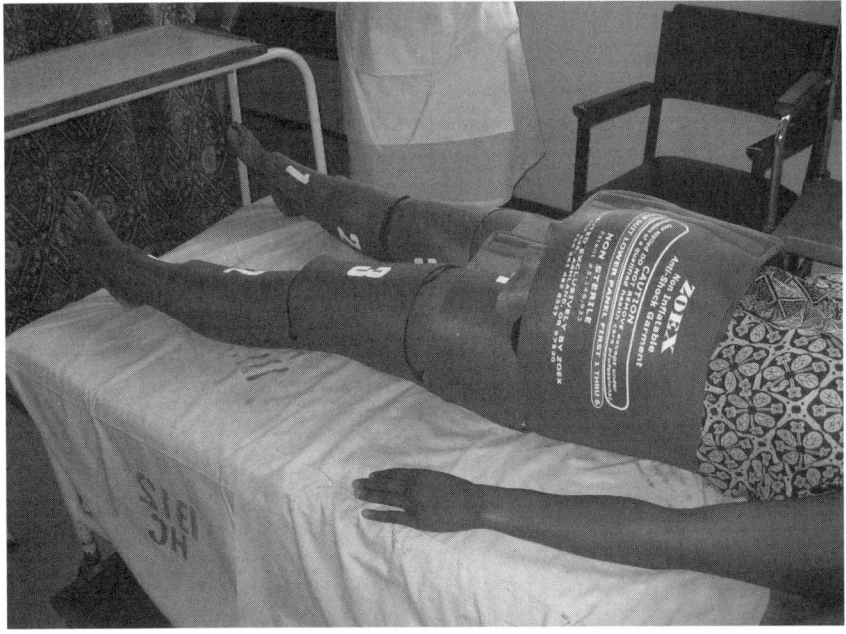

Figure 16-1 A woman in a nonpneumatic anti-shock garment.
Source: Courtesy of Safe Motherhood Program, UCSF.

access definitive treatment and care. The NASG can very quickly and effectively arrest the shock that arises from heavy blood loss, restoring consciousness and normalizing vital signs (Hensleigh, 2002; Miller, Hamza, et al., 2006).

As is often the case in low-resource settings, most maternal deaths from obstetric complications are related to delays. The woman or her family delay making the decision to seek care at a facility; after the decision is made, transportation is often difficult to obtain; and upon her arrival at the facility, there may be a delay before adequate care is given (Society of Gynaecology and Obstetrics of Nigeria, 2004; Thaddeus & Maine, 1994). These delays are particularly pernicious in the case of obstetric hemorrhage—due to the physiology involved, a woman can easily bleed to death in just 2 hours (Li, Fortney, Kotelchuck, & Glover, 1996). When it is wrapped tightly around a women's body, the NASG reduces blood loss and shunts pooled blood from the lower to the upper body, restoring oxygen and blood to the core organs. Through this stabilization process, a woman suffering hemorrhage and shock can survive the delays.

CHAPTER 16 The Nonpneumatic Anti-Shock Garment in Nigeria

Though the NASG is not a definitive treatment for obstetric hemorrhage, it offers strong advantages for use in Nigeria and other low-resource countries. It is simple to use, and with a few hours of training, anyone can competently apply it (although removal should be done only under medical supervision after treatment is complete). The NASG is low-tech, inexpensive (approximately US$4.25 per use), and reusable (up to 40 applications).

Prior to the beginning of this project, the NASG had only been used for obstetric hemorrhage cases in Pakistan by Drs. Paul Hensleigh and Carol Brees, who published a small case series on their work (Brees, Hensleigh, Miller, & Pelligra, 2004; Hensleigh, 2002). Dr. Suellen Miller of UCSF met Dr. Hensleigh, and they collaborated with Dr. Oladosu Ojengbede, University College Hospital, Ibadan, Nigeria for this project.

THE PROJECT

Stakeholders

The project, a pilot study and scale-up, had multiple stakeholders involved. The principal investigator, Dr. Suellen Miller, is the director of the Safe Motherhood Program, Bixby Center for Global Reproductive Health at UCSF. Dr. Miller is a certified nurse–midwife with many years of experience in international research and a long-standing frustration with the lack of tools to decrease maternal mortality. The John D. and Catherine T. MacArthur Foundation funded the study with the hope of lowering maternal mortality in Nigeria through projects that result in concrete and replicable outcomes.

The primary in-country partner was Dr. Oladosu Ojengbede from the Centre for Population and Reproductive Health at the UCH, College of Medicine, University of Ibadan and is an obstetrician–gynecologist and national trainer of Life Saving Skills (Basic Emergency Obstetric Care) for midwives. The study was reviewed and supported by the Federal Ministry of Health, whose drive to lower maternal mortality is further fueled by Millennium Development Goal number 5 and the lack of progress being made toward reducing maternal mortality. The study was carried out in hospitals across Nigeria where providers witness women dying from hemorrhage and eclampsia on a daily basis. Ministries of Health for each of the four states in which the project was set were also stakeholders, as were members of professional obstetrical (Society of Gynaecology and Obstetrics of Nigeria) and midwifery organizations. Hospital directors and heads of departments of obstetrics were involved in the expansion.

Design

The project was designed to improve on the evidence provided by Dr. Hensleigh's original case series. However, since reports of NASG use indicated that it could have a dramatic and obvious effect on resuscitation, it was clear that a randomized design was neither practical nor ethical. Thus, it was agreed to do a period of observation of cases in the hospitals without using the NASG (preintervention phase) followed by a period of observation of cases with the NASG (intervention, or NASG phase). Work began first in four hospitals in southern Nigeria, but it was eventually expanded to include 12 hospitals covering four states in the north and south of the country. Nigeria is a diverse country with important differences between north and south, so there was a strong commitment by stakeholders to address both regions.

Staff Training

Obstetric hemorrhage is, by definition, an emergency that can occur at any time to patients in various wards within a hospital. Hiring and retaining a round-the-clock research staff was not feasible, so it was necessary to train existing staff members to identify patients for the study and enroll them. Before initiation of preintervention data collection, staff trainings were held at each study facility to sensitize the staff to the issue of maternal mortality, review standard management of obstetric hemorrhage, and orient the staff to study data collection forms. The staff was also trained in the use of a blood collection drape for measurement of blood loss for patients enrolled in the study. These trainings occurred at the different study sites and were facilitated by lead staff from UCH and UCSF for both the preintervention and intervention phases. After 3 to 6 months of collecting preintervention data, the staff at the different facilities were trained in the use of the NASG and its integration into the standardized treatment protocol for obstetric hemorrhage. Thereafter, the staff collected data on each case of obstetric hemorrhage in which the NASG was applied. Research team members conducted regular follow-up visits and retrainings at hospitals for new staff members as needed.

Data Collection

Data collection forms included the following information:

- Basic obstetric history
- Details of the labor and delivery

- The cause(s) and initiation of hemorrhage
- Hemorrhage treatment and outcomes, including regular monitoring of vital signs, all blood, fluid, and uterotonics administered, and procedures and surgeries performed to treat the cause of hemorrhage
- NASG side effects
- Maternal and child outcomes

Expansion

Our research team was the first to use the NASG for obstetric hemorrhage in low-resource settings. In addition to collecting data, our research partners gained firsthand experience in treating women with the NASG. Providers had become accustomed to the difficulties of trying to treat women in shock who were slipping away. With the NASG, women in dire condition now became stable and treatable, and the providers and researchers became advocates of the NASG. As the project progressed, emerging results confirmed the physicians' experience. These results were duplicated in a similar study that our team carried out in Egypt with local partners (Miller, Hamza, et al., 2006).

Thus, as the project progressed, the stakeholders' commitment to expansion grew. The second funding cycle included an expansion into northern Nigeria. The maternal mortality rates in northern Nigeria are higher than those in the south, and the conditions are considered more challenging. Some of the facilities that were added later were deemed to have inadequate staffing for rigorous data collection and were not required to do the observational preintervention phase. In the last year of the project, interest by stakeholders in seeing the NASG reach as many patients as possible led the team to pilot the inclusion of several Primary Health Centers (PHCs) in the same catchment areas as the hospitals using the NASG. These PHCs are often the first stop for patients coming from the community. The PHC cases were not included in the study data, but the experience of working with and training them was valuable.

RESULTS AND REACTIONS

Acceptance of the NASG by providers was overwhelming. Doctors and midwives describe the device as a "life saver" (Oshinowo et al., 2007). One nurse described it this way: "It is very, very effective. Especially when there was low blood pressure—blood pressure which could not be recorded. When you apply it, you start to pick [up] the blood pressure" (Liu, 2009). Patients who were given up for dead by their relatives, regained consciousness and walked away from the hospital a few days later. One woman who gave birth at home arrived at the emergency room bleeding heavily. She had no pulse, no blood pressure, and was pale and cold. Her relatives left her bedside to go outside and grieve her death. The doctors in the hospital had just received the NASG, and they placed it on the woman. Within 2 minutes, her eyelids began to flutter and she began murmuring. The doctors called to her relatives to tell them that she was alive. The relatives returned, elated, and said to her, "You need a new name. From now on you are Ayorunbo—she who has been to heaven and returned."

Another woman who was treated with the NASG had this to say: "I beg the government, both state and federal hospitals, the [NASG] garment should be available. This thing is really saving life. The way women here give birth these days it takes women's lives . . . if this is available many women will not die" (Liu, 2009).

The results of the trial showed enormous promise. Statistically significant reductions were found in blood loss and extreme adverse outcomes, and these results emerged in peer-reviewed publications, where they have been presented in greater detail (Miller, Hamza, et al., 2006; Miller, Ojengbede, et al., 2009; Miller, Turan, et al., 2007).

As a result of this study, the Federal Ministry of Health in Nigeria has approved the NASG for use within Nigeria and is actively seeking funds to get it distributed nationally. The United Nations Population Fund (UNFPA), Pathfinder, and other nongovernmental organizations (NGOs) have expressed interest in using the NASG in national programs. Pathfinder included the NASG as one of the interventions in a large implementation project, Continuum of Care for Postpartum Hemorrhage, to address postpartum hemorrhage in Nigeria and India. Other NGOs have expressed interest in using the device, and local investigators are working with other states that want to implement the NASG.

The study has also been an important catalyst for building local capacity. It has reinforced the proper management of hemorrhage and shock and has given providers a new tool in the face of daunting maternal mortality rates. As one Nigerian doctor said, "the NASG to me is emergency preparedness. Because if you don't have it, you can't use it and you can't salvage life. That's the truth. To, me, it should be made available" (Liu, 2009).

The NASG has generated a lot of positive publicity, and media response has been strong. Local and international investigators have been interviewed by local television and newspapers, and the potential of the NASG has gained a lot of exposure within the region (Ejiogu & Adejokun, 2008; Nigerian Television Association, 2006; Oguntola, 2005; Orji, 2006). However, as important as these research findings and reactions are, of equal importance have been the challenges identified during this project that will need to be addressed when larger scale implementation in Nigeria or another low-resource setting is undertaken.

CHALLENGES

Institutional Capacity

The NASG is a remarkable device. It reduces blood loss, stabilizes vital signs, and prevents women on the brink of death from slipping away. However, it is only a first line of defense and *not a definitive treatment*. Full treatment of obstetric hemorrhage may include uterotonics, suturing, Cesarean section, repair of a ruptured uterus, blood transfusion, or any additional indicated treatments for the condition. In addition, though the NASG allows more time for the woman to seek care, it is critical that the facility have adequate, trained staff to monitor and deliver critical interventions, as well as adequate supplies of oxygen and normal saline for resuscitation, and additional medications and materials for definitive treatment. Finally, the timely availability of blood remains crucial for these patients, although fewer transfusions may be required due to the application of the NASG.

Staff Rotation

Training staff members to use the NASG is not particularly difficult or time consuming. However, as with all critical skills, if there is no repetition or continued use of the NASG, retrainings are required at fairly regular intervals. During the study period, we found it was critical to conduct regular retrainings mainly because the NASG was a new and unfamiliar device in these settings, and new staff members who had rotated in after the initial trainings rarely received a thorough orientation to the use and clinical applications of the NASG without retrainings.

Ultimately, in a national program, a significant part of NASG training will be part of preservice training and become the responsibilities of schools of medicine and midwifery to ensure an early and more structured integration of the NASG into the language and curriculum of healthcare providers. Full competency comes only with experience, so continued hands-on training in facilities will also be imperative.

Need for Supportive Supervision

Until the NASG is incorporated into preservice training, introduction of the device requires a period of intensive supportive supervision. Providers need feedback and a venue to discuss cases as they integrate the NASG into their practice. Because the NASG is most useful and needed during emergency cases—such as when a bleeding woman arrives with no pulse and no blood pressure—it needs to become completely ingrained in the emergency care routine. The NASG needs to be kept easily accessible, and staff members need to be trained to apply it immediately for a patient in shock. The device can ameliorate common problems such as the difficulty in securing a critical IV line in a woman who has already gone into shock. However, for this to occur, the staff must be trained to immediately apply the NASG before securing a line, which means applying the NASG instinctively as part of treating a patient in shock. This can be best achieved through practice and with intense, supportive supervision in all sites where the NASG has been introduced.

Referral Protocols

To date the NASG has mainly been used in tertiary facilities and a few secondary centers. Most of the facilities have been able to provide the definitive treatment that women may need. However, for the NASG to be employed to save the most women possible, its use should be extended to primary care facilities, which may not have the ability to perform emergency Cesarean sections, give blood transfusions, or provide other definitive treatment.

In order to employ the NASG in these situations it is essential that clear referral protocols be put in place, and *all* higher-level facilities to which a patient might be transferred must be trained in managing patients with the NASG. While the NASG is very easy to place, the greatest risk is premature and inappropriate removal. Staff members at a referral center who are not trained in its use might simply remove it as an unknown foreign object, thus causing the woman to rapidly return to a state of shock.

Our limited experience to date in introducing the NASG at the primary care level is a case in point. In spite of a clear emphasis during trainings that all patients must be transferred to specific higher-level facilities already trained in the use of the NASG, two of the first three referrals were made to a private mission hospital, which had not been trained in the use of the NASG. These referrals were made because the designated project facilities were on strike. Although in these specific cases the primary care facility staff reported accompanying the woman to the referral facility and supervising the removal of the NASG, these cases illustrate the potential risk of introducing the NASG at the community level when tertiary facilities are not prepared for such patients.

Finally, any system that requires the transfer of a women in an NASG also requires a system for tracking, cleaning, and returning the NASG to the center from which it came. In an environment where even the transport of a critically ill patient can be challenging, setting up such a system is no small feat.

Care and Maintenance

The NASG is made of neoprene and Velcro. With proper care, a single NASG can be used for up to 40 women. Washing is straightforward and follows the same procedure as other soiled hospital linens: decontamination with diluted bleach solution followed by scrubbing, washing, and hanging to dry. However, neoprene is an unfamiliar material to most hospital cleaning staff. It is bulky and will float, so it needs to be forcibly submerged in water to allow it to soak. In addition, the folding technique—while simple and easy to learn—is very specific; if it is not followed correctly, the NASG may be found in a tangled ball unable to be used with the speed required in an emergency. The issues around care and maintenance can easily be overcome with training, retraining, and supportive supervision. It is important to keep those who will be responsible for the care and maintenance in mind, especially since this may entail training laundry or cleaning staff, a group that is not usually included in large training sessions for healthcare providers. Separate smaller trainings in the local language are key to success with this group.

Community Acceptance

The NASG, for all its life saving properties, is not yet widely known. Therefore, it is not uncommon to have a woman brought back from unconsciousness only to request that the healthcare provider remove the very device that is keeping her stable! Until the NASG becomes more widely known, it is critical that providers educate patients and family members about its lifesaving properties and work to ensure that someone is always on hand to counsel a woman who has regained consciousness to find herself in an unfamiliar device lest she open the segments and lapse into shock again.

Research Versus Implementation

This project began as a research project to test a device with no previous rigorous testing in an obstetric population. As the project evolved, however, local researchers and other stakeholders became advocates for increased expansion and implementation. Faced with high maternal mortality and few strategies to combat it, after physicians saw the effect of the NASG, their goal was to get it to as many providers as possible. Although the funders were ultimately flexible and supportive of this goal, the researchers were challenged by the resulting data and observations from disparate facilities, with imbalanced comparison groups, and struggled to document enough cases to get statistically significant findings that could measure up in the peer-reviewed press. Publication in widely read journals would lead to broader support for research and dissemination as well as acknowledgement by international institutions, such as the World Health Organization, that have the power to implement the device at the global level. However, implementing this research in resource-poor settings with few other tools to reduce maternal mortality meant that saving lives took precedence over collecting complete and accurate data.

LESSONS LEARNED

The NASG is certainly a useful tool in combating maternal mortality in Nigeria. Any wide-scale implementation of its use, however, will have a number of challenges to overcome. We have presented here a few of the most salient challenges, noted by our team in the stepwise expansion from high-level teaching facilities accustomed to carrying out research to state-run secondary and tertiary facilities in lower-resource settings.

Primary among the important considerations for large-scale implementation is the caution that the NASG, as good as it may be, is no substitute for definitive treatment. Treatment requires facilities with trained personnel and necessary supplies. If a woman is unable to get medications, surgery, or blood after she makes it to a facility, the NASG is limited in how long it can keep her alive. When using an untested device such as this in a research model, it is important to establish clear, rigorous standards for facilities. In low-resource settings, research will often be given a lower priority than the immediate need to save lives. Assessing the capacity of facilities to participate in research, creating clear expectations for participating facilities, and simplifying data collection methods is essential.

Research in emergency settings requires a large staff or extensive training and retraining of facility staff, especially as staff rotate in and out of facilities. Intensive supportive supervision is also critical to assuring protocol compliance as staff members master new skills and integrate new protocols into their standard care.

Maternal mortality is a significant problem in Nigeria and throughout sub-Saharan Africa. Any solution must involve a multifaceted approach, and the NASG is one more important tool to put into the hands of providers.

Discussion Questions

1. List some requirements for the development and use of medical technology for labor and delivery in low-resource settings.
2. Explain the reasons for the rapid uptake of the NASG throughout different health settings and geographical regions of Nigeria.
3. What are the medical limitations of the NASG, and what are the other resources needed for it to be effective? How does this impact its scalability?
4. The use of medical technology is limited by human resources, both with regard to numbers of people and their professional capacity. Outline the human resource requirements for successful implementation of the NASG as presented in this chapter.
5. Discuss the interaction of the empirical demands of scientific research, with the resource needs of poor communities using the NASG as an example. Explore how the needs of both the research community and the client community can be met concurrently.

REFERENCES

Brees, C., Hensleigh, P. A., Miller, S., & Pelligra, R. (2004). A non-inflatable anti-shock garment for obstetric hemorrhage. *International Journal of Gynecology and Obstetrics, 87*(2), 119–124.

Ejiogu, E., & Adejokun, B. (2008, January 1). Miracle garment that saves women. *Daily Sun*. Retrieved from http://www.sunnewsonline.com/webpages/features/goodhealth/2008/jan/01/goodhealth-01-01-2008

References

Hensleigh, P. A. (2002). Anti-shock garment provides resuscitation and haemostasis for obstetric haemorrhage. *British Journal of Obstetrics and Gynaecology, 109*(12), 1377–1384.

Khan, K. S., Wojdyla, D., Say, L., Gülmezoglu, A. M., & Van Look, P. F. (2006). WHO analysis of causes of maternal death: A systematic review. *Lancet, 367*(9516), 1066–1074.

Li, X. F., Fortney, J. A., Kotelchuck, M., & Glover, L. H. (1996). The postpartum period: The key to maternal mortality. *International Journal of Gynecology and Obstetrics, 54*, 1–10.

Liu, L. A. (2009). *Mixed methods study of two interventions implemented to reduce maternal mortality in Ibadan, Oyo State, Nigeria* (Unpublished master's dissertation). University of Liverpool, England.

Miller, S., Hamza, S., Bray, E. H., Lester, F., Nada, K., Gibson, R., . . . Hensleigh, P. (2006). First aid for obstetric haemorrhage: The pilot study of the non-pneumatic anti-shock garment in Egypt. *British Journal of Obstetrics and Gynaecology, 113*, 424–429.

Miller, S., Ojengbede, O., Turan, J. M., Morhason-Bello, I. O., Martin, H. B., & Nsima, D. (2009). A comparative study of the non-pneumatic anti-shock garment for the treatment of obstetric hemorrhage in nigeria. *International Journal of Obstetrics and Gynecology, 107*(2), 121–125. doi:10.1016/j.ijgo.2009.06.005

Miller, S., Turan, J. M., Dau, K., Fathalla, M., Mourad, M., Sutherland, T., . . . Hensleigh, P. (2007). Use of the non-pneumatic anti-shock garment (NASG) to reduce blood loss and time to recovery from shock for women with obstetric haemorrhage in Egypt. *Global Public Health, 2*, 110–124.

Miller, S., Turan, J. M., Ojengbede, A., Ojengbede, O., Fathalla, M. F., Morhason-Bello, I. O., . . . Hensleigh, P. (2006). The pilot study of the non-pneumatic anti-shock garment (NASG) in women with severe obstetric hemorrhage: Combined results from Egypt and Nigeria. *International Journal of Gynaecology and Obstetrics, 94*(2), S154–S156.

Nigerian Television Association. (2006, July). Health reports: Maternal mortality and the NASG featuring Oladosu Ojengbede and Suellen Miller. Lagos, Nigeria.

Oguntola, S. (2005, December 8). Simple garment promises to safe [sic] lives of women dying due to bleeding. *Nigerian Tribune*, p. 3.

Orji, B. (2006, January). NASG device: A low cost intervention for severe obstetrics bleeding. *Current Reproductive Health and Population News, 1*(1).

Oshinowo, A., Galadanci, H., Awwal, M., Ojengbede, O., McDonough, L., Butrick, E., & Miller, S. (2007, November). *Overcoming delays in childbirth due to hemorrhage: A qualitative study of the non-pneumatic anti-shock garment (NASG) in Nigeria*. Panel presentation at the 135th annual meeting of the American Public Health Association, Washington, DC.

Society of Gynaecology and Obstetrics of Nigeria. (2004). Status of emergency obstetric services in six states of Nigeria—a needs assessment *report*. Abuja, Nigeria: Author.

Thaddeus, S., & Maine, D. (1994). Too far to walk: Maternal mortality in context. *Social Science and Medicine, 38*, 1091–1110.

Ujah, I. A., Aisien, O. A., Mutihir, J. T., Vanderjagt, D. J., Glew, R. H., & Uguru, V. E. (2005). Factors contributing to maternal mortality in north-central Nigeria: A seventeen-year review. *African Journal of Reproductive Health, 9*(3), 27–40.

United Nations. (2000). *United Nations millennium declaration, resolution*. New York, NY: Author.

World Health Organization. (2007). Maternal mortality in 2005: Estimates developed by WHO, UNICEF, UNFPA, and the Word Bank. Retrieved from http://whqlibdoc.who.int/publications/2007/9789241596213_eng.pdf

Index

Note: Italicized page locators indicate photos/figures; tables are indicated with *t*.

A

Abortions
  in Guatemala, 27
  incomplete, maternal deaths and, 304
  in Uganda, 75
Açaí palm (*Euterpe oleracea*), 226
Açaí products, marketing of, 226–227
Accountability
  Moms Mentoring Moms program and, 165, 166
  sustainability and, 267
Addiction, Moms Mentoring Moms program, Victoria, BC and, 154–155, 156–167
Adhikari, Urmila, 92
Afghanistan, maternal mortality in, 176
Africa, maternal mortality in, 176
Agency, Moms Mentoring Moms program and, 165, 166
Agriculture, Guajá of Brazilian Amazon and, 219–220
AHWs. *See* Assistant health workers
AIDS, 85
  in Democratic Republic of Congo, girls and women with, 134
  infant mortality in Uganda and, 75
AIDS care providers, in Uganda, 81
AJWS. *See* American Jewish Worldwide Services
Alcoholics Anonymous, 151
Alcohol use, pregnant women and, issues related to, 154–155
Altamira, Brazilian Amazon, 216
Amaranth growing, microfinancing loans for, from MHCD: MCH program, Democratic Republic of Congo, 143, 144
Amazon region
  development in
    altered lifestyles in Pará state and, 223
    globalization and, 228
  eastern, indigenous communities in Pará and Maranhão states, 214
  regional ecology of, 215
Amazon River, water volume flow of, 215
American Association of Birth Centers, 173
American Jewish Worldwide Services, 39
ANAHI. *See* Program for the National Support of Humanitarian Actions for Indigenous Populations
Anatomical apron, Timor-Leste
  family planning film discussion and use of, 112
  midwife leading family planning discussion, 113
ANC. *See* Antenatal care
Anemia
  home deliveries in Uganda and, 78, 78*t*
  Mbyá people and, 234
ANMs. *See* Assistant nurse midwives; Auxiliary nurse midwives
Antenatal care
  Community-Based Newborn Care Package in Nepal and, 297
  in Humla, Nepal, 92
  MINI in Nepal and, 290
  in Monrovia, Liberia, 130
  at Namwezi Health Center, Uganda, 82, 82
  in Timor-Leste, 105, 115
Antibiotics, MINI in Nepal and administration of, 287, 290, 293
Antigua, Guatemala
  Guatemalan context, 26–28
  Ixmucané Birth and Women's Health Center in, 28–45
  traditional and professional midwifery in, 25–48
Anxiety disorders, women who use alcohol and history of, 154
Argentina
  Mbyá people in, 233
  National University of La Plata in, 231
Armed conflict, outcome of, 101. *See also* War
Art activities, in Moms Mentoring Moms program, 160
ASECSA, 37
Asphyxia management, Community-Based Newborn Care Package in Nepal and, 297
Assimilation
  of Guajá into mainstream society, 221
  "weapons of the weak" and, 224

317

INDEX

Assistant health workers, in Nepal, 281, 284
Assistant nurse midwives, in Morang District, Nepal, 284
Audiovisual materials, for family planning program in Timor-Leste, 111–112, 113, *113*, 114, 118
Aukland University of Technology, Centre for Midwifery and Women's Health Research, 189
Australian Agency for International Development (AusAID), 103, 115, 145
AUT. *See* Aukland University of Technology
Autonomy, Moms Mentoring Moms program and, 165, 166
Auxiliary nurse midwives, in Humla, Nepal, 91, 92, 93
Awareness, Mobilization, and Action for Safe Motherhood: A Field Guide, 80

B

Balbina Dam, Brazilian Amazon, 217
Bangladesh, infection management in, 282
Barlake system, in Timor-Leste, fertility rate and, 106
Barriers to health care, lifting, Moms Mentoring Moms program and, 154, 157, 161, 165, 167
Basic essential obstetric care, 45
Basnet, Pushpa, 92
Bed nets, malaria control and, 77
Behavior change, incentives for, within health systems worldwide, 93
Behavior Change Initiative, Humla, Nepal, 89–97
Belém, Brazilian Amazon, 215, 216, 222
Belize, Central America, 5, 7–8. *See also* Toledo District, Belize, Central America
place of birth and attendant (2002), 8*t*
population of, 8
Belizean medical system, childbirth in, 9–10
Belizean Ministry of Health (MOH), 14
disjuncture between GIFT's TBA program and maternal health services of, 15, 16, 17, 18, 19, 20, 21
maternal and child health initiatives and, 6, 7, 9
Belize Creole linguistic structure, 15, 23*n*10, 23*n*12
BEOC. *See* Basic essential obstetric care
Betrothal of young girls, among Guajá, 218
Bhatta, Sandhya, 92
Bill and Melinda Gates Foundation, 275, 282
Biomedical knowledge, Mbyá granddaughter on traditional knowledge and, 247–248, 249
Birth centers
in Haiti, 173
in New Zealand, 174
Birth complications, lifelong disabilities due to, 184

Birth defects, alcohol consumption during pregnancy and, 155
Birthing centers, growth of, 173
Birth kits, for women in third trimester, Uganda, 81
Birth Kits Foundation Australia, 134
Birth rates, at Warkworth from 2005 to 2008, 190*t*
Birth(s). *See* Childbirth(s)
BKFA. *See* Birth Kits Foundation Australia
Bolivia, 26
Bone health, sedentarization and, 220
Book for Midwives, A (Klein, Miller, & Thomson), 36–37
Boy soldiers, in Sierra Leone, rescuing, 123
Brain damage to infants, fetal alcohol spectrum disorder and, 155
Brain drain, 3
Brazil, 273
economic miracle of 1970 in, 216–217
global economy and status of, 227–228
Indian service in (FUNAI), 214
Mbyá people in, 233
northeast, human development index of, 225
Brazilian Amazon
maternal-infant care in, 213–228
regional ecology, history and development of, 215–217
Breastfeeding
Mbyá grandmother's account of, 240–241
Mbyá mother's account of, 241
MINI in Nepal and information on, 290, 296
of pets, by Guajá women, 221
public health campaigns in Brazilian Amazon on, 223
in Uganda, problems/issues/solutions, 78*t*, 79
at Warkworth Birthing Centre, New Zealand, 193
women in foraging bands and, 219
Brees, Carol, 306
Bride price, in Timor-Leste, 114
Bright Actors, Uganda, 80, 81
British Columbia, Moms Mentoring Moms Program, Victoria, 153–167
Buddhism, in Nepal, 278
Bukavu, Democratic Republic of Congo, 142
Bush doctors, in Toledo, Belize, 9, 13, 22*n*7
Business training, Community-Based Safe Motherhood Advisor program, Malawi, 66

C

caída de mollera (fallen fontanel), 254*n*5
Calendar method, use of, in Timor-Leste, 113–114
Canada, holistic, community-wide interventions for mothers at risk in, 154
Canada Mortgage and Housing Corporation, 158

Index

Carajás Mining Project, Brazilian Amazon, 217
Cardiopulmonary resuscitation, in Timor-Leste, 115
CARE/Peru, 37
Catholic church, as effective ally in Timor-Leste, 117–118
Catholic population, in Timor-Leste, 106, 108, 109, 116
CB-IMCI. *See* Community-Based Integrated Management of Childhood Illnesses
CB-NCP. *See* Community-Based Newborn Care Package
CBOs. *See* Community-based organizations
CBSMA program. *See* Community-Based Safe Motherhood Advisor program
Cell phones, Maison de Naissance community health workers and, 182
Cell phone towers, in Guatemala, 267
Central nervous system impairment, fetal alcohol spectrum disorder and, 155
Centre of Excellence for Women's Health, 155
Certified nurse midwives, program directors in Guatemala as, 263. *See also* Midwives
Cesarean sections, 310, 311
 rate of, at Ixmucané Birth and Women's Center, Guatemala, 33
 rate of, in United States, 190
Change, sustainability and, 267–268
Charles Sturt University, Australia, School of Nursing and Midwifery at, 146
Chichewa language, Malawi, 60
Chicken Soup Factory, Monrovia, 127
Chief nursing officers, in Malawi, Africa, 58
Childbearing patterns, foraging bands and, 219
Childbirth(s). *See also* Delivery(ies); Labor
 in Belizean medical system, 9–10
 in Haiti, social context of, 176, 177, 178–179, 183, 184, 185
 at Ixmucané Birth and Women's Center, Guatemala, 31, 33
 in Liberia, 124
 Mbyá grandmother's account of, 239
 medicalization of, 193
 recording, MINI in Nepal and, 293, 294, 297
 in Uganda, 75
Child care responsibilities, in Guajá society, gender and, 220, 222
Child health. *See also* Infant mortality; Neonates; Newborns
 Mbyá granddaughter's observation on, 248
 war and, 101
Childhood mortality. *See also* Infant mortality
 in Democratic Republic of Congo, 139
 in Haiti, 176
 leading causes of, 3
 in Maranhão, Brazilian Amazon, 225
 in Nepal, 279

 trends in, 280
 in Torbeck Plain, Haiti, 178
Child rearing
 Guaraní ethnic groups and, 236
 Mbyá grandmother's account of, 240–241
Child soldiers
 recruitment of, in Democratic Republic of Congo, 138
 rescued, in Democratic Republic of Congo, 134
Child spacing, integrating with maternal care, Timor-Leste, 108–118. *See also* Contraception; Family planning
Chimaltenango, Guatemalan highlands, MFM trained traditional midwives in, 38
Chimutu, Chief, 58, 59, 71
China, 273
Chiwamba, Malawi, Africa, 55
Chiwamba, Traditional Authority Chimutu, Lilongwe District, Malawi, Africa, meeting literacy challenge in, 57
Chiwamba Area Traditional Authority (TA) Chimutu, 57
Cholera, in Democratic Republic of Congo, 135
Christian minorities, in Nepal, 278
CHWs. *See* Community health workers
Citizens of the World program, 257
Civil unrest, in Timor-Leste, 116
Civil war, in Guatemala, 262. *See also* War
Classroom discussions, in Malawi, 60–61
Clinical tourism, 258, 262
Clinton, Bill, 259
Clothing
 distribution through PHASE Nepal, 95–97, 96
 in Guatemala, 267
 service learning in Guatemala and, 265
CNMs. *See* Certified nurse midwives
CNOs. *See* Chief nursing officers
Cole, Richard, 123
College of Medicine/University College Hospital, University of Ibadan, Nigeria, 303–304, 306
Colostrum, 36
Comadronas (traditional midwives), 26, 29, 34, 35, 36, 48*n*1, 257
Commodification, global, subsistence resources and, 226–227
Communication style, service learning in Guatemala and, 265–266
Community-Based Integrated Management of Childhood Illnesses, in Nepal, 296
Community-Based Newborn Care Package, in Nepal, components of, to decrease neonatal mortality, 297
Community-based organizations, in Uganda, 80, 81

319

INDEX

Community-Based Safe Motherhood Advisor program, Malawi, 55
  achievements of, 71
  adult functional literacy training, 65–66
  background on, 57–58
  business training and income-generating activities, 66
  community recognition of CBSMAs, 64–65
  key challenges faced by, 56–57
  singing in class: what songs and why, 61–63
  targeted activities to raise women's status/self-concept, 63–64, 71
  volunteers for, motivational factors, 66–69
    attendance of more TOTs in the city, 69
    contact and follow-up, 68
    friendship, mutual respect, and partnership, 67–68
    gaining new knowledge, 67
    high status of being visited by health worker traveling by vehicle, 68–69
    trip to city for training, 67
    work-related gifts and incentives, 69
Community development
  microfinancing loans from MHCD: MCH program, Democratic Republic of Congo, 143–145
  in Uganda, 75
Community-empowerment model, in Uganda, MOSMI and, 77, 79, 82
Community health workers
  at Maison de Naissance, Haiti, 181
  in Torbeck Plain, Haiti, 177–178
  in Uganda, 77
    summary of maternal and child health priorities, 78–79, 78*t*
Community service, service learning and, 259
Community Team for Ordinary Peoples, Argentina, 235
Complementary Survey of Indigenous Peoples, 233
Condoms, 80
Confidence building, at Warkworth Birthing Centre, New Zealand, 192–193
Conflict management, Moms Mentoring Moms program and, 164
Conflict zones, healthcare workers in, 101. *See also* War
Congo. *See* Democratic Republic of Congo
CONICET. *See* National Council for Scientific and Technical Research
Continuing education, Midwives for Midwives Training Program, Guatemala, 42
Continuum of Care for Postpartum Hemorrhage, 309
Contraception. *See also* Family planning
  contraceptive implant insertion, HAI midwifery staff, Timor-Leste, 110
  contraceptive prevalence rate, in Guatemala, 27

knowledge about, in Timorese villages, 112–114
Cord care. *See* Umbilical cord care
Corporation for National and Community Service, 259
Cosminsky, Shelia, 48*n*1
Cotrim, for neonate pneumonia, in Nepal, 284
Cotrim Pediatric, MINI in Nepal and administration of, 287, 290, *292*
Courtesy, service learning in Guatemala and, 266
Couvade period, Brazilian Amazonian cultural protocols and, 218
Cowshed deliveries
  discouraging, clothing incentive through PHASE Nepal and, 93–97, 96
  in Humla, Nepal, 93
Crimes against humanity, in Democratic Republic of Congo, 134, 135, 138–139
Crops, staple, Guajá of Brazilian Amazon and, 219. *See also* Diet; Food; Nutrition
Cross-cultural interaction, ethics of, 211
Cultural awareness, service learning and, 259–260
Cultural competency
  cultural humility vs., 259
  defined, 258–259
Cultural humility
  being present and, 267
  nuanced meanings and, 266
Cultural understanding, international student experiences and, 268
Curriculum
  for comadronas, Guatemala, 34
  nursing education, international perspective in, 258
Custody of children, regaining, Moms Mentoring Moms program and, 166

D

Dancing, in TOT workshops, Malawi, 61
Dawson, Peggy, 288
"Death without weeping," in Brazilian northeast, 225
Decision-making, service learning in Guatemala and, 265
Deforestation, in Brazilian Amazon, 217
Delay in care
  neonatal death and, 282
  obstetric hemorrhage and, 305
Delivery(ies). *See also* Childbirth(s); Labor
  in the community, Mbyá grandmother's account of, 239
  Community-Based Newborn Care Package in Nepal and, 297
  in Humla, Nepal, 91
  at Ixmucané Birth and Women's Center, Guatemala, 31
  Mbyá intragenerational/intergenerational agreement and disagreement on, 251

Index

Mbyá mother's account of, 245, 246
medical intervention in, 273
war and, 101
Democratic Forces for the Liberation of Rwanda, male and female sexual victims of, 142
Democratic Republic of Congo
  Mission in Health Care and Development in, 133
  rape as weapon of war in, 133–147
  stories of women and girls in, 139–144
  unverifiable statistics relating to health outcomes in, 145
  war fatalities in, 138
Demographic and Health Survey, in Timor-Leste, 114
Dental health
  carbohydrate-dense crops and, 219, 221
  caries in Guajá children, 221
Department of International Development (UK), cash incentives for institutional deliveries through, 93
Developing countries
  birthing centers in, 173
  maternal deaths from pregnancy-related complications in, 56
  mother–infant health practices in, importance of, 213–214
Developmental disabilities, alcohol consumption during pregnancy and, 155
DFID UK. *See* Department of International Development (UK)
Dharma, FCHVs in Nepal and, 287
Diarrhea, 244, 245, 248, 249. *See also* Gastrointestinal diseases
Diet. *See also* Food; Nutrition
  food pyramid guidelines, Amazonian experience and, 226, 227
  for Guajá of Brazilian Amazon, 219–220
  Mbyá husband on taboos related to, 243
Dietsch, Elaine, 146
Dietsch, John, 146
Dili, East Timor, HAI maternity services in, 106
Dirección de Asuntos Guaraníes, Argentina, 234
Disappearances
  in Democratic Republic of Congo, 138
  in East Timor, 104
  in Guatemala, 28
District Public Health Office, Nepal, 281, 284, 297, 299
Domestic realm, Mbyá women and, 236, 237
Donations, inappropriate, service learning in Guatemala and, 264
DPHO. *See* District Public Health Office
DRC. *See* Democratic Republic of Congo
Drug use during pregnancy, incidence of, in Vancouver's Downtown Eastside, 155

E

East Timor, 90
Eclampsia, 35, 127, 179, 304, 306
ECPI. *See* Complementary Survey of Indigenous Peoples
Electronic medical record system, at Maison de Naissance, Haiti, 181
El Salvador, 26
Emerging economies, medical interventions and, 273
Empowerment of women, traditional midwifery in Guatemala and, 26
ENC. *See* Essential newborn care
England, safety of maternity service in, 205
Enteroparasitoses, 243
EPI. *See* Expanded Program on Immunization
Episcopal Church of Haiti, 183
Espaso Oan (child spacing), Timor-Leste audiences and, 109, 112, 114
Essential newborn care, MINI in Nepal and, 289, *291*
Ethics, of cross-cultural interaction, 211
Ethnomedicine
  Guajá and, 221, 223
  non-Indian Amazonians and, 223
Eurocentric model, service learning and cultural understanding relative to, 262
Expanded Program on Immunization, Liberia, 129

F

Facial abnormalities, fetal alcohol spectrum disorder and, 155
Facility-based Community Health Workers, in Nepal, 288, 289, 290
Faculty
  preparation for, in Guatemala, 263
  service learning and role of, 268
Family empowerment, Moms Mentoring Moms program and, 162–163
Family planning. *See also* Contraception
  in Nepal, 92, 287
  in Timor-Leste, 108–118
  in Uganda, 75
FASD. *See* Fetal alcohol spectrum disorder
FB-CHWs. *See* Facility-based Community Health Workers
FCHVs. *See* Female Community Health Volunteers
FDLR. *See* Democratic Forces for the Liberation of Rwanda
Federal Ministry of Health, Nigeria, Nonpneumatic Anti-Shock Garment and, 309
Feeding practices. *See* Mother–infant feeding practices
Female Community Health Volunteers, Nepal, 276, 281

321

INDEX

antenatal care and, 290
classification card, 291
field staff and, 288–289
incentives for, 299
lessons learned, 299–300
MINI model and, 285
  as champions for, 287–288
  program model, 292
in Morang District, Nepal, 284
training and supervision of, 289
UNIJECT administration and, 298
Female Volunteer Health Workers, in Humla, Nepal, 92, 93, 97
Fertility
  enhanced food security and increase in, 218–219
  rate of, in Timor-Leste, factors related to, 105–106
  regulation of, in Timor-Leste, 103–118
Fetal alcohol spectrum disorder, 154, 160, 167
  diagnosing, criteria for, 155
  prevalence of, in Canada, 155
  prevention strategy for, 156
Fetal Alcohol Spectrum Disorder Community Circle, 153, 156
Feto Nia Funu (A Woman's War), HAI-produced film, 111, 112
Film, as health promotion tool in Timor-Leste, 111–112, 118
Financial cost, medical intervention in low-resource countries and, 273
Fish farms, microfinancing loans for, from MHCD: MCH program, Democratic Republic of Congo, 143–144
Fontanel, late closing of, in Mbyá child, 244
Food. *See also* Diet; Nutrition
  Brazilian Amazonian cultural protocols and taboos tied to, 218
  enhanced food security, increased fertility and, 218–219
  Mbyá women and preparation of, 236
  restrictions, Mbyá grandmother's account of, 240
Foraging societies
  fewer children borne by women in, 219
  gender relations in, 220
Forced sex for procreation, in Guatemala, 36
Formula feeding, in Guatemala, 36
Foster care system, 154, 158
  Moms Mentoring Moms program and reducing involvement with, 163
  Moms Mentoring Moms program for women once part of, 167
Four Cleans course (UNICEF), 36
Frenkel, Gal, 39
FRETILIN. *See* Revolutionary Front for an Independent East Timor

Friewald, Hannah, 29
Frontal fontanel, subsidence of, in Mbyá child, 244
Fruitful accommodation concept, 32
FUNAI, Brazil, 214, 219, 220, 224
FUNASA. *See* National Health Foundation, Brazil (FUNASA)
FVHWs. *See* Female Volunteer Health Workers

G

Gastrointestinal diseases, Mbyá child morbidity and mortality and, 234, 238, 244. *See also* Diarrhea
Gender
  discrimination and, in Guatemala, 27, 28
  Mbyá, care of sick children and, 250
  Mbyá culture, traditional roles and, 236–237
  violence based on, 38
Gender inequity
  in Guajá society, 220
  in Malawi, 63–64
  in Timor-Leste, 114
  in Uganda, 75
Gennaro, Susan, 58
Genocide
  in Democratic Republic of Congo, 139
  in Rwanda, 136
Gentamicin
  intramuscular injections, FCHVs in Nepal and, 293
  for neonatal sepsis, MINI in Nepal and, 294
  syringes, MINI in Nepal and funding for, 297, 298
  UNIJECT field trials in Morang, Nepal and, 298
Geographic information system (GIS) software, Maison de Naissance, Haiti and use of, 181–182
Geohelminths, infections among Mbyá people with, 234
Gift giving, service learning in Guatemala and caveat on, 264
Giron, Jelin Yadira Carranza, 26
Giving Ideas for Tomorrow (GIFT), traditional birth attendant training and, 5, 6, 7, 8, 12, 14, 15, 17, 18, 19, 21
Globalization
  maternal-infant feeding practices and, 227–228
  small environments and, 262
Global maternal child health, students of health professions with interest in, 258
Global maternal health care, service learning and, 268
Google Earth, 182
GPS locations of homes, in Torbeck Plain, Haiti, 178, 181–182

Index

Graduation ceremonies, Community-Based Safe Motherhood Advisor program, Malawi, 64–65
Ground nut project
 microfinancing loans for, from MHCD: MCH program, Democratic Republic of Congo, 144
Growth deficiencies, fetal alcohol spectrum disorder and, 155
Guajá Indians, 213
 case study of, 214
 rapid transition from foraging to farming and, 214, 218, 219–220
Guaraní women
 on mother–child health care, 238–253
  lessons learned, 249–253
  Mbyá granddaughter, 246–249
  Mbyá grandmother, 238–241
  Mbyá mother, 241–246
Guatemala
 civil war in, 28, 262
 distrust of health professionals in, 224
 institutional delivery in, 47
 organizing midwives in, 47
 population of, 27
 rural, introducing nursing students to childbearing practices in, 257–268
 social inequities in, 31–32
 traditional and professional midwifery in, 25–48
Guatemalan Ministry of Health, MFM training program intertwined with, 43–44
Guaymi, 238
Guinea pig farms, microfinancing loans for, from MHCD: MCH program, Democratic Republic of Congo, 144
Gurung, Mamita, 92
Gwenigale, Walter, 122

H

HAI. *See* Health Alliance International
Hai (mother-breeder), Guraní women's role as, 236
Haiti, 26
 Maison de Naissance in, 175, 180–185
 MamaBaby center in, 173
 maternal mortality in, 176
 social and economic disparities in, 176
HDI. *See* Human development index
Health Alliance International, Timor-Leste, 103, 105
 civil unrest and, 116
 cultural and religious barriers and, 116
 description of, 106
 family planning program through, 108–118
 film as health promotion tool and, 111–112, 118
 findings from community discussions in villages, 112–114
 information systems, 116
 lessons learned, 117–118
 primary mission of, 107
 program districts, Timor-Leste, 107
Health assistance, in Argentina, indigenous communities and access barriers, 235
Health Canada, 155
Health conditions
 Mbyá children and women and access to sanitary services and programs, 233–235
 Mbyá grandmother's account of, 239–240
Health disparities, reducing, service learning and, 259–260
Healthline Medical Clinic, New Georgia Area, Monrovia, Liberia
 description of, 128–129
 financial accounting at, 128, 130
 membership in LifeLine Network, 129–130
 opening of, 128
Health Ministry of Misiones Province, Argentina, 234
Health posts, in Nepal, 281
Health Professions Schools in Service to the Nation program, 259
Health Sector Strategic Plan (2007), Health Alliance International and, 108
Hemorrhage
 maternal deaths in low-resource settings due to, 305
 maternal deaths in Uganda and, 79
 reducing, Nonpneumatic Anti-Shock Garment and, 304–314
Hensleigh, Paul, 306, 307
Hesperian Foundation, 36
Hinduism, in Nepal, 278
HIV, 85
 in Democratic Republic of Congo, 135, 139, 142
 infant mortality in Uganda and, 75
HIV care providers, in Uganda, 81
HIV-positive mothers, USAID agriculture project in Haiti and, 183
Holistic view of patient, sociocultural preferences for care and, 259
Home births
 in prosperous countries, 273
 in Uganda, problems/issues/solutions, 78, 78*t*
Homeless women, in Moms Mentoring Moms program, 158
Homosexuality, stigma attached to, in Democratic Republic of Congo, 141–142
Hope, Moms Mentoring Moms program and, 159–160
Hospital de Jardín América, Argentina, 234

323

INDEX

Hospital delivery, Mbyá women and, 239, 245
Housing affordability issues, in Victoria, British Columbia, 158, 164
Houston, Jenna, 28, 29, 30, 31
Howler monkeys, Guajá women and breastfeeding of, 221
HRW. *See* Human Rights Watch
Huehuetenango, Guatemalan highlands, MFM trained traditional midwives in, 38
Huipile blouses, Guatemala, 267
Human Development Index
    Brazilian northeast and, 225
    Nepal's ranking in, 276
Human rights abuses
    in Democratic Republic of Congo, 134, 135, 138–139
    in Timor-Leste, 104, 108
Human Rights Watch, 138
Humla District, Nepal, 89, 91
Hunting and gathering societies, partible paternity and, 218–219
Husbands. *See also* Men
    FCHVs in Nepal and, 287
    Mayan, childbirth and role of, 9
    as sexual assault survivors, in Democratic Republic of Congo, 141–142
    at Warkworth Birthing Centre, New Zealand, 194
Hutus, in Democratic Republic of Congo, 136
Hygiene issues, maternal and child health in Uganda and, 78*t*, 79, 80
Hypothermia management, Community-Based Newborn Care Package in Nepal and, 297

I

IGA. *See* Income-generating activities
Illiteracy
    in Guatemala, 27
    in Malawi, 60
    in Nepal, 279
    in Timor-Leste, 105
Illness
    Mbyá, dichotomy between traditional vs. biomedical knowledge and, 250–251
    Mbyá granddaughter's account of, 248–249
    Mbyá grandmother's account of, 238
    Mbyá mother's account of, 243–244
    Mbyá women, intergenerational resources, decision making and, 252
Immigrants in U.S., meeting health needs of, 258
Immunization programs
    in Liberia, 125
    in Nepal, 287
IMPAC manual. *See* Integrated Management of Pregnancy and Childbirth manual
Incentives for behavior change, 93, 95–97
Incest, in Guatemala, 28, 36

Income-generating activities, Community-Based Safe Motherhood Advisor program, Malawi, 66
India
    medical technology and, 273
    SEARCH trial in, 282
Indigenous communities
    Argentina, sanitary programs for, 235
    Brazilian Amazon, 215–216, 217, 223–226
    Mayans in Guatemala, 27
    Western societies, power relations and, 220
    women's role in, 251–252
Indirect communication, service learning in Guatemala and, 266
Indonesia, East Timor occupied by, 104
Infant mortality
    clothing incentive in Humla, Nepal and reduction in, 95–97
    in Guatemala, 26, 27
    in Liberia, 122
    TTMs and reduction in, 125
    in Nepal, 279
    in Timor-Leste, 105
    in Uganda, 74, 76
    major causes of, 75
Infants. *See* Infant mortality; Neonates
Infections. *See also* Possible severe bacterial infection
    maternal mortality and, 179
    MINI in Nepal and treatment of, 287, 290, 293, 294, 297
    neonatal deaths and, 282
Influenza, Guajá Indians and, 214
Institute of Medicine (U.S.), 45
Integrated Management of Pregnancy and Childbirth manual, 37
Interahamwe soldiers, Hutu militia, Democratic Republic of Congo, 136, 142
Internal displacement camps, in Timor-Leste, 116
Internally displaced persons, in Democratic Republic of Congo, 134, 138, 141
International programming in health services, service learning applied to, 259–260
Internet cafes, in Guatemala, 267
Internet service, at Maison de Naissance, Haiti, 181
Intrauterine device (IUD) insertion, HAI midwifery staff in Timor-Leste and, 110
ipirui, 244
Iron-folate supplements, FCHVs in Nepal and administration of, 287
Ixmucané (Mayan goddess), 29
Ixmucané Women's Health and Birth Center, Guatemala, 25, 26
    beginnings of, 28–30
    as clinical practice model, 30–34
    "fruitful accommodation" at, 32

graduate thesis on Chicago home birth service and births at, 32–33
Guatemalan context, 26–28
lessons learned at, 45–46
training traditional midwives at, 37–38
unraveling and closure, 44–45

J

Jachuka (Mbyá mother), 237, 241–246
JHPIEGO. *See* Johns Hopkins Program for International Education in Gynecology and Obstetrics
Jimenez, Melida, 43–44
Jinja Hospital, Uganda, 76
Jinja School of Comprehensive Nursing, Uganda, partnering with Namwezi Health Center, 76, 85
Johns Hopkins Program for International Education in Gynecology and Obstetrics, 37
Jordan, B., 32
JSI Research and Training Institute, Nepal, 275, 284–285, 299
jurua, 251

K

Ka'aguy Poty community, Argentina, 234
Ka'a-Kupe community, Argentina, 234
Kambewa, Mary, 57, 58, 60, 68, 70
kamby ryru jere
  local healers and, 244
  Mbyá mother's account of, 245
"Kantayo" (song in Malawi), 62, 63
KAPs. *See* Knowledge, attitudes, and practices
Karai status, Mbyá and, 236, 254n2
Karakia (prayer), Maori culture, New Zealand, 205
Karki, Rita, 92
Kathmandu, Mrigendra Samijhana Medical Trust in, 91
Kathmandu Valley, 276
Katumba, Fred, 81
KB. *See Keluarga Berencana*
Kekchi-speaking Maya, in Toledo District, Belize, 8, 9, 13, 22n5
Keluarga Berencana, 108
Kenya, Mission in Health Care and Development in, 133
Kerechu (Mbyá grandmother), 237, 238–241, 252
Kivu provinces, Democratic Republic of Congo, 134, 136
Knowledge, attitudes, and practices, Safe Motherhood and, 58
Kristeller technique, at hospital in Punta Gorda, Belize, 10
Kuña Karai status, Mbyá and, 236, 254n2
"Kuphunzira Nkusintha" (song in Malawi), 61

L

Labor. *See also* Childbirth(s); Delivery(ies)
  cultural misconceptions about, in Malawi, Africa, 56
  at Ixmucané Birth and Women's Center, Guatemala, 31
  Mbyá grandmother's account of, 239
  Mbyá mother's account of, 246
  medical intervention in, 273
  obstructed, home deliveries in Uganda and, 78
  at Warkworth Birthing Centre, New Zealand, 193, 195–197
Ladinos/Ladinas, in Guatemala, 27, 31
Lamprecht, Virginia, 39
Landscapes, of Amazon region, 216
Land settlement projects, in Brazilian Amazon, 216–217
Language(s)
  gaining fluency in, 212
  service learning in Guatemala and, 261, 263–264, 265–266
Latin America, immigrants in United States from, 258
LBW. *See* Low birth weight
Leaf doctors, in Torbeck Plain, Haiti, 177, 178
Leisure time, gender and, in Guajá society, 220, 222
Les Cayes, Haiti, hospitals in, 177
Liberia
  background statistics on, 122
  childbirth in, 124
  civil war in, 122, 125–126
  reducing maternal and infant mortality in, 121–130
  training traditional birth attendants in, 124–125
Liberian Ministry of Health, 125, 129
Life cycle characterization, Guaraní ethnic groups and, 236
Life expectancy
  in Democratic Republic of Congo, 139
  in Uganda, 74
LifeLine Community Healthcare Program, Liberia, 121
LifeLine Network
  aims of, 129
  Healthline Medical Clinic, Monrovia becomes part of, 129–130
Life planning, Moms Mentoring Moms program and, 162, 163, 164, 167
Lilongwe District Health Office, Malawi, 66
Literacy
  effective medical intervention at community level and, 273
  Moms Mentoring Moms program participants and, 158
  rate of, in Nepal, 91, 279, 283

INDEX

training, Community-Based Safe Motherhood Advisor program, Malawi, 65–66
Lobbying, dietary guidelines, subsistence resources and, 226, 227
locro (Argentinian stew), 240, 254n3
Low birth weight infants
    Community-Based Newborn Care Package in Nepal and, 297
    infant mortality and, 75
    MINI in Nepal and, 290
Luganda language, in Uganda, 76
Lula da Silva, Luiz Inácio, 227

M

Maama Omwaana, meaning of, 76
Maama Omwaana Safe Motherhood Initiative, Uganda, 73–86
    community assessment and mobilization, 77–79
    data collection for, 84
    endnote, 86
    founding of, 76
    goals and objectives of, 76–77
    key to success of, 84
    outcomes, 82
    utilization of antenatal care, 82, 82
    in White Ribbon Alliance for Safe Motherhood, 81
Machismo, 38
Mai Ita Koko! (Come Let's Try!) campaign, in Timor-Leste, 111
Maila, Humla, Nepal
    community meeting in, 94
    PHASE health workers in, 91, 92
Maison de Naissance, Haiti, 175, 180–185
    case study review, 185
    community-based services, 181
    discussion, 184–185
    facility-based services, 180–181
    funding challenges of, 173
    home visits through, 185
    monitoring and evaluation, 182–183
    results, 183
    supporting technology, 181–182
Malaria
    control of, in Uganda, 75, 77, 80
    in Democratic Republic of Congo, girls and women with, 135
    Guajá Indians and, 214, 224
Malawi, Africa
    maternal mortality ratio in, 56
    Safe Motherhood program in, 55–71
Malawian Adult Literacy Trainers, certified, 65
Mallinga, Stephen, 81
Malnutrition
    in Humla, Nepal, 91, 92
    in Kivu provinces, Democratic Republic of Congo, 134, 142

Mbyá people and, 234
MamaBaby, Haiti, founding of, 173
Manaus, Brazilian Amazon, 216
Manioc (*Manihot esculenta*), Guajá of Brazilian Amazon and cultivation of, 219, 227
Maoist Communist Party, Nepal, 277
Maori culture, New Zealand, 205
Maranhão, Brazilian Amazon
    child mortality in, 225
    maternal-infant care in, 213
Marketing, of açaí products, 226–227
Marriage practices, among Guajá of Brazilian Amazon, 218–219, 220
Maternal and Child Health (MCH) program. *See* Mission in Health Care and Development: Maternal and Child Health Program, Democratic Republic of Congo
Maternal health care
    global, learning about through service learning, 268
    integrating child spacing with, Timor-Leste, 108–118
    Mbyá mother's account of, 243–244
    war and, 101
Maternal-infant feeding practices, globalization and, 227–228
Maternal mortality
    in Democratic Republic of Congo, 139
    formative research on, in Haiti, 177–179
        data, 178–179
        methodology, 177–178
    globally, 53
    in Guatemala, 26, 27
        for nonliterate vs. literate women, 27–28
    in Haiti, 176
    international, lack of improvement in, 258
    leading causes of, 3
    in Liberia, 122
        TTMs and reduction in, 125
    in Lilongwe District, Malawi, Africa, 58
    Maison de Naissance, Haiti and results related to, 183
    methods and strategic goals related to, in Haiti, 179–181
    in Nepal, 91, 92–93
    from obstetric complications, 305, 306
    ratios (MMRs)
        in Malawi, Africa, 56
        in Nigeria, 304, 314
    northern vs. southern, 308
    "Three Delays" and, 178
    in Timor-Leste, 105
    in Uganda, 74, 76
        major causes of, 75
    working toward elimination of, 304, 306
Maternity
    cultural of, 211–212

Index

Mbyá view of, 236
Maternity homes, in New Zealand, 193
Maumete, Timor-Leste, rural village in, *106*
Mayans
    domestic conflicts in Guatemala and, 262
    indigenous population, in Guatemala, 27
    traditions of, colonialism, imperialism and, 28
mbogua, 239, 248
Mbyá Guaraní communities, Misiones Province, Argentina, 231, 232, 233
Mbyá Guaraní women
    health conditions and access to sanitary services and programs, 233–235
    intracultural variability and generational changes among, 237–249
    Jachuka, traditional mother participating in changes, 237, 241–246
    Kerechu, elderly lady from the past, 237, 238–241
    Para, granddaughter articulating the inside and the outside, 237, 246–249
Mbyá language, 233
Mbyá women, in ethnographic literature, 235–237
MCFD. *See* Ministry of Children and Family Development, Canada
MDGs. *See* Millennium Development Goals
Medical intervention in labor and delivery, varying standards for, 273
Médicins Sans Frontières, 101, 126, 142
Melchham, Humla, Nepal, PHASE health workers in, 91, 92
Men. *See also* Husbands
    Guajá, nutritional status, leisure time and, 220
    Mbyá, care of sick children and, 250
    Mbyá culture and, 236
Mental illness, war and, 101
MHCD. *See* Mission in Health Care and Development
Microfinancing loans, in Democratic Republic of Congo, 143–144, 145
Midwives
    in Guatemala, 25–48
    in Liberia, need for, 122
    Mbyá grandmother's account of, 239
    Mbyá mother's account of, 246
    at Warkworth Birthing Centre, New Zealand, 188–189, 191, 192, 197, 198, 199, 200, 201, 202, 203, 204, 205
Midwives for Midwives (MFM) Training Program, Guatemala, 25, 26
    fabric for the future, 46–47
    formation of, 30
    intertwining with Ministry of Health, 30, 43–44
    lessons learned at, 45–46
    linguistic nuances relative to midwifery, 48*n*1

    model for midwifery training and, 32
    monitoring and evaluation of training, 38–43
        demonstrated knowledge during training, 41, 42
        final exam, 40, 41
        tools for, 39, 40
    traditional midwives trained through, 34–38
    training curriculum developed by, 36–38
Migration, war and, 101
Millennium Development Goals (UN), 75, 136
    MHCD: MCH objectives articulated with, 136, 137*t*
    newborn health in Nepal and, 279–280
    reduction of maternal mortality and, 304, 306
Miller, Suellen, 306
MINI. *See* Morang Innovative Neonatal Intervention
Ministry of Children and Family Development, Canada, 155, 163
Ministry of Gender, Youth, and Community Services, Malawi, 65, 66, 70
Ministry of Health and Population, Malawi, 70
Ministry of Health and Population (MoHP), Nepal, 280, 284, 286
Mission in Health Care and Development: Maternal and Child Health Program, Democratic Republic of Congo, 133, 135
    microfinancing loans through, 143–144, 145
    Millennium Development Goals and objectives of, 136, 137*t*
Mississippi River, 215
mitã pyta, 242, 243, 254*n*4
mitã yrui, 242
MN. *See* Maison de Naissance (Haiti)
Mobility during labor, at Warkworth Birthing Centre, New Zealand, 196
Molinos population, Salta Province, Argentina, 231
Moms Mentoring Moms Program, Victoria, British Columbia, 153
    benefits of, 167
    closing prayer, 167
    data sources for, 159
    facilitators, mentors, and assistants, 156–157
    funders for, 153, 156
    goal of, 154–155
    lessons learned and recommendations, 165–167
    meeting program objectives, 160–164
        educating participants about health, 161
        family empowerment, 162–163
        reducing intake during pregnancy, 162
    participants in, 157–159
        overall effect on, 159–160
        ratings for, 160
    reducing unnecessary involvement with foster care system, 163
        building mentoring capacity, 164

INDEX

building positive community relationships, 163–164
topics addressed during one-to-one meetings, 157
Moniliasis, Guajá infants and, 221
Monrovia, Liberia, displaced persons in, 126–127
Monte (rainforest), Mbyá men and sphere of, 236, 250
Mopan-speaking Maya, in Toledo District, Belize, 8, 9, 13, 22n5
Morang District, Nepal, *283*
   District Public Health Officer in, 297, 298
   ethnic groups in, 284
   MINI site in, 283–284
   per capita income in, 283
Morang Innovative Neonatal Intervention, Nepal, 275, 276
   achievements, 294
   challenges and opportunities, 297–298
   decreased supervision model, 294
   demonstrating a model for scale-up, 295–296
   evidence base, 282
   FCHV classification card, 291
   field staff, 288–289
      training and supervision, 289
      treatment and management of sick young infants, 289–290, 293
   funding for, 282–283
   harnessing strength of existing programs, 296
   human resources, FCHVs, 287–288
   idea and motivation behind, 285
   impact indicators, 294–295
   implementation, 285
      existing government infrastructure, 286
   indirect benefits: social and economic impact, 296–297
   information management, 293
   leadership, 288
   lessons learned, 298–300
   partners, 284–285
   program model, 292
   snapshot: UNIJECT, 298
   supply chain management, 293–294
MOSMI. *See* Maama Omwaana Safe Motherhood Initiative
MotherCare, 37
Mother–child health care
   Mbyá granddaughter's account of, 246–249
   Mbyá grandmother's account of, 238–241
   Mbyá mother's account of, 241–246
   Mbyá women's beliefs, role transformations, new opportunities and, 252–253
Motherhood, culture of, 211–212
Mother–infant feeding practices
   among Guajá of Brazilian Amazon, 219–222
   Brazilian state, reflections and recommendations, 225–227
   conceptualizing, within scope of Brazilan Amazon, 215
   nuances of native and peasant communities and, 223
   PAHO health study in Brazilian Amazon, 222–225
Mothering, commitment to, at Warkworth Birthing Centre, New Zealand, 198
Mothers' clubs, in Haiti, 183
Mothers Memorial quilt project, London, 86
Mount Everest, Nepal, 276
Mrigendra Samijhana Medical Trust (MSMT), 91
Muhl, Cornelia, 44
Mulimbalimba-Masururu, Luc, 145, 146
Multiple paternity, among native Amazonians, 218
Muslim minorities, in Nepal, 278
Myths, of Amazon region, 216

N

Namwezi Health Center, Uganda, 81
   antenatal care services at, utilization of, 82, *82*
   deliveries at, 83
   outpatient attendance at, 83
   partnerships with, 76
NASG. *See* Nonpneumatic Anti-Shock Garment
National Council for Scientific and Technical Research, 231, 254n1
National Health Foundation, Brazil (FUNASA), 221, 224
National Indian Foundation (FUNAI), 219
National Neonatal Health Strategy, Nepal, 280
National University of La Plata, Argentina, 231, 254n1
Natural birth, at Warkworth Birthing Centre, New Zealand, 195–197
Natural resources, of Brazilian Amazon, 215–216
Ndokakuaachy, 249
Neolithic hunter-gatherers, cultural practices and, 219
Neonates
   neonatal deaths
      globally, 53
      at Ixmucané Birth and Women's Center, Guatemala, 34
   sepsis and, 282, 284
   neonatal health in Nepal
      data on, 279
      MINI story, 282–300
   neonatal mortality rate, in Torbeck Plain, Haiti, 178
Nepal
   development of, 278–279
   literacy rate in, 91
   map of, 283
   maternal mortality in, 176

Index

MINI story: leading the way for neonates in, 282–300
neonatal health in, 279
political history of, 277
political mobilization in, 279–280
population of, 276
poverty in, 90
public health system in, 280–281
    district public health office, 281
    health posts, 281
    payment for health services, 281
    primary healthcare outreach services, 281
religion and culture in, 278
trends in childhood mortality in, 280
Nepal Demographic and Health Survey, 279
Nepalese Children's Foundation, 89, 91
Nepal Family Health Program, 285
Nepal Family Health Program II, UNIJECT and, *298*
Nepal Health Sector Implementation Plan, 280
Newborns. *See also* Infant mortality; Morang Innovative Neonatal Intervention; Neonates
    newborn child care, Mbyá mother on, 243–244
    newborn health
        in Bangladesh, 282
        in India, 282
        maternal health and, 74
        war and, 101
New Zealand
    birth centers in, 174
    maternity system in, 187–188
    Warkworth Birthing Centre in, 187–206
New Zealand Ministry of Health, 174
NFHP. *See* Nepal Family Health Program
NGO-ization of birth, in Belize, 12–18
NGOs. *See* Nongovernmental organizations
Nguliro, Freddy, 145, 146
Nigeria
    maternal mortality in, 304, 308, 314
    Nonpneumatic Anti-Shock Garment use in, 303–314
Nile Breweries, Uganda, MOSMI partnership with, 84
Nile River, 215
Njeru, Uganda, 73–86
Njeru Public Health Department, Uganda, 79
Njeru Town Council, Uganda, partnering with Namwezi Health Center, 76
Nkunda, Laurent, 136
Nongovernmental organizations, 4, 268
    in Liberia, 122
    Nonpneumatic Anti-Shock Garment and, 309
    traditional midwives training in Guatemala and, 36
Nonpneumatic Anti-Shock Garment, 303, *305*
    description and function of, 304–305
    in Nigeria, reducing obstetric hemorrhage with, 303–314
    care and maintenance, 312
    community acceptance, 312
    data collection, 307–308
    design, 307
    expansion, 308
    institutional capacity, 310
    lessons learned, 313–314
    need for supportive supervision, 311
    referral protocols, 311–312
    research vs. implementation, 313
    results and reactions, 308–310
    staff rotation, 310–311
    staff training, 307
    stakeholders, 306
North Kivu province, Democratic Republic of Congo
    murders in, 138
    sexual assaults in, 136
    stories of women and girls in, 139–144
November, Lucy, 121
Nuclear families
    Mbyá, 246
    Western societies, indigenous societies and, 220
Numeracy skills, Community-Based Safe Motherhood Advisor program, Malawi, 65–66
Nurse midwives, at Maison de Naissance, Haiti, 180. *See also* Midwives
Nursing education, international perspective for curriculums in, 258
Nursing students
    introducing to childbearing practices in rural Guatemala, 257–268
    assuming that no one understands English, 263–264
    avoiding unintentional harm, 263
    beware of gift giving, 264
    course work, 261–262
    faculty preparation, 263
    inappropriate donations, 264
    pretrip promotion, 260–261
    respectful behavior, 265–266
    scope of work, 263
    selection of students, 261
    self-reflection, 266
    slowly watching and waiting, 266–267
    sustainability and change, 267–268
    use of scarce resources, 265
Nutrition. *See also* Diet; Food
    Mbyá mother's account of, 241–242
    Moms Mentoring Moms program and, 162

INDEX

O

Obstetric complications, maternal deaths and, 304, 305, 306
Obstetric hemorrhage
  emergency nature of, 307
  full treatment of, 310
  reducing in Nigeria, with Nonpneumatic Anti-Shock Garment, 303–314
Obstetric hospitals, 193
Ojengbede, Oladosu, 306
ojeo ke'a, local healers and, 244
Old World diseases, indigenous peoples of the Americas and, 214
Optimality Index-U.S., 33
Opyguá, 244, 247, 249, 254*n*2
Oral rehydration therapy, FCHVs in Nepal and administration of, 287
Organisation for Economic Cooperation and Development, 173
Orphans
  in Democratic Republic of Congo, 134, 135
  teenage girls in Uganda and, 75

P

PAHO. *See* Pan American Health Organization
Pai, 254*n*2
Pakistan, Nonpneumatic Anti-Shock Garment used in, 306
Pan American Health Organization, 213, 214, 215, 222–225
Panema, 216
Paraguay, Mbyá people in, 233
Para (Mbyá granddaughter), 237, 246–249, 252
Parasites, 244
Parasitoses, 244
Pará state, Brazilian Amazon, PAHO health study in, 222–225
Parenthood, Mbyá view of, 236
Parenting strategies, Moms Mentoring Moms program and, 162, 163
Partible paternity, among native Amazonians, 218
PEAP. *See* Poverty Eradication Action Plan
Peasant communities, in Brazilian Amazon, 215–216, 217, 223–226
PEERS. *See* Prostitutes Empowerment Education and Recovery Society
Penn-Malawi Women for Women's Health project, 55, 57
Peripartum hemorrhage, maternal mortality and, 179
Personal digital assistants, Maison de Naisance community health workers and use of, 182
Pets, Guajá women and breastfeeding of, 221
Pew Health Professions Commission, 259
PGC. *See* Carajás Mining Project
PHA. *See* Primary health attention
Pharmacopeia, traditional, Guajá and, 221

PHASE Nepal
  background, 90
  clothing distribution to new mothers and babies, 95–97
  clothing incentive offered through, 94
  governmental health posts supported by, 91
  history, 92
  lessons learned, 97
  main objectives of, 89
  mother with newborn baby before behavior change initiative, 95
  outcomes, 97
  plan for incentives for behavior change, 93–94
  two babies in new clothes, 96
PHASE Worldwide UK, 89
PHCs. *See* Primary Health Centers
Phebe midwifery school, Monrovia, 123
Physical abuse, women who use alcohol and history of, 154
Physician-patient relationship, Moms Mentoring Moms program and, 161
PIN. *See* Projeto de Integração (Program for National Integration)
Plan Nacer, Argentina, 235
Pneumonia
  MINI in Nepal and management of, 290, 293
  neonatal deaths and, 282
Poetry, in TOT workshops, Malawi, 61
Polio vaccinations, FCHVs in Nepal and administration of, 287
Polyandrous marriages, Guajá social organization and, 218, 220
Polygynous marriages, Guajá social organization and, 220
Popol Vuh, 29
Population losses, mechanisms for recovering, among Guajá, 218
Portugal, foreign colonies of, 104
Possible severe bacterial infection
  approval of clinical algorithm for, 290, 300*n*2
  diagnostic algorithm for, 300*n*1
  FCHV classification card, 291
  MINI in Nepal, and identification of, 295
  in Nepal, injectable antibiotics for, 289–290
  SEARCH trial on, 282
Postconflict settings, family planning in Timor-Leste, 108–118
Postnatal care
  Community-Based Newborn Care Package in Nepal and, 297
  at Warkworth Birthing Centre, New Zealand, 188, 193, 194
Postpartum depression, Mbyá grandmother's account of, 240
Postpartum period, cultural misconceptions about, in Malawi, Africa, 56

330

Post-traumatic stress disorder, women who use alcohol and history of, 154
Poverty
    in Brazilian northeast, 225
    in Democratic Republic of Congo, 135
    in Guatemala, 27–28
    in Liberia, 122
    in Nepal, 90, 279
    in Timor-Leste, 105
Poverty Eradication Action Plan, in Uganda, 75
Power relations
    in Guajá society, 220
    Western societies, indigenous societies and, 220
Powoe, Henry, 121, 128, 129
Practical Help Achieving Self-Empowerment. *See* PHASE Nepal
Practical Midwifery Course for Nannies, Belize, 11
Preeclampsia, 35, 79
Pregnancy
    cultural misconceptions about, in Malawi, Africa, 56
    due to rape, in Democratic Republic of Congo, 139, 141, 144
    maternal morbidity and complications tied to, 56, 74
    Mbyá granddaughter on illness episodes during and after, 247
    Mbyá mother's account of, 242
    reducing substance use during, 162
Pregnant women, war and, 101
Prenatal care
    in Haiti, 178, 184
    in rural Guatemalan communities, 257
Primary health attention, for Mbyá population, Argentina, 234
Primary Health Centers, in Nigeria, 308
Primigravidas, at Ixmucané Birth and Women's Center, Guatemala, 33–34
Program for the National Support of Humanitarian Actions for Indigenous Populations, Argentina, 234, 235
Project Hope, 183
Projeto de Integração (Program for National Integration), Brazil, 216–217
Prostitutes Empowerment Education and Recovery Society, 153, 156, 157
PSBI. *See* Possible severe bacterial infection
Puberty initiation ceremonies, Guaraní ethnic groups and, 236
Puerperal infections, in Humla, Nepal, 97
Punta Gorda, Belize, 14
    hospital in, 10, 19*t*

Q

Quetzaltenango, Guatemalan highlands, MFM trained traditional midwives in, 38

R

Rabbit farms, microfinancing loans for, Democratic Republic of Congo, 144
Rape
    in East Timor, 104
    in Guatemala, 28, 36
    as weapon of war in Democratic Republic of Congo, 101, 133–147
Rectovaginal fistulas, rape and torture in Democratic Republic of Congo and, 135, 141
Refugees
    in Democratic Republic of Congo, 134, 135, 141
    in Guinea, 125, 126
Registered nurse midwives, Malawian, TOT Safe Motherhood workshops for, 57
Relationship building, service learning and, 268
Reproductive rights, in Guatemala, lack of, 28
Resource allocation, service learning in Guatemala and, 265
Respect
    Moms Mentoring Moms program participants and, 159–160
    service learning in Guatemala and, 265–266
Respiratory illnesses, in indigenous populations, 234, 244
Retained placenta, in Chiwamba, Malawi, 62
Revolutionary Front for an Independent East Timor, 104
Ritual behavior, Brazilian Amazonian cultural protocols and, 218
River Ridge Birth Center, New Zealand, 174
RNMs. *See* Registered nurse midwives
Rodney, New Zealand, Warkworth Birthing Centre and commitment to, 190–192
Role modeling, in TOT workshops, Malawi, 61
Rwanda
    genocide in, 136
    money demanded by border officials for donated goods transported to, 145

S

Sacatepéquez, Guatemalan highlands, MFM trained traditional midwives in, 38
Safe Motherhood initiative, 304
    global challenges related to, 53
    launching of national secretariat for, 86
    on maternal mortality, 74
Safe Motherhood Program, Bixby Center for Global Reproductive Health, University of California, San Francisco, 303, 306
Safe Motherhood TOT workshops, Malawi
    activities targeted to raise women's status/self-concept, 63–64
    community recognition of CBSMAs, 64–65
    creative teaching methods, 60–61

331

INDEX

lessons learned, 69–71
overview of content, 59
primary aim of program, 58–59
singing in class: what songs and why, 61–63
welcome and introductions, 59–60
Safe practice, at Warkworth Birthing Centre, New Zealand, 204–205
Sahumados, 239
Salesian Catholic Sisters, in Timor-Leste, 106
Salter scale, 290
Sanitary agents, for Mbyá community, Argentina, 234
Sanitary programs, for indigenous communities in Argentina, 235
Sanitation, in Uganda, 75
San Juan catchment area, Belize, rural health center data for (2003–2005), 19*t*
San Lucas Mission, Solola, Guatemala, 257
Satellite linkage, Internet service via, at Maison de Naissance, Haiti, 181
Save Newborn Lives, 275, 282
Save the Children–USA, 275, 282, 285
SEARCH, 282
Seattle University, Namwezi Health Center, Uganda, partnership with, 76, 77, 79, 81, 84
Sedentarization, health risks with, 219–220
Self-confidence, for women in Malawi, 63–64, 71
Self-reflection, service learning in Guatemala and, 266
Sepsis
    maternal deaths and, 304
    MINI in Nepal and prevention of, 296
    neonatal deaths and, 282, 284
    newborn, in Humla, Nepal, 97
Service learning
    learning about global maternal health care through, 268
    for reducing health disparities, 259–260
    in western highlands of Guatemala, practical strategies, 260–268
Sexual abstinence, Brazilian Amazonian cultural protocols and, 218
Sexual abuse, women who use alcohol and history of, 154
Sexual intercourse prohibition, Mbyá grandmother's account of, 240
Sexually transmitted diseases
    in Democratic Republic of Congo, 135
    in Liberia, 122
    prevention messages, Uganda, 80
Sexual violence, in Democratic Republic of Congo, 134, 138, 139–143
Sex workers, in Uganda, 75
SIAS. *See* Sistema Integral en Atención en Salud
Sick child care, Mbyá, gender roles and, 250
Sierra Leone, rescuing boy soldiers in, 123
Singing, in TOT workshops, Malawi: what songs and why, 61–63

Sistema Integral en Atención en Salud, 47
Skilled birth attendants, 45
    in Humla, Nepal, 97
    Nepalese national average for, 92
    in Timor-Leste, 115
Social support network, through Moms Mentoring Moms program, 166–167
Sociocultural preferences for care, holistic view of patient and, 259
Socioeconomic status, in Brazil's eastern Amazon region, 225–226
Solar power system, at Maison de Naissance, Haiti, 182
Sololá, Guatemalan highlands, MFM trained traditional midwives in, 38, 43, 47
Songs, Safe Motherhood, Malawi, 61–63
South America, Guaraní people of, in ethnographic literature, 235–237
South Kivu province, Democratic Republic of Congo
    murders in, 138
    story of women and girls in, 139–144
Spanish speaking skills, service learning in Guatemala and, 261, 263–264, 265–266
St. Francis Health Services, partnering with Namwezi Health Center, 76
St. Luke's Hospital Center for Women and Infants (University of Missouri–Kansas City, School of Medicine), 175
Standard Days Cycle Beads, use of, in Timor-Leste, 113
Status awareness, for women in Malawi, 63–64, 71
STDs. *See* Sexually transmitted diseases
Stigma, substance-using women and, 154, 166
Stillbirths
    globally, 53
    in Liberia, 124
Storytelling, in TOT workshops, Malawi, 61
Student experiences in international health, designing programs for, 268. *See also* Nursing students
Subordinated peoples, resistant forms of behavior among, 224–225
Subsistence agriculture, staple, Guajá of Brazilian Amazon and, 219
Subsistence economy, of Mbyá people, 233–234
Substance-using women
    Moms Mentoring Moms program, Victoria, British Columbia and, 154–155, 156–167
    stigma and, 154, 166
Success, measuring, service learning in Guatemala and, 267
Sulfamethoxazole
    MINI in Nepal and administration of, 290, 293
    for neonate pneumonia, in Nepal, 284

Index

Supervision, effective medical intervention at community level and, 273
Support groups, worldwide use of, 151
Sustainability, change and, 267–268
Swallie, Ezekiel, 121, 129, 130
Swallie, Ruth, 121, 122, 123, 124, 125, 126, 127, 128, 129
Swallie, Tage, 121, 122, 123, 124, 125, 126, 127, 128, 129
Sweden, childbirth in, 197
Sylhet, Bangladesh, infection management in, 282

T

Taps-taps (Haitian buses), 177
TBAs. *See* Traditional birth attendants
Techaî Mbyá, Argentina, 235
Technical working groups, MINI implementation in Nepal and, 290
Technology
 in Guatemala, 267
 Maison de Naissance, Haiti and, 181–182
 medical intervention in labor and delivery and, 273
Tembé indigenous community, Pará state, Brazilian Amazon, mother–infant feeding practices in, 215
Tetanus, neonatal, preventing in Uganda, 77
Tetanus vaccinations
 at Maison de Naissance, Haiti, 182–183
 for pregnant women in Uganda, 77, 80
 rate for, in Humla, Nepal, 93
"Three Delays," maternal mortality and, 178
Thyangathyanga, Daima, 58, 60, 61, 62, 68, 70
Timor-Leste
 background on, 104–105
 health in democratic republic of, 105–109
 integrating child spacing with maternal care in, 103, 109–118
 map of, 107
 national maternal health indicators for 2003 and 2009, 115
 population of, 105
Timor-Leste Ministry of Health, 103, 105, 106, 107, 110, 115, 116, 117
TiPa TiPa tool, monitoring/evaluation in Haiti and, 182, 183
Toledo District, Belize, Central America, 5
 background, 6–7
 childbirth in Belizean medical system, 9–10
 concluding analysis of GIFT's TBA program in, 21
 description of region, 7–8
 deserted development initiatives in, 16
 enduring misunderstandings in, 19–21
 generations of traditional birth attendants in, 11–12
 NGO-ization of birth in, 12–18

persistent patterns with births in, 18–19
place of birth and attendant (2002), 8*t*
rainfall readings in, 22*n*2
total fertility rate for, 22*n*4
traditions in, 8–9
Torbeck Plain, Haiti
 formative research conducted in, 177–179
 improving pregnancy outcomes among women in, 183, 184
 Maison de Naissance in, 175
Torture
 in East Timor, 104
 of women and girls, in Democratic Republic of Congo, 135, 139, 141
Total fertility rate, in Guatemala, 27
Totonicapán, Guatemalan highlands, MFM trained traditional midwives in, 38, 43
TOT workshops. *See* Training of trainer workshops
Tradition
 tribal, women's role in, 251–252
 women's role in indigenous societies and, 251–252
Traditional Authority Chimutu, Lilongwe District, Malawi, Africa, meeting literacy challenge in Chiwamba, 57
Traditional birth attendants
 generations of, 11–12
 GIFT's training program for (Belize), 5, 6, 7, 12–14, 15, 17, 18, 19, 20, 21
 goal of health interventions linked with, 4
 in Guatemala, 48*n*1
 in Liberia, training, 124–125
 in Torbeck Plain, Haiti, 177, 178
 untrained, in Liberia, 124
 vital functions of, 3
Traditional midwives
 in Guatemala, 27
 knowledge gaps for, 35–36
 training, 34–38
Trained birth attendants
 at Namwezi Health Center, Uganda, increased utilization of, 82
 in Uganda, lack of, 75, 78
Trained Traditional Midwives, in Liberia, 124–125
Training, effective medical intervention at community level and, 273
Training of trainer Safe Motherhood workshops, for Malawian registered nurse midwives, 57
Traje, 29
Transfers, at Warkworth Birthing Centre, New Zealand, 204–205
Trimethoprim
 MINI in Nepal and administration of, 290, 293

333

INDEX

for neonate pneumonia, in Nepal, 284
Tropical forest products, marketing of, 226
TTMs. *See* Trained Traditional Midwives
tuguy roicha, 247
Tuks tuks (motorcycle taxis), in Guatemala, 267
Tutsis, war in North Kivu province of Democratic Republic of Congo and, 136
TWGs. *See* Technical working groups
Two Children Are Enough campaign, East Timor, 108
Typhoid, in Democratic Republic of Congo, 135

U

Uganda
    Maama Omwaana Safe Motherhood Initiative in, 73–86
    population of, 74
Uganda Ministry of Finance, Planning, and Economic Development, 74, 75, 76
Uganda Ministry of Health, 86
Umbilical cord care
    MINI in Nepal and information on, 290, 296
    in Uganda, 77, 79
Umbliguero, use of, in Guatemala, 36
UMFPED. *See* Uganda Ministry of Finance, Planning, and Economic Development
Undergraduate education, service learning and, 259
UNDP. *See* United Nations Development Programme
UNFPA. *See* United Nations Population Fund
UNICEF
    Belize office childbirth survey through, 12, 15, 19
    Four Cleans course, 36
    traditional birth attendant program in Southern Belize and, 5, 6, 11, 13, 14, 15, 16, 17
Unidad Sanitaria Aristóbulo del Valle, Argentina, 234
UNIJECT, MINI (Nepal) snapshot, *298*
Unintentional harm, avoiding, service learning in Guatemala and, 263
United Nations, 101
    Development Programme, 90
    East Timor as non-self governing territory of, 104
    Millennium Development Goals, 75, 136, 279–280, 304, 306
    Office on Drugs and Crime, 154
    Population Fund, 116
        Nonpneumatic Anti-Shock Garment and, 309
    on war fatalities in Democratic Republic of Congo, 138
United States
    birth centers in, 173

Cesarean section rate in, 190
Guatemala history and, 262
maternal mortality rate in, 27
percentage of foreign-born immigrants in, 258
Universal precautions, service learning in Guatemala and, 265
Universidade Federal do Pará, Brazil, 222
University of California, San Francisco (UCSF), Safe Motherhood Program, Bixby Center for Global Reproductive Health, 303, 304, 306
University of Ibadan, University College Hospital, Ibadan, Nigeria, 304, 306
University of Washington, Seattle, Department of Global Health, 106
University of Washington School of Nursing, 257
UNLP. *See* National University of La Plata
UN peacekeeping force (MONUC), in Democratic Republic of Congo, 136, 138
Untouchability tradition, deliveries in Nepal and, 93, 95
U.S. Agency for International Development (USAID), 74, 103, 106, 115, 183
U.S. Census Bureau, 258
USAID–Nepal Family Health Program, 275
Uterine massage, hemorrhage prevention in Uganda and, 79
Uterine prolapse, among Nepali women, 91
Uterotonics, 310

V

Vaccinations, for Mbyá children, 245. *See also* Tetanus vaccinations
Vaginal birth after Cesarean, at Ixmucané Birth and Women's Center, Guatemala, 33
Valle del Arroyo Kuña-Piní, Misiones Province, Argentina, 233
VBAC. *See* Vaginal birth after Cesarean
VDCs. *See* Village development committees
Vesico-urethral-vaginal fistulae, rape and torture in Democratic Republic of Congo and, 135
Victoria, British Columbia, Moms Mentoring Moms Program in, 153–167
Victoria Foundation, British Columbia, 156
Village development committees, Nepal, 276
    Female Community Health Volunteers visit remote corners of, 278
    in Morang District, Nepal, 284
    pharmacy inventory and dosages on display at, 277
Vinck population-based survey, Democratic Republic of Congo, 138, 140
Violence against women
    in Democratic Republic of Congo, 133–136, 138, 139–143
    in Guatemala, 27, 28

Index

Vitamin A supplements, FCHVs in Nepal and administration of, 287
Volunteers. *See also* Female Community Health Volunteers, Nepal
  motivations for, Community-Based Safe Motherhood Advisor program, Malawi, 66–69
  service delivery in rural areas and role of, 273
Voodoo priests, in Torbeck Plain, Haiti, 177, 178

W

War
  in East Timor, 104
  in Liberia, 122, 125–126
  rape as weapon of, in Democratic Republic of Congo, 134–147
Warkworth, Rodney district, New Zealand, self-employed midwives in, 188–189
Warkworth Birthing Centre, New Zealand, 187–26
  birth rates at, 2005–2008, 190t
  case study, 189–206
  commitment to local community and, 190–192
  commitment to mothering at, 198–201
  commitment to the whole at, 201–204
  confidence building at, 192–193
  as excellent maternity case study, 189
  feeling like home at, 193–195
  natural birth upheld at, 195–197
  safety at, 204–205
Watching and waiting, service learning in Guatemala and, 266–267
Water births, at Ixmucané Birth and Women's Center, Guatemala, 33
Waterford Center, New Zealand, 174
Weaning
  childhood ailments in Brazlian Amazon and, 226
  Guajá women, toddlers and, 221
  PAHA health study in Pará state, Brazilian Amazon, 222–223
Weighing scales, MINI in Nepal and funding for, 297
Western influences, Mayan traditions and hegemony of, 28

Western Institutional Review Board, U.S., 284
Western societies, power relations, indigenous societies and, 220
Western-style clothing, in Guatemala, 267
Western volunteers, service learning and examining role of, 262
Wet nursing, Guajá infants and, 221
WFP. *See* World Food Programme
White Ribbon Alliance for Safe Motherhood, 4, 80
  Maama Omwaana celebrates membership in, 81
  Mothers Memorial quilt project, 86
WHO. *See* World Health Organization
Wilson, Sally, 189, 191, 199, 200, 204
Wives, Mbyá women in ethnographic literature, 235–237
Women
  in Democratic Republic of Congo, rape as weapon of war and, 133–136, 138–143
  Guajá, nutritional status, leisure time and, 220
  indigenous societies and role of, 251
  Mbyá culture, traditional roles and, 236–237
Wood, Samantha, 12, 13, 14, 15, 16, 17, 20
World Food Programme, 91
World Health Organization
  advocacy for TBA training by, 11, 21
  Nonpneumatic Anti-Shock Garment and, 313
  Safe Motherhood campaign and, 53
  skilled birth attendant defined by, 27
  on war fatalities in Democratic Republic of Congo, 138
World War II, 138
Wynyard, Sue, 189, 191, 203

Y

Yopara (Paraguayan Guaraní), 233
Yvy Pytã community, Argentina, 234

Z

Zaire. *See* Democratic Republic of Congo
Zinc tablets, FCHVs in Nepal and dispensing of, 287